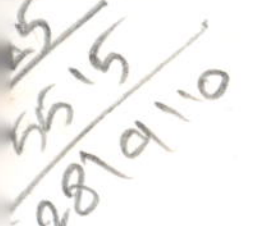

MEDICAL TOURISM AND HOSPITAL SERVICES

MEDICAL TOURISM AND HOSPITAL SERVICES

(Encyclopaedia of Hospital Management—7)

DR. S.L. GOEL
Professor of Public Administration (Retd.),
Panjab University, Chandigarh
Editor, Indian Journal of Public Administration, IIPA, New Delhi
Former Member, UGC, Former Member Distance Education Council
Former Member All India Board of Management, AICTE
Member, Executive Council, IIPA, New Delhi.
Former Vice-President, IIPA, New Delhi.
Emeritus Fellow, University Grants Commission
Former Director, State Bank of India (Local Board) Chandigarh
Former Director, National Horticulture Board, Ministry of Agriculture,
Government of India, New Delhi.

and

DR. R. KUMAR
MBBS, MS, Ex. PGI
President, Chandigarh Ophthalmological Society, 2000-01,
Columnist on Health Education and Management,
Advisor on Health Care and Medical Tourism,
Member Tourism Advisory Forum,
Chandigarh Administration, Chandigarh

DEEP & DEEP PUBLICATIONS PVT. LTD.
F-159, Rajouri Garden, New Delhi-110027

MEDICAL TOURISM AND HOSPITAL SERVICES
(Encyclopaedia of Hospital Management—7)

ISBN 978-81-8450-222-0

Typeset by S.S. COMPOSERS
3190, Mohindra Park, Shakur Basti, Delhi-110034.

Printed in India at MAYUR ENTERPRISES
WZ Plot No. 3, Gujjar Market, Tihar Village, New Delhi-110018.

Published by DEEP & DEEP PUBLICATIONS PVT. LTD.
F-159, Rajouri Garden, New Delhi-110027.
Phones: 25435369, 25440916
E-mail: ddpbooks@yahoo.co.in • ddpubs@gmail.com
Showroom:
2/13, Ansari Road, Daryaganj, New Delhi-110002 • Telefax: 23245122

Contents

Preface

Every year thousand of visitors are coming to Indian hospitals from around the world for medical check up/surgeries related to bone or liver or eye and others. India is giving Thailand stiff competition in health care services for overseas patients with cost of surgery lower by over 30% and in fact cheapest in entire Southeast Asia. Health tourism in fast emerging as a big opportunity for India with its low cost advantage, high quality health care and an English speaking populace. The notion that catering to the needs of foreigners or rich Indian patients will be at the cost of poor Indian citizens appears misplaced. In fact these are private facilities and are created as a business venture by the Indian industry for a niche market. The government can set-up a good public health system, which can be facilitated by the revenue earned from taxes and royalty from the private sector. If India makes medical tourism a success, it will spur more investment in health care, greater research and development in medical field and reversal of brain drain. This will also promote Indian pharmaceuticals and also make India a hub of International conventions.

The thought of the health holiday is to offer you a chance to get away from your daily habitual and come into a dissimilar calming neighbouring. Here you can take pleasure in being close to the beach and the mountains. At the same time you are able to accept a compass reading that will assist you advance your life in terms of your health and general well-being. It is like reconstruction and cleans up process on all levels—physical, psychological and expressive. However, a nice blend of top-class medical expertise at attractive prices is helping a rising number of Indian corporate hospitals attract foreign patients, including from developed nations such as the UK and the US. The things are going to change radically in favour of India, particularly in view of the high eminence expertise of medical professionals, backed by the fast improving tools and nursing amenities, and above all, the cost-effectiveness of the pack up.

Hospitals and health care facilities can show an improvement

The entrepreneurs of Indian hospitals argue that a high-paying Western clientele can subsidize the cost of providing services for the local population. There are 47 million uninsured Americans; there are 120 million Americans who are underinsured. Health care costs in the United States are prohibitive. Even in Europe and Canada, the wait list for elective surgery is too long. The private health care system in those countries is so expensive that many have little option but to seek medical services from low-cost Asian countries such as India. The cost for heart bypass in India is just 7.7 per cent of the cost in the U.S. The costs for other surgeries including spinal surgery are about 10 per cent of that in the U.S. Even after adding first class airfare and five star hotel facilities, Westerners are better off seeking medical services in India. Obviously, Indian hospitals are ready to exploit such opportunities and the massive cost differentials. Numerous state-of-the-art hospitals are popping up in major Indian cities to service foreign clientele. Many more are needed. If we have to follow Thailand model, we have to provide adequate health care to our own people first of all. That entails massive investment in health care infrastructure with public-private partnership (PPP). Once that is achieved it will lead to all round development and prosperity of the country.

India has the potential to become the world leader

With internationally recognized health care professionals, holistic medicinal services and low cost of treatment, India has the potential to attract over one million "health tourists" (equal to Thailand) every year, according to the Confederation of Indian Industry (CII). The country offers a unique mix of modern medical treatment at world class hospitals along with indigenous systems such as yoga, ayurveda and meditation techniques. This, along with the presence of top medical experts and the cost advantage, can help earn $5 billion every year. While a heart surgery costs $100,000 in the US, it costs $6,000 in India. Similarly, a bone marrow transplant costs $26,000 here compared to $250,000 in the US. A study by CII-McKinsey estimates that the country could earn Rs. 5,000-10,000 crore by 2012. Ambika Soni, the Minister of Tourism, stated recently that the capacity of medical tourism to earn foreign exchange is greater than even the IT sector.

Visitors, especially from the West and the Middle East find Indian hospitals a very affordable and viable option. Karnataka, Andhra, Tamilnadu, Maharashtra and Gujarat are in the forefront of medical tourism promotion. Kerala is God's own health paradise. However, the country would have to improve its health care infrastructure, connectivity between major cities and streamline visa procedures for medical visitors.

Accreditation of hospitals is essential

Accreditation of Indian hospitals is also essential for attracting such tourists. Apart from receiving patients from those parts of the globe that have poor medical facilities viz. SAARC countries, India has been getting some medical visitors from the West for a variety of reasons, including the long waiting period for treatment in Government hospitals in those countries. There are plenty of challenges that need to be addressed for India to become the world's preferred health care destination. Prominent among them is the need for proper accreditation and the putting in place of requisite standardization systems. A tripartite synergy between hospitals, tour operators and the government would need to be created. There might be need for a separate regulatory authority viz. National medical tourism authority. Standardization of a price band for graded hospitals and a quality assurance model should be taken up immediately to take medical tourism ahead.

Massive investment in hospitals is basic requirement

Most basic of all is huge investment in the health care infrastructure that is required to provide adequate facilities to our own people as well as the visiting patients. Stark contrasts are no surprise in urban India, and in the health care sector, the difference between what is available—world-class techniques and service, at a price—and what the common man is missing in terms of even basic facilities in the health care system, is sizable. Private sector health care centers are gleaming islands of excellence, all too often surrounded by seas of medical neglect and overcrowding in the public health sector. Look at the possibility of the public hospitals being technologically upgraded to world-class standards with the additional source of income from foreign medical visitors. So the beneficiary of such growth will be the country's desperately overburdened public health system, say industry associations such as CII and FICCI.

Hospital industry is booming

The hospital boom in India was fueled by India's growing middle-class who demanded access to quality health care. Now, the country known for exporting doctors is trying hard to import patients as well as get back its trained medical manpower. The most important player is the Apollo Group, the largest hospital group in India, and the third largest in the world. Many more are ready to jump in the fray. It makes sense to establish India as a world destination for health care, since it will lead to enhanced image of the country in the comity of nations, besides earning precious foreign exchange.

But why should foreigners come here despite the familiar images of the country (teeming, dusty streets, infections and poverty)? Anne Bell, a patient from UK who had a baby and says she's glad she was here, and not in England: "There's been no pressure to go home after the delivery. We've been welcomed to stay as long as we want. They're looking after the baby. They're looking after me, giving me enough time to get settled and get confident enough to go back home. Often in the UK, you might be out of the hospital within five hours if you've had a normal delivery." And in the UK, she wouldn't have had a private room and a private bath. Not to mention massages, and yoga, too. And the doctors? Indian doctors are known worldwide, they speak English, and they're often the very same doctors you may have had in Europe or America, where many of them practiced before returning to India.

India's Health Care system is dismal, but...

Those who are against health tourism in India argue: World Health Organisation (WHO) identifies India as having the greatest shortage of doctors. India is short of one million of hospital beds. In comparison, the U.S. has 2.56 per 1000 (India 0.60) and most Western nations have at least four times higher density of doctors than India. India has a large number of patients with tuberculosis, malaria, AIDS/HIV, leprosy, and other infectious diseases. India has low public health care spending, i.e. only 0.9% of GDP as per 2001 census. Latest figure of 1.39% of GDP of centre and states combined; is also abysmally low. In India, more than 75 per cent of the health care spending is in the private sector. The percentage of out-of-pocket spending on private health care is a whopping 97 per cent. In the U.S., it is just 24.5 per cent and in most European countries it is even lower. Private cost of health care services in India may rise with the advent of medical tourism, since this will amplify the gap between the demand and the supply. Since doctors' reputations attract patients, there will be a bidding war for well-known doctors. All this can be expected to increase the cost of health care services for the local population. Is it then in the best interests of the nation? There are stories of families spending their life savings to keep their loved ones alive. That is, health care is something that cannot be negotiated. As the percentage of senior citizens continues to increase, there will be a greater demand for health care services that can impact the cost in India. Should India allow export of essential food grains for enormous profits, when the local population is starving? You need to accept a ban on medical tourism given the abysmal health care access? The entrepreneurs, the medical profession, and all the enablers such as industry associations and State governments need to tread carefully.

Further, foreign clientele will expect more than the required resources since the long-term risks involved are higher. Thus, hospitals and doctors will spend disproportionately more resources for foreign (or wealthy) patients. It is hard to conceive how resources can be allocated for poor patients under severe deficit. Is this is a case for socially responsible governance?

However, the fact remains that if we have world class hospitals it will benefit our own people first and then give opportunity to serve international community as well. No doubt the world is now a global village in terms of health care.

Chandigarh

S.L. GOEL
R. KUMAR

1

Accreditation of Hospitals: *Sin qua non* of Quality

Quality of services comes first; before the cost. This is specially true to attract international patients to the hospitals of host country, like India. Hospitals services are vital components of any well-ordered and humane society, and will indisputably be the recipients of societal resources. The hospitals should be places of safety, not only for patients but also for the staff and for the general public, is of the greatest importance. Quality of hospitals and health care services is also of great interest to many other bodies, including governments, NGOs targeting health care and social welfare, professional organisations; representing doctors, patient organisations, shareholders of companies providing health care services, etc. However, accreditation schemes are not the same thing as government-controlled initiatives set-up to assess health care providers with only governmental objectives in mind—ideally, the functioning and finance of hospital accreditation schemes should be independent of governmental control. Then what is accreditation? Accreditation is not just about standard-setting: there are analytical, counseling and self-improvement dimensions to the process. Hospital accreditation means "A self-assessment and external peer assessment process used by health care organisations to accurately assess their level of performance in relation to established standards and to implement ways to continuously improve" as per Dr. Chandrima B. Chatterjee and Dr. Sudha Sheth. Accreditation can also be defined as "A public recognition of the achievement of standards by a health care organisation, demonstrated through an independent external peer assessment of that organisation's level of performance in relation to the standards". Thus assessment and accreditation go hand in hand. The quality has to be assessed and accredited not only to satisfy the demands and needs of the natives or the different wings of media, it has to be world class, so as to inspire confidence in the international community.

Health services in many developed countries have come under severe scrutiny in recent years. Positioned against the backdrop of globalization, there is an intense move towards accreditation of hospitals. Accreditation of hospitals is a voluntary process by which an authorized agency or organisation evaluates and recognizes health services according to a set of standards describing the 'structures and processes that contribute to desirable patient outcomes. Accreditation can be understood as an indicator of professional achievement and quality of care. Accreditation is opposed to licensing or regulation of health care facilities, which is usually mandatory and state-imposed. Central to accreditation are two features: the principle of external review and the use of standards (Dr. Sudha Sheth).

THE ACCREDITATION SCHEMES

Broadly speaking, there exist two types of hospital accreditations:

(1) Hospital accreditation which takes place within national borders.
(2) International health care accreditation.

Accreditation schemes well-recognized as providers of national as well as international health care accreditation services include:

1. National board of hospital accreditation, India.
2. Trent Accreditation Scheme or TRENT (based in UK-Europe and Hong Kong).
3. Joint Commission International or JCI (based in the USA).
4. Australian Council for Health Care Standards International, or ACHSI (based in Australia).
5. Canadian Council on Health Services Regulation, or CCHSA (based in Canada).

History of Accreditation

Accreditation of hospitals is not new to the health system. The first initiative towards accreditation was taken in the United States of America as early as 1910. Over a period of time, the Joint Commission on Accreditation of Health Care Organisation (JCAHO), a national accreditation programme, established itself as an esteemed accreditation body by 1987. JCAHO has high standards of quality assurance and rigorous process of evaluation, which makes it a much-esteemed agency for accreditation. Health services certified by JCAHO are given 'deemed status'. In 1960, with the introduction of Medicare and Medicaid, hospitals which were accredited by JCAHO were considered to have met the conditions for participating in Medicare. At present, 42 States allow hospitals exemption from their own regulatory process if they have received accredited status of JCAHO.

The onset of accreditation in different countries

Canada

In Canada, the move towards accreditation started in 1952 with the initiative from the medical profession. Presently, the Canadian Commission on Hospital Accreditation is the sole agency to accredit hospitals and enjoys complete monopoly.

Australia

In Australia, accreditation was introduced in 1926, with the state initiative but it was only in the early seventies that the Australian Council on Hospital Standards was set-up. It assures interested groups that health professionals consider it a responsibility to monitor their standards of performance. It has with other medical colleges, developed a set of clinical outcome indicators for accreditation.

United Kingdom

There are many accreditation systems like the King's Fund Organisational Audit, the Hospital Accreditation Programme, Trent Community Hospital, South Western Health Records, etc. The regional health authorities have supported some of them.

China

Development of accreditation system in China has received the Ministry of Public Health's support since inception in developing standards of regulation in four areas of treatment, namely, prevention, health care reconstruction, support and participation in disease prevention and care and health care activities.

Latin America and Caribbean Countries

Accreditation in Latin American and the Caribbean countries have begun in the early nineties with the release of certain set of hospital standards by the Pan American Health Organisation and the Latin American Federation of Hospitals. The standards have two dimensions: compulsory minimum standards and the non-compulsory standards. Compulsory minimum standards have five areas of evaluation namely the organisation of medical care, technical and support areas, building documentation, functional physical structure and installations. Non-compulsory standards include such things as critical care, neo-natology, nuclear medicine, etc.

Other countries that have accreditation system and some that is in the process of setting up one are Spain, France, Pakistan, South Africa, Italy, Taiwan, Netherlands, and Israel among others. Over a period of time accreditation systems have moved away from single system focusing on entire hospitals to more complex patterns.

India

The rising demand for quality care, the limited health care investment, the growing number of private players in health care and insurance sector, the opening-up of the health-sector to global patients makes the search for quality an imminent reality. The accreditation process should begin with minimum or moderate level standards and, over a period of time expand to higher, "ideal" level standards. In India, the initial premises of introducing accreditation were based on the overall objective to ensure the quality of care. The Bureau of Indian Standards (BIS) had laid down standards for hospitals having 30, 100 and 250 beds. The National Institute of Health and Family Welfare (NIHFW) had such rules laid for more than 50-bed hospitals and only for equipment. Most of the standards laid down by both BIS and NIHFW were criticized for having an urban bias. There have been attempts in some states to institutionalize uniform standards for hospitals. In Maharashtra, the government hospitals follow the Hospital Administration Manual. The Andhra Pradesh Vaidya Vidhana Parisad has laid down standards for secondary-level hospitals in the government sector, which comes under it. Apart from this some efforts have been made by consumer bodies, groups of health professionals, hospital organisations and non-governmental organisations to evolve standards for accreditation.

At the threshold of globalization and increasingly opening-up of the Indian health sector, attempts are being made at various quarters to draft systems of accreditation. What does accreditation mean for India? The answer to this question would help us to know which model can be adopted for accreditation of hospitals in India. If it follows the ranking-model based on quality of services provided, accreditation will have very little to contribute to the improvement of the overall health system in India. In contrast, the facility-survey model can be partially pertinent in putting in place the basic facilities required for providing care. The most relevant model of accreditation for the Indian health system is the people-centric model, which would ensure the presence of 4 A's, namely Acceptability, Accessibility, Accountability and Allocative efficiency.

An accreditation body has to have a restrictive relation with the State to be effective in regulating the health system. It can have observers from the government but largely it has to be an autonomous body constituted of health professionals, experts and various stakeholders. The nature of relationship of the accreditation bodies with the to-be accredited institutions would also determine its relevance for the health systems in India. In the backdrop of the opening-up of the Indian health system to foreign patients and the increased pressure from the insurance sector seeking grading of the hospitals, there would certainly be an exceeded emphasis on quality of hospitals and other health institutions providing health care. Under such circumstances, the role of accreditation systems may be expected to be more stringent than mere consultative.

Let us take into account various factors in which the nursing homes function:

- India is one of the few countries where the concept of small private nursing homes, owned either in a proprietary or a couple partnership fashion is largely prevalent and delivers good percentage of health care. Many have been running for years with good track record of medical services and health care delivery. Besides it is their only means of decent livelihood. A thought can be given to consider them as a small scale industry and give protection and encouragement. May be they can be charged water and electricity at non commercial rates? May be property tax can be levied at non commercial rate? Standards set will have to take into consideration the paucity of space and very high premium on the space available in the nursing homes. Small nursing home may not be an income generating unit if strict standards are adhered to.
- It is argued that if the accrediting body has no legal sanctions its certification will have no meaning. Besides if one has to go through the same regulations under Nursing Homes Registration Act, what is the idea of duplicating the same procedure?
- Problem of getting qualified nursing staff is universal for small nursing homes, every one is aware of it. However no efforts are being made to make qualified staff available. Environment in which small nursing homes are forced to work should be kept in mind.

It is feared by some that with accreditation there will be grading of the nursing homes. This will reduce the nursing homes to the level of hotels. A lower grade may be given only because the space standards are not met with.

Models of Accreditation

Accreditation across the globe followed three models. The first model of assessment gives priority to standards related to available facility norms, equipment requirements, human resources and space specifications. Here, the criterion of accreditation is based on the availability of basic health facilities.

The second gives importance to quality assurance and sets standards for those institutions striving to arrive or improve quality of care, hence accreditation is based on satisfying some basic indicators of quality and involves ranking based on levels of quality.

The third model is based on the ground that health systems should be accessible and acceptable to health-seekers. It gives importance to the health-seeker with an emphasis on evaluating health systems from indicators such as user-friendliness, providing information to users about the services available, setting up procedures for redressing grievances, etc. In the third model, the criterion of assessment is explicitly geared towards people-centric indicators and brings accountability of the health system to the health-seekers to the table.

Globalization and accredited hospitals

Globalization is the watchword of the current generation, giving rise to new phenomena day-by-day. One such phenomenon is "medical tourism" which has given patients the option to shop for affordable health care worldwide. Patients who cannot afford expensive treatment, or who do not have health insurance; or are wait-listed for procedures in their own countries are compelled to travel to developing countries for other treatment options. These options are now greatly sought after because of the immense benefits they offer. Not only is the cost of treatment greatly reduced, the medical tourists recuperate in style at a health spa or resort as part of the treatment-*cum*-vacation package. Five star hospitals with expatriate doctors (either board certified in the United States or specialists with advanced degrees from the United Kingdom) are a must-have for these hospitals in order to rope in the trust of the medical tourists who come here to get western quality health care at third world prices. In order to meet the growing demand for hospital accreditation overseas, Joint Commission International (JCI) has been launched to accredit hospitals worldwide. As per the international accreditation standards, special attention is paid to core aspects of patient care, together with such essential requirements as admission policy that has in place for access to and continuity of care, discharge procedure, referral, follow-up and transfer of patients. These policies are in the interests of the medical tourists who provide a medical history consisting of on-line health questionnaires, faxed medical records and perhaps telephone communications with the doctor's office prior to actually arriving at the hospital for treatment. Accreditation requires the hospital to identify and evaluate the medical needs of the patient before being admitted and this in itself is highly reassuring. Once the treatment is over, the issues of follow-up care arises, as the patient needs to be back home within a week or two. An accredited hospital should therefore have a policy to provide to all the patients with a complete discharge history and recommended follow-up care to take back home to their physicians.

Accredited hospitals also take special care of drinking water facilities and other issues of cleanliness and safety. An accredited hospital has instituted policies requiring the use of gloves, masks, soap and disinfectants, has developed infection reduction strategies, and supports programs designed to improve patient care and safety. Often medical tourists opt for accredited hospitals. Besides, it will also be able to monitor the patient according to established procedures while in surgery or when anesthesia is administered prior to and during the procedure. Medications administered to patients during and after their stay in the hospital may also be safer in accredited hospitals, as accreditation standards require that medications be prepared, stored and dispensed according to set norms. See attached appendix to this chapter for a case study of Bangkok International hospital and the accreditation therein.

Reining the private Hospitals

How does one make the widespread and unethical private sector accountable, ask Sunil Nandraj, Anagha Khot and Sumita Menon in their thought provoking article. The deliberate nurturing of this sector has made it financially and politically powerful. As a consequence even, simple attempts by some state governments to enact legislation for registration of private NHs/hospitals have evoked angry protests from the medical establishments. In the study by the researchers mentioned above, 113 NHs/ hospital owners, eight medical associations, two consumer organisations and 100 patients were studied and following observations made:

- Almost all the stakeholders surveyed in the course of this study favoured accreditation. Five probable reasons could be identified:
- There has been great increase in competition.
- Those not observing good standards were taking unfair advantage and lowering credibility of the profession.
- The apprehension that the opening up of the health insurance sector would force providers to accept the standards set by the insurance companies.
- An Accreditation system would help the providers not only to set its own standards, but also facilitate selection of providers by the insurance companies for their schemes.
- The growing consumer awareness and increasing litigation against the providers have shown that people are becoming more vigilant. Interestingly, the 100 indoor and outdoor patients interviewed in this study overwhelmingly supported accreditation.
- Of the 113 hospital owners/administrators interviewed, 93 said that an accreditation body was essential to assess hospitals for compliance with physical and functional standards. 87 of them said such a body should assist hospitals in continuous quality assurance. 42 of the owners interviewed held that it should also serve as a forum for consumer redress. 31 wanted the body to take punitive action against hospitals. 101 agreed that the body should monitor physical aspects such as operation theatres, space, wards, etc., and only 44 of them felt that it should monitor the quantum of fees charged.
- While hospital owners/administrators wanted the government to keep out of the process, all other stakeholders felt that its participation would provide much needed legitimacy to accreditation.
- Most stakeholders felt that insurance companies should not be involved in accreditation.

ORGANISATIONAL FRAMEWORK FOR HOSPITAL ACCREDITATION SYSTEM IN INDIA

This is the report of the sub-panel (SUNIL NANDRAJ, SRI VIDYA ANAGHA KHOT) on organisational options for quality assurance submitted in February 2001 to Ministry of Health and Family Welfare Government of India. This document provides organisational options for national and state accrediting organisations and considers important issues in operationalising the proposed system.

THE ESTABLISHMENT OF A NEW HOSPITAL

The new quality organisation could be a company limited by guarantee and registered as a charity; or be an autonomous body of the Central Government to be empowered later by legislation. There would be national and state level organisations for implementing accreditation and national institutes for quality and standards could also be constituted. The national level organisation could be the body to build partnership and reach a consensus with the stakeholders—

- Generating policy and accreditation design by the above process. The state level organisations would act as the executive and training/support bodies at the local levels, and would mobilize support and resources for their functioning at the local level.

The key objective is to attain effective, efficient and rational care in all hospitals in India. The role of the body has been envisioned to be facilitator, supportive and educative, rather than inspectatory.

THE QUALITY ASSURANCE

To build up a system that enables provision of quality health care based upon principles and practices of ethics, equity, redress, access, integration, partnership, sustainable use of resources, and cost-effectiveness. The process of assessment should have significant benefits for health care institutions and its customers and should be sufficiently flexible to accommodate wide variations in types of services provided. Standards of excellence should assure the management of ethical, humane, rational and competent care. The basic objective of the strategy of accreditation is to ensure that areas of critical importance to the delivery of quality health services are evaluated by appropriate methods and methods are developed to confirm their efficacy, validity and reliability. Taken as a whole, the process will assess the extent to which health care organisations are delivering safe health care effectively. It would indicate areas of strength and weakness, including aspects requiring attention; involve an evaluation of the validity and reliability of an institution's internal review procedures, and provide reassurance that each institution has in place effective arrangements for assuring optimal standards in the organisation and has procedures securely in place which will enable it to continue to do so.

BACKGROUND

Since quality is a crucial factor in health care in hospitals, initiatives to address quality of health care have become world-wide phenomena. Many countries are exploring various means to improve the quality of health care services. In India the quality of services provided to the population by both public and private sectors is questionable. The current structure of the health care delivery system does not provide enough incentives for improvement in efficiency. The for-profit private sector accounts for a substantial proportion of health care in India (50% of inpatient care and 75% of outpatient care), but has received relatively less attention from the policy-makers as compared to the public sector. Thus the private sector health care delivery system in India has remained largely fragmented and uncontrolled, and there is a clear evidence of serious quality deficiencies in their practices. Problems range from inadequate and inappropriate treatments, excessive use of higher technologies, and wasting of scarce resources, to serious problems of medical malpractice and negligence. Current policies and processes for health care are inadequate or not responsive to ensure health care services of acceptable quality and prevent negligence.

A commitment to quality enhancement throughout the whole of the health care system involving all professional and service groups is essential to ensure that high quality in health care is achieved, while minimizing the inherent risks associated with modern health care delivery. One of the methods that is being proposed is accreditation system. The focus of accreditation is on continuous improvement in the organisational and clinical performance of health services, not just the achievement of a certificate or award or merely assuring compliance with minimum acceptable standards. Quality Assurance should help improves effectiveness, efficiency and in cost containment, and should address accountability and the need to reduce errors and increase safety in the system. In India concerns about how to improve health care quality have been frequently raised by the general public and a wide variety of stakeholders, including government, professional associations, private providers and agencies financing health care. There attempts to establish systems and processes that would ensure quality of care by the health providers. Many state governments are in the process or have drafted legislations that incorporate standards for private institutional health care providers.

LIMITATIONS

Various factors affecting the functioning of an accreditation system, such as the group dynamics among the stakeholders as well as the existing social, political and economic ground realities need to be taken into account while implementing it. Much would depend on the involvement and initiative of the stakeholders. The accreditation system itself should be an outcome of discussions and debates on issues of concern among all the stakeholders. Collaboration, transparency between related parties and open communication are the hallmarks of the system. Only then would it be meaningful and viable. This document is an attempt to lay down principles and guidelines for implementing the formation of an accrediting body that is credible, and transparent. The policies and processes related to the development of a credible, effective and transparent system of accreditation has been discussed in the various sections of the document. Within this framework, the group has sought to identify critical areas of weakness. Key action areas that would allow weaknesses to be addressed have been identified for implementation.

POLICY FRAMEWORK

Current policies and processes for health care are inadequate to ensure that health care delivery is of high quality and malpractice is prevented. The years of neglect and the lack of a comprehensive system for addressing quality issues in the health sector are quite well known. The Government's commitment to quality health care for all needs to translate into sustainable mechanisms for the delivery of effective health care. It is the intention of this policy framework to put in place a system that will begin to make quality health care a reality for all who require it.

The main purpose of our policy is to help planners to promote, implement, monitor and evaluate robust practice in order to ensure that occupies a central place in the development of the health care system. In doing so it recognizes the roles to be played by a multiplicity of stakeholders from the public (state), non-governmental and private and economic sectors. Quality should be an integral part of the overall national health policy. It is believed that accreditation if sensibly designed can have a significant impact on improving quality and safety in health care; improving health outcomes; ensuring more equitable health service provision; enhancing management practices; and improving decision-making. Such a system must be founded on equity, it must respect diversity, it must honor learning and strive for excellence, it must be owned and cared for by the communities and stakeholders it serves, and it must use all the resources available to it in the most effective manner possible.

Assessment Process

A balanced system of assessment would involve on-site hospital surveys, both announced and unannounced; an ongoing capacity to respond quickly and effectively to complaints and adverse events; development and application of standardized performance measures; and, a mechanism for conducting retrospective reviews of the appropriateness of hospital care. It would also ensure that current systems of audit are maintained. It should promote internal evaluation and assessment processes as well as external assessment processes.

Ethics

Patients are increasingly and appropriately aware of health care issues, and desire participation in decisions affecting their health. The ultimate responsibility of a health care system is to the patient. Adherence to high standards, such as those related to timeliness of treatment, diagnostic accuracy, clinical relevance of the tests performed and interventions, qualifications and training of personnel, and prevention of errors, is an ethical responsibility of all hospital staff. Accreditation of health providers should ensure that the owners, managers and staff comply with ethical standards, such as maintenance of confidentiality of patient information, adherence to appropriate technical and professional standards regardless of cost pressures and avoidance of personal, financial and organisational conflicts of interest .

ORGANISATIONAL MECHANISMS

This accreditation organisation is committed to and exists to provide leadership in enhancing health care quality and to promote accountability and rationality in health care. This mission will be achieved through—

(a) Accreditation.
(b) Partnership and Collaboration—Promoting networking, partnership and collaboration between disciplines and organisations at regional, national and international level.
(c) Research and Dissemination—Promoting research which is of a quality and scale to achieve a national reputation in all fields and an international reputation in quality areas encouraging and facilitating the development of multi-disciplinary research groups which are of sufficient size and quality.
(d) Training.
(e) Quality culture—Promoting innovative and flexible policies in the employment and development of staff.

The organisation believes in furthering the process of quality consciousness and accreditation by maintaining rigorous quality standards and by being a rigorous learning organisation with the highest regard for efficiency, effectiveness. The organisation should strive for effectiveness and innovation in standard setting and monitoring for the sustained impact of these on the improvement of quality.

This organisation believes in being fully accountable and transparent in it's functioning. The organisation should develop systems for excellence, accountability and learning. The organisation's role should be that of a promoter, facilitator and evaluator, rather than a regulator. It should provide high quality leadership in matters relating to health care quality and in ensuring accountability. It has to be highly responsive and sensitive to various issues regarding health.

It is suggested that the organisation of the accreditation system be at two levels, namely at the state and national level. Recognizing the need for and working towards the realization of the mission and vision of the organisation and its accompanying policies and plans require the building of appropriate infrastructure at the national and state levels. The roles and responsibilities at the national and state levels have been identified initially to facilitate the structuring of the organisation.

The key objectives of the accreditation organisation

1. To have an organisation, which can deliver high quality leadership in matters relating to accreditation, quality and in relevant research in a cost effective way.
2. To have an administrative organisational structure, which can provide the necessary support to the organisation's core activity in a cost effective way.
3. To have in place procedures for making strategic decisions which enables all relevant views to be taken into account without being unnecessarily unwieldy or protracted.
4. To maintain a culture of openness and transparency where information is made widely available.

The state level accreditation body: Objectives

1. Conduct comprehensive assessments of health care organisations in consonance with the national framework, for the promotion and maintenance of quality and standards.
2. To engage and train conscientious surveyors and to develop training systems generally for accreditation surveyors.
3. To promote accreditation, including its values, purpose and results to health care organisations, medical profession, patients and the community.
4. To collaborate with relevant organisations.
5. To regularly monitor and evaluate all aspects of the accreditation system and accreditation decisions and provide feedback on the standards and Address issues related to grievance redress.
6. To do anything else which is incidental or conductive to attaining these objectives.

The national level accreditation organisation: Objectives

1. Policy-making at the national level, support state level accreditation bodies in education and establishing training institutions and modules for the accreditation process and liaison with other accrediting bodies.
2. It could develop national level standards, guidelines and protocols.

3. It could conduct research, documentation, information dissemination and evaluating the state level accreditation bodies. It could function in a supportive role and as a federation of the state accreditation bodies.
4. The accountability and audit of the accreditation bodies in terms of its functioning, relevance needs to be incorporated within the existing system.
5. Develop a national quality framework. Co-ordinate the development and implementation of national standards in relation to the National Quality Framework that are developed in consultation with relevant stakeholders.
6. Develop a comprehensive, credible and transparent system of voluntary accreditation, considering the medical, social, economic and legal implications to health care organisations.
7. Support state level accreditation organisation in all possible manners.
8. Develop and continually refine methods of assessment and incorporate measures in the accreditation process to rationalize health care (to reduce irrational and unethical practices), establish, encourage and foster high professional standards.
9. Promote the involvement of the private sector in national initiatives and in offering preventive services.
10. Monitor and affect public policy affecting the provision of quality health care; and promoting quality as a coherent national health policy, and of the integrated health care system, which allows and enhances rational and equitable care with a commitment to quality and ethics.
11. Provide a national education program as the basic foundation that enables trainers to develop their full potential and to engage in further education and training and lifelong learning.
12. Facilitate partnerships between government departments; the member institutions, the insurance sector and others in order to stimulate accreditation design development and training.
13. To ensure timely publication of reports on quality and standards and the effective dissemination of appropriate information to members and others concerned.
14. Conduct essential research to promote the above objectives.
15. The provision of advice to government as and when requested.
16. Any other matter that is conducive to the attainment of the above objectives.

SCOPE, ROLES AND RESPONSIBILITIES OF ORGANISATIONS

National Level Organisation would be the ultimate authoritative central body responsible for health care quality in India. It would where possible involve and evolve it's strategies in consultation with the stakeholders. It would monitor quality improvement in the country and would support and guide the functioning of the state level organisations. It could also function as the body, which accredits and audits the functioning of the state level organisations. The organisational structure must accommodate machinery to provide close management relationships between the two levels. The national level organisation could be the body build a consensus with the stakeholders and generating policy and accreditation design.

Membership Entitlements

Personal

- Provide continuing professional development opportunities for relevant persons;
- Provide channels of communication through the publication of a journal;
- Entitlement to become surveyors on demonstration of competence Institutional;
- Serve as a centre for information on quality and related activities; and
- Encourage and promote regional and international co-operation between institutions and between the professional organisations and interests representing them..

Health Care Institution interested in accreditation

The membership fees should be based on the size and complexity of the organisation. However, as a non-profit independent organisation, the membership fees will be as low as possible. Membership could provide support to health organisations in achieving accredited status. The options could be the following:

Self-assessment support

1. Quality planning workbooks
2. Tailored self-assessment tools

Public relations support

Access to the information services offered

Internet membership support network

Additional surveys and education sessions are at the member organisation's cost. Membership could entitle the organisation to one survey in a two year period. If no accreditation is awarded after the survey and another survey is required within the two year period, that survey will be at a cost to the organisation equivalent to an additional one year's membership fee. This will cover the direct costs of the survey only.

ORGANISATIONAL STRUCTURE AND MANAGEMENT

The organisation of the accreditation system would be at two levels namely at the national and state level. Recognizing the need for and working towards the realization of the mission and vision of the organisation and its accompanying policies and plans require the building of appropriate infrastructure at the national and state levels.

The roles and responsibilities at the national and state levels have been identified initially to facilitate the structuring of the organisation. As mentioned earlier the national level accreditation body would be entrusted with overall policy-making at the national level, support state level accreditation bodies. Develop and evolve in establishing training institutions and modules for the accreditation process and liaison with other accrediting bodies. It could develop national level standards, guidelines and protocols. It could conduct research, documentation, information dissemination and evaluating the state level accreditation bodies. It could function in a supportive role and as a federation of the state accreditation bodies. The national level could consist of representatives from the state accreditation bodies. The accountability and audit of the accreditation bodies in terms of its functioning, relevance needs to be incorporated within the existing system. The state level accreditation body would have the primary responsibility of accrediting. It is envisaged that there would be a Governing Board (GB) that would have representation from various associations and organisations as well as the government and other stakeholders. In its composition, care should be taken to allow each of the stakeholders to be equally represented. This would prevent the GB from being monopolized and overtaken by dominant stakeholders. The composition of the GB could be changed periodically. The main function of the accreditation body would be to assess whether hospitals comply with set standards, to assist them to upgrade their standards and to play an educative and informative role. To carry out these functions such as assessment, educational, marketing, administration and so on staff would be employed. The staff could work either full time or part time depending on the resources available. The staff at various levels would responsible and report to the governing board.

Governing Board

The governing board would be the supreme authority, which would be the statutory body, entrusted with the responsibility of managing the organisation. The basic premise of this framework is that it would be a result of discussions, debates on areas of concern, collaboration and transparency between related parties, and open communication among all the stakeholders. It would be the final authority in decision-making and an arbiter of major issues. It would provide a platform for the various stakeholders to meet. Democratic participation of all members that allow expression of differing points of view is essential, with each member given equal voting rights. The participation of all stakeholders is to be ensured and mechanisms could be worked out for meaningful participation of consumer representatives also.

Any member may raise issues of importance; issues may be graded in importance and be taken up in their order of importance.

Evolving a consensus would be the guiding principle of all decisions. When serious differences of opinion occur, however, the decision of the majority would stand. The governing body would have to meet at least four times a year, with invited observers from the Government Health Departments, including Public Health.

At the state level the board would be composed of nominees of representative associations and organisations as well as the government and other stakeholders. In its composition, it would allow each of the stakeholders to be equally represented. This would prevent the board from being monopolized-and overtaken by dominant stakeholders. The composition of the board should be changed every year with a fresh set of nominations.

The composition of the governing board would be the following:

Totally there would be 12 members. A chairperson and a secretary elected by this group would have tenures of 3 years each.

One representative each from hospital owner's associations;

One representative from a medical association of the area;

One representative each from two specialists associations;

One representative from a consultant's association;

One representative from the nurses association;

One representative each from two consumer's associations;

One representative each from two NGOs;

One representative from the local government; and

One representative from the state government.

Other than the representatives of the hospital owner's associations, none of the other nominees are associated with private hospitals. The chairperson and secretary's terms of office would be limited, as would the number of times they might be re-appointed.

Balance of membership of the board

In respect of both initial and subsequent appointments to the board, we believe that it will be important to ensure that a balance is achieved, and maintained, among the various stakeholders. With this in mind a representative sub-committee could be appointed by the board, chaired by a member of the board, to be responsible for ensuring wide consultation concerning the appointment of members to the board.

At the National level the governing board would consist of the representatives from the state level accrediting bodies. Each state would be able to have two members at the national level organisations.

Advisory committees and Task force

The Board is also served by advisory committee specially formed with specific terms of reference as per the need. It could be to define and review standards, assess applications, recommend surveyors and advise on major decisions. For matters relating to accreditation design, there could be discipline-specific Specialist Advisory Committees (SACs), constituted by the governing board as and when required. The Advisory Committees would provide advice to the Board as and when necessary. For matters relating to research and development, there is a multi-disciplinary Advisory Committee fulfilling a similar role. These committees rely on a major input from relevant specialist societies which have the right to nominate members. The specialty committee Chairmen are appointed by the Board. These committees report to the governing board and their recommendations would have to be approved by the governing board, which could also make the necessary clarifications and recommendations.

The purpose of these is to serve as task forces to bring together members with relevant knowledge and expertise to help to formulate policies and to provide advice on the conduct of activities. Ideally they will draw on the reservoirs of expertise represented in the local specialist groups. These national level sub-organisations should be linked with the main board through cross-representation of memberships. The size of the committees, sub-committees, task Forces will depend on the work they are established to perform.

FINANCING OPTIONS

Stable financial resources are critical to the existence of the body and for the proper functioning of the body. Therefore, it is important that the organisation operates programs with sustainability in mind. Initial funding for the organisation could come from grants. Ongoing financial support could include Survey fees for assessment paid by participating providers. The advantage of this option is that it would capitalize on the private sector initiative and interest. Disadvantages of this option include potential problems with funding.

Possible public funding

A combination of private and public sector involvement could be essential for any system of accreditation of hospitals.

Membership fees

Contributions from medical associations, member pharmaceutical companies, leading corporate hospitals? Such contributions raise important questions about the influence that such bodies may have on the accreditation process.

Third party payers

In the near future, third party payers would be interested in paying for relevant information. Also, if the accreditation system proves itself to be credible and reliable, insurance companies may use accreditation as tool to decide which health care organisations to reimburse. Therefore it could be a priority that such information that could inform these also should be available and its quality should be ensured.

- Grants from various bilateral/multilateral funding agencies, state governments, philanthropic organisations, corporate sponsorships, etc.
- Other options could include Public shareholding, alliance with international quality organisations and income generating activities.

OPERATIONAL ISSUES IN IMPLEMENTATION

A strategy is in effect, the underlying basis for the design and implementation of any coherent system for functioning of an organisation. Strategies reflect desired policy directions and ideas on how best to move in those directions. Without a conceptually clear strategy, any system will suffer from inconsistencies and unclear objectives. The strategy is based on identifying core activities and addressing operational issues for establishing the accreditation organisations.

STAFFING

The staffs whether honorary or unpaid are important elements in the organisation. The number, their functions and responsibilities will vary according to the size and nature of the organisation. Equally important are paid staff—their number will depend on finances available and the tasks to be performed and will vary also according to the size and nature of the organisation. In an organisation where all, or the greater part, of the staff are honorary they should, be involved in the day-to-day administration of the organisation and therefore on its executive committee. To ensure that all staff are effective in their roles, and have opportunities to develop their capabilities. To make available, and encourage staff to participate in a wide range of staff development programmes which meet the job-related training needs of all staff, encouraging a lifelong learning culture and providing qualifications and accreditation where appropriate, with the aim of ensuring that all staff are effective in their current posts, equipped to cope with change, and to advance their careers. To improve their capacity in interpersonal relations, training, to document and disseminate information and other identified needs and to develop the principle of lifelong learning and improve self-confidence There is a need to identify specific strengths of people, utilize and develop them.

The structure and systems of the organisation is the key to human resource development. Democratic and decentralized functioning will strengthen the organisation. Development of appropriate systems and procedures at work will enhance work efficiency.

Training methodologies

The training methodologies should be participative, in common with the training of professionals.

1. Active learning and interactive approaches.
2. Collaboration and co-operation.
3. Contextually relevant learning.
4. Exploratory learning.
5. Reflective learning strategies.
6. Learner-centredness, relevance, critical and creative thinking, flexibility and progression better the outcome of the process.

Accreditor Methodologies

JCAHO—Adult learning technique; classroom; audio (telephone) conferences, written material, audiotapes, computer-based training.

CC—Didactic..., teleconferences, video, workshops, mock surveys, role play exercises, instructional guide.

ACHS—Workshops seminars, written material, satellite and video conferencing.

KFOA—Information giving (lectures, Q and A), role play, master classes.

HAP—Review of documentation, lectures, role playing, mock surveys.

NZC—Small group work, role plays, overheads, interactive groups.

Precepting experience is also employed by some accreditors.

JCAHO—3-4 surveys.

ACHS—Access to preceptor indefinite.

HAP—6 surveys (3 surveys as a trainee, 3 with experienced surveyors).

NZC—5 years.

Content of Training

Surveyors should have a general conceptual foundation on quality, Quality procedures, Quality systems, Quality control and Standardisation.

Training content should include the following areas:

1. Standards knowledge.
2. Surveying processes.
3. Communication, interviewing and report writing skills.
4. Training in relation to legal and regulatory requirements.

Accreditor experiences: Most accreditors use the observation of real surveys as a part of the training.

Training topics

JCAHO—Standards interpretation, survey process, laptop technology; Life Safety Code; Core competencies, i.e. interpersonal skills and consulting techniques, performance measurement.

CC—Strategic directions, quality, standards, survey process, (i.e. team interviews, report writing), recognition (award) guidelines, surveyor skills.

ACHS—Understanding standards, role of the surveyor, survey process, survey report writing.

KFOA—Information giving (lectures, Q and A), standards framework, team work, interview skills, report writing, feedback skills, KFOA process details.

HAP—Documentation review, understanding data, interpretation of the standards, team interaction, observation skills, the survey process, report writing techniques.

NZC—New standards/processes, standards where surveyors are having difficulty; overseas developments, up to date knowledge in specific areas, e.g. infection control; report writing; how to assess.

Surveying experience and activity

The average days a surveyor works each year give an idea of the activity undertaken by a surveyor. A minimum number of days are usually required in order to assure surveyors maintain and develop their knowledge of the standards and their surveying skills. The maximum days can give an idea of the maximum workload a surveyor can undertake yearly. When the surveyors are volunteers working in other health organisations, there may be a maximum number of days per year in order not to disturb the normal job of the surveyor. These three figures are important when planning the surveyor resources required.

The voluntary systems, and the British ones in particular, require less commitment owing to the fact that the surveyors are employed by their organisations. These systems require a proportionately higher number of surveyors to deal with the workload.

Training Outcomes

It is vital is that the training process should give assessors a proper sensitivity to the aims and objectives of the organisation to which they belong and also recognize the high degree of diversity in the organisations which they will assess. It is axiomatic that assessors should go about their business with tact and proper consideration for their colleagues who are undergoing assessment and, clearly, the importance of good communication skills cannot be over-emphasized.

Specifically, the training must enable individuals to:

1. Work effectively with others as a member of a team, group, organisation.
2. Organize and manage oneself and one's activities responsibly and effectively.
3. Communicate effectively using visual, mathematical and/or language skills in the modes of oral and/or written presentation.

4. Develop a general conceptual foundation, technical and practical skills, knowledge and understanding necessary for carrying out or directing accreditation and training activities in the field.
5. Collect, analyze, organize and critically evaluate information.
6. To develop core skills required to become effective trainers and learners.

All surveyors to undertake training at the beginning of their surveyor careers. Classroom training is to be sponsored by the organisation who bears the costs of the training. Usually the first surveys are followed by a senior surveyor and its results are a part of the selection process.

Accreditor Experience

Most accreditors require 2 to 4 days of initial training, an exception being the Joint Commission which requires surveyors 15 days orientation and training. Thereafter surveyors receive ongoing update and education between 1 and 5 days per year.

Development of training strategies: The implementation of the national curriculum framework will be informed by needs assessment, research and monitoring and evaluation of pilot programmes, to ensure its ongoing refinement.

Assessment of training needs

Effectively contextualize the learning outcomes based upon an accurate analysis of the surveyor's training needs and an assessment of their capabilities and prior knowledge. Such an analysis should inform the process of assessing and selecting or developing materials for use within the training programme.

The needs assessment can be carried out by interview technique, by the technique of job analysis or by field observation.

A national curriculum framework should thus be drawn out and it should equip learners with the knowledge, attitudes, skills and critical capacity to attain expertise in quality processes and systems, training and rating procedures if so required.

The curriculum framework should emphasize the outcomes of learning rather than the means or way of learning, so that learners will be able to attain the learning outcomes through a wide range of experiences encountered in a variety of contexts and settings. Learners will be able to attain these outcomes at different rates of learning in a wide and rich variety of programmes developed at national and state levels. An outcomes-based approach is characterized by the following features:

- An emphasis on the results of learning (outcomes).
- A focus on learning by doing, and on what learners can do as well as learning of content.
- An emphasis on the applications of learning in new and different contexts.

Training Options

- A central training unit could train all lead assessors on assessment methodologies.
- Core team of assessors (experts on quality) who train other assessors to be full time workers.
- Training of the other members of the team can be decentralized by building the capacity to train within the state, by exploring the establishment and/or development of existing national and state training units as internal agencies to provide overall and sustainable co-ordination and management of training and capacity building.
- The training could otherwise be sub-contracted.

Planning training programs

A timetable should be drawn out for training lead assessors throughout the country in a time-bound manner and should be widely circulated and adhered to.

Professional and technical support

A back-up system of professional and technical support needs to be built. The professional resources of society located at local, state, national and international levels must be identified, accessed and used to provide professional services and support.

Development of training Materials

Well designed learning programmes and materials that can help learners to attain the required outcomes are essential. They are better modularized rather than presented as a full course. Thus, potentially, there will be a great variety of modular units of learning materials, either discrete, or integrated, that meet the needs of a diversity of learners and institutional settings and which can be combined in the most effective way.

With materials that are used in distance education or self-instructional programmes there may be a shortage of time for trainees to engage with the materials. This, together with recognition that adults have different levels of knowledge as well as learning rates, necessitates that materials be carefully structured into appropriately sized modules or units of material. All learner materials, where appropriate, should have a strong self-instructional component built into them.

Cost is another key consideration in choices for materials developers: learners often have to pay for their own materials if they want anything more than basic course books. The organisation should provide leadership on the provision of low-cost, innovative and well designed materials.

Training of Assessors

Training of lead assessors could be conducted at the national level

- By the national level body. This option could be unwieldy as thousands of assessors would have to be trained in a limited time frame.
- Training could be carried out by collaboration with other national or international organisations. This would require a high level of networking and collaboration.
- Self study by potential assessors of quality assessment and proving of their competence by passing an assessor selection examination could simplify the process of training. The modules to be disbursed to eligible candidates selected through a process of application and screening have to be prepared in advance.

Training of the other members of the assessment team could be carried out at the state level organisations by the lead assessors themselves. The lead assessors could be full time workers while the other members of the assessment team could be part time or voluntary workers, who carry out assessment for a specified time period in a year. Regular reaffirmation of competence could be assured by re-exams.

RESEARCH AND DISSEMINATION

Research would be an essential activity in order to ensure credibility of the assessment process and to keep abreast to the changes in the regional and international health, technology and quality scenario. The dissemination of issues regarding accreditation would play a vital role in the development of quality consciousness in the health care system of the country.

Objectives

- Develop and refine methods of assessment including scientific, economic and social tools.
- Develop and refine tools of assessment.
- Detect changes in medical practice, consumer perceptions, and give renewed direction to the assessment process.
- Conduct comprehensive assessments of medical technologies considering their scientific, economic, social, ethical and legal implications and to perform evaluations at the request of providers and third parties.
- Surveillance of use of drugs, devices and medical interventions.

Develop an agenda of problem-oriented research topic alternatives on which the members could vote and prioritize. This should lead to a comprehensive research agenda. Advisory councils/Research committee may be set-up for research into priority areas, with representation of the specialists associations, may be set-up for on-going research responsive to needs.

Working in partnership with a range of research agencies and institutions:

Objectives

- To provide, in explicit public format, information on the quality assurance program, standards, their development, etc.
- Creating a reliable database on identified quality issues to facilitate interventions
- To enable staff, members and trainees to have access to all sources of published information on quality to support their learning, teaching and research activities, using a range of means including access arrangements with other institutions, electronic access, and any other appropriate means.
- To encourage the development and use of more extensive resource-based learning.
- Production of high quality publications on identified issues.
- Develop book and journal stock in quality and areas of particular need
- Develop electronic resources in order to extend range and coverage by providing a high quality and fast network infrastructure
- Provision of access to electronic resources in the form of bibliographic, numerical, scientific and full text databases, either locally or remotely located. The active management of the collections (acquisition, withdrawal, stocktaking and optimal deployment), by Information Services and academic staff in partnership, to ensure that the resources are relevant and appropriate to the training and research programme.

Web Site

Responsibility for maintaining and developing the hardware and software environment of the web site lies with Information Services, who also train departmental contributors. Departments are responsible for maintaining their own entries. The immediate priorities are to have a wide base of contributors while maintaining and improving the quality and currency of the information content, to encourage use of the web as a platform for innovative learning and teaching applications, and to develop the web site as a powerful external marketing tool for the courses, research activity of the organisation.

Publications

To develop comprehensive audio-visual media and communication materials for the support of all educational, meeting and conference activities, and training in they're effective use.

- Accreditation manual and survey protocols for all programs recognized and notification of revisions;
- Self-assessment manuals and workbooks;
- Listings of accredited providers, including accreditation status and survey due date;
- Access to data contained in performance reports (organisation survey) score and comparison with other organisations;
- The publicness of this information to be decided after deliberations with the various stakeholders;
- Immediate notification of serious situations that may jeopardize patient safety identified upon survey;
- Notification of organisations placed in conditional, preliminary accreditation, or non-accreditation status, including follow-up plan of correction;
- Educational opportunities, staff and/or provider briefings;
- Input into standards development process and representation on the organisation's Task Forces or work groups as available;
- Active information-sharing practices that can include survey findings, complaint tracking and so forth; and
- Serious complaints or sentinel event information.

MONITORING AND EVALUATION

Assessment and review of performance is essential, because knowledge of performance stimulates improvement. Monitoring and evaluation of institution's efforts to integrate quality systems will be monitored by regional monitoring teams. There could be a minimum necessary MIS which could guide the process. It would involve selection of key indicators and also submission of the involved health care providers of minimum essential information to the organisation on a periodic basis.

Objectives

- Oversee implementation of quality systems; and
- Monitor the quality of accredited organisations through the prioritization and investigation of complaints received from various sources, reports of sentinel events, and out of compliance notifications.

Regional monitoring team will oversee quality systems implementation in hospitals. Whilst the institutions will assess their own performance, the regional team monitors performance over time and therefore can compare institutions, rank them and give feedback at the regional forum.

Monitoring should be carried out using a comprehensive checklist. The regional monitoring team will provide supportive supervision by:

- Frequent monitoring of institutions,
- Assisting in problem identification, analysis and solution,
- Advising on implementation strategies,
- Responding to new problems, and
- Encouraging high performance by comparing institutions and promoting best practice.

Members of the regional monitoring team should be trained as QA facilitators. Members of the team should be drawn from the regional levels so that there are resource people available in the districts.

Key performance indicators which will be submitted by the accredited hospital on a periodic basis will be a mandatory requirement to renew accreditation. This will:

- Confirm that institutions' internal quality assurance procedures are working effectively.
- Focus on those issues necessary for the funding bodies to secure their responsibilities for public accountability and public information.

MANAGEMENT INFORMATION SYSTEMS (MIS)

A comprehensive MIS for the storage and retrieval of descriptive and evaluative data and information flowing from participating institutions is useful and is a priority. The MIS could also pull together the fragmented and duplicated health-related data collection activities currently practiced.

MIS for:

- Documentation and information systems,
- Drug information system for doctors,
- Newsletters, journal publications, conferences organize regular fora for quality,
- Information skills training to staff, and
- Organizing seminars and conferences.

Performance Indicators

A set of minimum indicators of the achievement of the goals of the organisation should be defined to ensure a standardization and uniform analysis of data collected by an MIS.

Influencing Public Policies

- Carrying out policy research and analysis on issues identified for influencing, which have a major bearing, positive or negative, on quality, rationality and accountability in health care.
- Networking, coalition building.

- Capacity building.
- Information dissemination.

MARKETING

Objectives

- To advance the mission and aims of the organisation through marketing and public relations activities, including internal communications, media.
- to develop a marketing policy which is coherent, targeted and customer-focused, ensuring best value for money.
- To develop coherent marketing and promotional strategies based on a clear definition of the organisation's market positioning and image.
- To identify the different markets within which the organisation is operating, and within an overall strategy, develop effective targeted promotional campaigns. Evolve strategies to involve new market players in the quality initiative.
- To develop a strategic approach to fundraising.
- To coordinate resources and activities related to promotion, to ensure the most cost-effective level of activity.
- Produce printed and electronic promotional materials.

Market positioning and target markets

- Identify potential markets and their segmentation.
- Evaluate the appropriateness of marketing mix.
- Consider the effectiveness of marketing materials and promotional approach.

Marketing policy Establish a marketing group to bring together all those involved in marketing to develop a marketing policy which is coherent, targeted, customer-focused and gives best value for money.

The group will work together to develop coordinated approaches to the promotion and marketing of the organisation's activities, to both the internal and external markets. This develops coordinated and combined activities

Marketing strategy to consider

- Marketability to participating hospitals.
- Accreditation to be a service development model rather than an inspection.
- Involvement of local clinical experts in the team of assessors
- Facilitation of networking.

- Public relations support.
- Marketing support by indicating accredited institutions in publications and web-site.

Marketability to consumers

- Addressing the interests of consumers regarding the process of accreditation.
- Their involvement in the assessment process.
- Making available useful information about participating hospital's quality standing in each area of function.
- Generating consumer interest and awareness by regularly publishing in local newspapers.

Marketability to insurance companies

- Collaboration with insurance companies and other market players in a systematic way.
- Generating data meaningful to the insurance companies.

Market research

A substantial amount of market research has to be undertaken in relation to different groups involved. Additional areas for research to be identified with a view to evaluating and helping to form promotional strategies in relation to the organisation's external image and profile.

COLLABORATIVE ALLIANCES

Objectives

- To improve communications with health care professional groups.
- The network ensures that the organisation gets important input when developing its services and products and helps maintain and strengthen the relationships between the organisations and these institutions.
- The intent is to build relationships with organisations in the network by sharing information about the quality of patient care.

Implementation

- Networking, coalition building.
- To facilitate the exchange of information, each organisation has an assigned.

Organisational staff Contact

- Liaison Network Forum to be held annually to inform its members about the current initiatives of the organisation and to solicit feedback from participating organisations on the latest trends affecting their organisations.
- Throughout the year, Liaison Network members should receive newsletters, field reviews, and informational materials to keep them up to date.

Possible Liaison Network Organisations

Academic bodies, Associations of various specialists, Blood Banks, Health Care Administrators, Occupational and Environmental Medicine specialists, Medical Technologists, Nurses, Pharmaceutics, Clinical Laboratory Science, Telemedicine Service Providers, Association of Managed Health Care Organisations, Social Work Administrators in Health Care, Voluntary service providers, Insurance administrators, NGOs, International Accrediting Agencies, National Institutes such as NABL, NTI, ICMR, JIPMER, AIIMS, etc.

Government

This deals with the interactions of the organisation with the government and key external constituencies.

- Expand the growth of the organisation's accreditation services by soliciting potential new customers, facilitating program growth through increased governmental recognition and reliance.
- Cultivate and enhance communications and collaborative relationships with state hospital associations and other health care associations in pursuit of increased recognition of the value of accreditation.
- Duplicative private accreditation and state performance measurement requirements could be reduced through the coordination of measurement and reporting

In any relationship between an external institution and the organisation, the ingredients to be obtained should be mutual trust, respect and a recognition that, on both sides, there are legitimate concerns that may not be easily harmonized. In the latter the reasons for these should be known and discussed even if harmonization proves immediately to be impossible. To permit positions of conflict to develop help neither side and will damage the credibility of the organisation. Engage in the relationship with tact and diplomacy.

FRAMEWORK AND PROCESS FOR ACCREDITATION

This section contains a more detailed discussion of the proposed system of quality assessment, and sets out a number of recommendations for its future operation. It is divided into the following sub-sections:

Assessment

- Principles of assessment
- Registration
- The pre-assessment program
- The self-assessment
- The documentation required for quality assessment
- The assessment visit
- Period of accreditation
- The assessment cycle
- Maintaining Accreditation
- Public disclosure
- Fee structure

The stakeholders should have significant benefits from the process of accreditation, the significant benefits being based on the priorities of each stakeholder. Priorities for the potential accreditee are that it should experience accreditation as helpful, it should have a continuous relationship with the accrediting body, and the process should be minimally intrusive and expensive (Schyve, 1995).

Getting quality of care on to the agenda in a shared arena which brings together policy-makers, professional bodies and service users. To facilitate continuous quality improvement by support health care institutions in discharging their responsibility for the maintenance and enhancement of the quality and standards of their health care provision to assure the safety and effectiveness of medical practice.

Assessment Principles

Sufficiently flexible to take account of the dynamic and diverse nature of health care institutions, the variety of sources of evidence, and the changing environment within which they operate.

The assessment process should recognize the positive aspects of the existing system, stimulate considerable debate on the strengths and weaknesses of practice, be a positive experience and identify areas where it can act to remedy particular problems or deficiencies.

Opportunity to improve should not be lost in a plethora of bureaucracy and grading

The quality assurance process itself should be under assessment and to ensure its continuing appropriateness to the achievement of the purposes of quality assurance set out above.

Operate as cost-effectively as possible in order to keep a minimum level of external demands on institutions.

The assessment experience should be developmental rather than judgmental and foster a sense of 'ownership' and 'partnership' among all those involved.

The assessment process should be integrative, relevant to all the stakeholders, and transparent. Systems should be available for moderation of assessment.

Registration

Application by hospital and dispatch of: application self-assessment materials, questionnaire (basic data on staff and activity, comprehensive checklist of criteria for compliance with standards).

Detailed report on preparation for the survey for achieving compliance with the standards (optional) and the set of internal documents to be submitted-resource and activity data, internal audits, policies, procedures.

Pre-assessment Program

To provide effective support required by hospitals to be able to implement the quality program. Induction programme which introduces them to quality and the assessment procedures.

Development of opportunities for experience

Provision of manuals, self-assessment workbooks, information sheets on key assessment areas, survey visit information.

Self-assessment support

Training of in-hospital staff to form a steering group/quality action team.

Provision of a professional service manager who provides support for survey preparation.

Mock survey

Progress visits by a surveyor to support ongoing quality improvements.

Self-assessment

Self-assessment is regarded within the discipline of accreditation as a critical first step and as a developmental instrument. It gives an organisation the opportunity to undertake a structured, critical and comprehensive assessment of its performance, improve the efficiency of its operations, enhance staff morale and teamwork and demonstrate to the facility's peers and the public a conscious and active effort to maintain high professional standards of care. Internal organisation and management needs can also be identified during this process. Self-assessment will therefore provide the basis for continuing quality improvement—an integral part of the accreditation cycle. In addition, as the second cycle of assessment begins, institutions should use the initial self-assessment to describe how they have responded to their earlier quality assessment experience.

Self-assessment of this sort is consistent with practice in industry and with total quality management. Self-assessment also has the potential to play an important part in the enhancement of quality by encouraging staff to identify opportunities for improvement and to reflect critically on their part in ensuring the quality of health care.

The self-assessment document should set out clearly the aims and objectives of the assessment and give an account of how these aims and objectives are met. The document should be structured using the aspects of provision contained in the National Quality Framework which will be used also in determining the form of assessment visits, and in governing the structure of assessment reports.

The self-assessment should give an opportunity to the institution to identify any problems which may exist in health care delivery in a particular area of care, and to describe how it is addressing these problems. There should be no invitation to institutions to assess the overall provision in the cognate area, or individual aspects of that provision, in terms of any rating scale as organisations usually tend to overrate themselves and it has no value in the overall rating process. The self-assessment should highlight recently introduced or proposed developments in the organisation of health care. The format of self-assessment should reflect institutional variations in each cognate area such as size, type and structure.

In the second cycle of assessment visits, institutions should be invited to use the self-assessment to provide an account of how they have responded to their earlier Assessment experience. The length of time between the submission of the self-assessment document and the assessment visit should be as short as possible. Support services may be provided during the period of self-assessment.

Taken as a whole, the process will assess the extent to which an institution is discharging its responsibilities for safe and effective health care effectively. It would indicate areas of strength and weakness, including aspects requiring attention; involve an evaluation of the validity and reliability of an institution's internal review procedures, and provide reassurance that each institution has in place effective arrangements for assuring academic standards in the institution.

Period of Accreditation

Accreditation is for two years, subject to continued implementation of the agreed Quality Action Plan (optional), and the maintenance of standards. If a survey reveals that there is a major risk to client, staff or visitor safety or there are significant deficits in a number of key areas, no accreditation status will be awarded. If there is an area of risk or a limited number of significant improvements needed to achieve the standards, and these can be put to action in a short timeframe, accreditation may be deferred until the risk is eliminated or the improvements have been made.

For those few applicants with major problems, approval of any sort is withdrawn until the difficulties have been corrected, and re-application is required. If a provider is not granted two year accreditation it may appeal this decision on the grounds that the survey report is inaccurate or incomplete and that those inaccuracies or omissions were not due to shortcomings on the part of the provider during the survey.

Progress Visits are made 12 months after the survey by a Quality Health Surveyor (larger services will require more than one surveyor) and are designed to support ongoing quality improvements, confirm standards are being maintained or exceeded, review the organisation's achievements and outcomes in relation to its quality action plan, and assist with interpreting the intent of the standards. It also provides an opportunity to advise the client on new or revised standards pertinent to their next survey, and discuss significant changes in service delivery. The organisation receives a report containing the findings of the progress visit and suggestions for improvement.

Accreditation Fees

The accreditation fee structure could be composed of four elements: the application fee, the annual fee, the cost of a comprehensive on-site survey every three years, and the on-site education session. These four elements are detailed below (adapted from CC).

Application Fee

An initial one-time fee upon submission of the application form. This amount covers the administrative overhead costs related to the processing of the application and the shipping of standards documents and CCHSA related material to the applicant. This fee also signals the seriousness of the intent of the organisation applying for accreditation.

Annual Fee

The annual fee paid by health service organisations is based on the operating budget that they submit to the organisation each year. This fee supports the cost of the activities involved in operating the accreditation program and is not directly related to the cost of conducting surveys. The activities associated with operating the program are: research and development, representation, and office overhead.

Survey Fee

Participating organisations undergo a full accreditation survey every three years design an approach to the survey to ensure that the objectives of both parties are met. As well, the type of organisation and the range of care and services provided determine the size and composition of the survey team and the time required to conduct the survey.

Education Session Fee

It is recognized by health service organisations that an education session is an essential component of achieving the most benefit from participation in the program. Participation in an education session, developed by the organisation in consultation with each institution undergoing assessment should be strongly encouraged. These sessions are provided on a cost recovery basis and include a small administrative fee for the development of customized materials and agenda.

SURVEYOR MANAGEMENT

The experience of the accrediting organisations across the world has also been provided along with the options that could be applied in India.

The surveyor is a health professional who is trained and skilled in surveying techniques and gathers the relevant information to enable hospital's compliance against a set of standards to be assessed. Surveyors are health professionals with basic training in medicine, nursing, administration and other related health care professions. Surveyors are practicing or have practiced in health services management. Surveyors around the world share many common features in terms of careers, training, profile and expectations. Surveyors are trained and retrained by the accreditors in the knowledge of the standards and in evaluation techniques. Surveyors see surveying as a role of helping health care institutions to improve their quality performance. These similarities probably arise from the objectives of the accreditors who try to make the survey process educational as well as a rigorous evaluation. The management of surveyors is a critical activity for an accrediting organisation. A great deal of the credibility and validity of the programme depends on this important function.

THE SURVEY REPORT

Following each survey a summary of the surveyors' findings is compiled to provide the participating health care provider with

- A detailed assessment of its performance against National standards and criteria,
- Identification of areas where performance is satisfactory or where further improvement is required,
- Commendations for areas of best practice, and
- Suggestions and recommendations for improvement.

Assessment reports will be based on evidence provided by an institution of the quality and standards, and on evidence gathered by the assessment team during the on the site survey.

The report could also consider:

- The institution's overall quality strategy,

- The arrangements by which it assures its standards,
- Its infrastructure, and its internal and external communications,
- Consideration of an institution's policies and arrangements for securing its objectives, and
- Management by it of its quality and quality assurance processes.

They will describe the extent to which an institution as a whole is discharging its responsibilities and has procedures securely in place, which will enable it to continue to do so.

Reporting Procedure

The format and style of reports should be such that they be easily interpreted and readable, and provide maximum developmental value. The content of reports should be readily accessible to all those to whom the reports are addressed.

The period of time between assessment visit taking place and the publication of the report should be as short as possible.

The lead assessor could be responsible for the compilation of the report or it could be the responsibility of an Accreditation Committee (URAC). The Accreditation Committee could consist of representatives from member organisations and experts and could recommend or delay accreditation.

Compilation and approval of reports

Objectives

- Eliminate flaws in the preparation of assessment reports.
- Address misperception, misinterpretation and factual errors.
- Provide an opportunity for the institution to present it's views on the assessment process.

Implementation

Preventing misperceptions and misinterpretations:

- An extended dialogue between assessors and assessed, so that the assessed see a draft of the report and are given a chance to comment.
- Sending institutions a copy of the draft report, together with a form on which the institution might report any factual and procedural errors. The institution could then receive confirmation that appropriate changes had been made to the report.
- The introduction to the assessment team of a facilitator who would work with the assessment team, have an active role in the provision of information and clarification to the team in the course of the visit and comment on the 'draft collated' report.

Preventing factual errors: The appointment of a 'professional assessor' by the accrediting organisation, to provide guidance on the assessment procedure and on the use of assessment criteria, rather than participate directly in judgments of quality. The professional assessor would be able, among other things, to ensure that the assessment team did not stray into examination of aspects of provision which were beyond their capacity for informed judgment. It would promote consistency in the approach taken by assessment teams and in the outcome of assessments.

The Assessment Scale

A four-point assessment scale could be as follows.

The definitions applied to each grading are: Excellent: Satisfactory in all and outstanding in most aspects.

Highly Satisfactory: satisfactory in all aspects and with areas of particular strength

Satisfactory: satisfactory in most aspects; overall, strengths outweigh weaknesses.

Unsatisfactory: unsatisfactory in several aspects; overall, weaknesses outweigh strengths.

The terminology of Excellent, Highly Satisfactory, Satisfactory and Unsatisfactory may stir considerable emotions. Leaving aside questions of whether such a scale can be applied consistently and reliably, it could be that it militates against developmental aspects of the assessment process, while emphasizing its judgmental nature.

NABH

National Accreditation Board for Hospitals and Health Care Providers (NABH) is a constituent board of Quality Council of India, set-up to establish and operate accreditation programme for health care organisations. The board is structured to cater to much desired needs of the consumers and to set benchmarks for progress of health industry. The board while being supported by all stakeholders including industry, consumers, government, have full functional autonomy in its operation.

Accreditation benefits all stakeholders. Patients are the biggest beneficiary. Accreditation results in high quality of care and patient safety. The patients get services by credential medical staff. Rights of patients are respected and protected. Patient satisfaction is regularly evaluated.

The staff in an accredited hospital is satisfied lot as it provides for continuous learning, good working environment, leadership and above all ownership of clinical processes.

Accreditation to a hospital stimulates continuous improvement. It enables hospital in demonstrating commitment to quality care. It raises community confidence in the services provided by the hospital. It also provides opportunity to health care unit to benchmark with the best.

Finally, accreditation provides an objective system of empanelment by insurance and other third parties. Accreditation provides access to reliable and certified information on facilities, infrastructure and level of care.

NABH standards for hospitals have been drafted by Technical Committee of NABH and contain complete set of standards for evaluation of hospitals for grant of accreditation. The standards provide framework for quality assurance and quality improvement for hospitals. The standards focus on patient safety and quality of care. The standards call for continuous monitoring of sentinel events and comprehensive corrective action plan leading to building of quality culture at all levels and across all the functions. The standards are equally applicable to hospitals and nursing homes in the government as well as in the private sector.

Outline of NABH Standards Access, Assessment and continuity of Care (AAC) Patient Rights and Education (PRE), Care of Patient (COP), Management of Medication (MOM), Hospital Infection control (HIC), Continuous Quality Improvement (CQI), Responsibility of Management (ROM), Facility Management and Safety (FMS), Human Resource Management (HRM), Information Management System.

The Accreditation process involves comprehensive review of hospital's compliance with NABH's standards. Cardinal principles of assessment are:

(i) Hospital operations are based on sound principles of system-based organisation.
(ii) NABH standards are implemented and institutionalize into hospital functioning.
(iii) Patient safety and quality of care, as core values, are established and owned by management and staff in all functions and at all levels.
(iv) There is structured quality improvement programme based on continuous monitoring of patient care services.

HOSPITAL/LABORATORY ACCREDITATION

It is now common knowledge that some form of accreditation/certification like NABL, NABH, ISO-9001:2000, ISO-14001:2001, etc. is required by clients, insurance companies, health administrators and embassies of foreign countries. Whether you wish to empanel in a reputed multinational company, or attract foreign patients coming for medical tourism, or be perceived as a forward-looking organisation with good systems in place, one or more of the above accreditations is becoming almost necessary for health care services. The doctors themselves cannot speak good about their competencies and service. Neither are they allowed to advertise. How should the word reach a wider market? A third-party certification to an international standard is one of the best ways to make your expertise and commitment known to thousands of people.

Having facilitated the accreditation/certification of over 50 nursing homes, hospitals, pathology labs, educational institutions, we are Mumbai's most competent advisors/facilitators of the process. Once you entrust your ISO or NABL certification job to us, you can be confident of getting the most effective and up-to-date advise, documentation, systemic improvements, training of para-medical staff, and certificate from India's most credible bodies approved by the Quality Council of India.

Accreditation for two private hospitals; MIMS and KIMS get accreditation

Two out of the eight private hospitals accredited by the National Accreditation Board for Hospitals (NABH) are in Kerala. Malabar Institute of Medical Sciences (MIMS), Kozhikode, and Kerala Institute of Medical Sciences (KIMS), Thiruvananthapuram, are among those hospitals, where the services offered have undergone a quality check. Three hospitals from Delhi, one each from Mumbai, Bangalore and Kolkata are the others which have been accredited out of the 42 applications received by NABH, which is a part of Quality Council of India. However, no government hospitals have been accredited so far. In Delhi, the Government-run Ram Manohar Lohia Hospital is being prepared to get accredited. Validity of accreditation is for three years, during which one follow-up is done. Another follow-up would be taken up if there was any parameter that was left at an unsatisfactory level, he said. The hospital should define the scope of service it provided. The NABH would soon come out with standards to be maintained by blood banks, small health care units, dental clinics and imaging centres. The NABH guidelines for medical laboratories already existed.

Joint Commission International (JCI) is a division of Joint Commission Resources (JCR), the subsidiary of the Joint Commission on Accreditation of Health Care Organisations (JCAHO). For more than 75 years, JCAHO and its predecessor organisation have been dedicated to improving the quality and safety of health care services. Today the largest accreditor of health care organisations in the United States, JCAHO surveys nearly 20,000 health care programs through a voluntary accreditation process. JCAHO and its subsidiary are both not-for-profit corporations. Joint Commission International has extensive international experience working with public and private health care organisations and local governments in more than 60 countries.

The Joint Commission is an independent, not-for-profit organisation, established more than 50 years ago. Joint Commission is governed by a board that includes physicians, nurses, and consumers. Joint Commission sets the standards by which health care quality is measured in America and around the world. In August 2005, the World Health Organisation (WHO) designated the Joint Commission and Joint Commission International (a component of JCR) as the world's first WHO Collaborating Centre dedicated solely to patients' safety as part of its major initiative-the World Alliance for Patient Safety.

Accreditation provides a visible commitment by an organisation to improve the quality of patient care, to ensure a safe environment and to continually work to reduce risks to patients and staff. Accreditation has gained worldwide attention as an effective quality evaluation and management tool.

Accreditation for 3 Apollo Hospital branches

The three branches of the Apollo Hospitals group in Chennai, Delhi and Hyderabad have been rated and accorded accreditation by an international hospital rating organisation, the Joint Commission International (JCI), based in Illinois, Chicago. The JCI granted accreditation after a process of external peer review to assess the hospitals' performance against established international standards. A team of three professionals attached to the JCI evaluated 1,033 measurable quality standards at the respective sites.

Stringent process

"We sought accreditation with the JCI because we wanted to provide the best possible care for our patients. The JCI audit was an extremely stringent process," Preetha Reddy, managing director, Apollo Hospitals, said. "Health Care organisations around the world want to create environments that focus on quality, safety and continuous improvement," Karen Timmons, Chief Executive Officer, JCI, said in a press release, "Accreditation meets this demand by stimulating continuous and systematic improvements in an organisation's performance and outcome of patient care."

NEW DELHI: Apollo Hospital, Delhi, has been accredited by the Joint Commission International (JCI) for its quality of care in a safe environment. JCI is known for health care accreditation worldwide. Apollo Hospital is one of the five hospitals in Asia to be accredited by the commission. The JCI standards focus on areas that directly impact patient care. These include access to care, assessment of patients, infection control, patient and family rights and education. Standards also address facility management and safety, staff qualifications, quality improvement, organisational leadership and management of information. Dr. Prathap C. Reddy, Chairman, Apollo Hospitals Group, said, "Safety and quality of care being provided to the patients is extremely important for any health care service provider."

Apollo Hospital, Chennai Accredited: 29 January 2006

Apollo Hospital, Hyderabad Accredited: 28 April 2006

Indraprastha Apollo Hospital, New Delhi, Accredited: 18 June 2005

Shroff Eye Hospital, Mumbai Accredited: 18 February 2006

Wockhardt Hospital, Mumbai, Accredited: 26 August 2005

JCI Introduces Revised International Accreditation Standards for Hospitals

(OAK BROOK, Ill., USA—August 30, 2007): Joint Commission International (JCI) today announced the release of the updated international accreditation standards for hospitals. The standards, published earlier this month in the manual Joint Commission International Accreditation Standards for Hospitals, Third Edition, will be the basis of JCI's on-site hospital accreditation survey beginning January 1, 2008.

The revised standards maintain JCI's focus on providing a framework for hospitals around the world to use to deliver, safe, high-quality care. Notable changes include the following: Additional importance has been given to the role of hospital leaders in overseeing all areas of performance, including the revision of some chapters to include standards related to the role leadership must take to set and implement priorities for ongoing organisational performance and improvement.

New chapters have been added for Anesthesia and Surgical Care, Medication Management and Use and Management of Communication and Information. These concepts were previously found in JCI standards, but are now grouped into content-specific chapters.

International Patient Safety Goals, which were introduced as part of the JCI survey process this year, are being published for the first time in the manual. There are six goals, along with intent statements and measurable elements.

"The revised hospital standards are an evolution of JCI's accreditation process in its mission to foster safe, high-quality patient care around the world," says Karen H. Timmons, president and chief executive officer, JCI. "We believe that the field will embrace these standards as a roadmap to organisational and staff improvement, with patients being the ultimate beneficiaries of our efforts to promote continuous standards compliance."

Additional changes for accredited hospitals include strengthened credentialing and privileging standards for health care professionals; and strengthened quality and patient safety standards that require root cause analysis for sentinel events, analysis for all adverse events and patterns of events, at least one proactive analysis process each year, and adoption and use of at least one clinical practice guideline and clinical pathway each year.

Select themes and issues found in the United States-based Joint Commission standards, such as the oversight of the health professional education, have also been moved into the JCI standards. Furthermore, the new manual features an organisational structure similar to that used by The Joint Commission in their standards chapters focused on Prevention and Control of Infections, and Medication Management and Use.

Revisions to JCI standards were based on feedback from Regional Advisory Councils in Asia Pacific, Europe and the Middle East, surveyors, accredited organisations, staff, and health care experts. Regional Advisory Councils represent an important constituency group from which JCI will regularly seek counsel as well as collaboration opportunities regarding accreditation, quality, patient safety, and performance measurement activities. The standards also were subject to a field review. JCI's Standards Subcommittee, with representatives from the Czech Republic, Italy, Singapore, Brazil, Saudi Arabia, Denmark, the People's Republic of China, South Africa, and the United States, was instrumental in the revisions to the standards.

JCI has been accrediting hospitals worldwide since 1999. Accreditation standards are based on international consensus standards and set uniform, achievable expectations for structures, processes and outcomes for hospitals. The accreditation process is designed to accommodate specific legal, religious and cultural factors within a country.

Fortis Hospital Mohali gets JCI accreditation

Fortis Hospital Mohali has received accreditation from US-based Joint Commission International (JCI). The accreditation, considered as the highest form of recognition in the health world, has been conferred in recognition of Fortis Hospital Mohali's empathetic patient care programme. JCI, the gold standard in global health care standards, focuses on areas that directly impact patient care. The focus areas include: Assessment of patients, utmost care of the patients, patient and family rights, strict infection control for the safety of the patients, education, and documentation.

Mr. Shivinder M. Singh, CEO and MD, Fortis Health Care, said, "Fortis has always been committed towards providing safe, high quality medical care to its patients. Receiving a JCI accreditation is a strong validation that we, at Fortis, have taken extra steps to meet the highest level of safety and quality care to our patients. We will continue to provide world-class health care at affordable prices and more units under the JCI Banner." Mr. Ashish Bhatia, COO, Fortis Hospital, Mohali, said, "This accreditation will add more value to Fortis Hospital Mohali and further enhance the confidence our patients have in our quality, safety of care, treatment and services." Dr. Ashok V. Chordiya, Medical Director, Fortis Hospital, Mohali, said, "With a JCI accreditation, Fortis Hospital Mohali will join an exclusive group of hospitals worldwide, which have passed JCI's stringent clinical quality standards."

The responsibility of the entire exercise to align processes and systems at Fortis Hospital Mohali with the stringent JCI requirements was ably led by the young Dr. Simmardeep Singh, Senior Manager Quality Assurance and Patient Care Services. Following this accreditation, new processes have been designed by Fortis Hospital Mohali to meet specific patient requirements and patients will continue to have access to the best treatments. Thus, patients will be the prime beneficiaries of the accreditation exercise.

Fortis Hospital Mohali uses "tracer methodology"—an evaluation method to "trace" a single patient's experiences within a health care organisation to ensure utmost comfort for the patient from the time s/he registers in till s/he is discharged.

The accreditation process has brought in significant changes in the way Fortis Hospital Mohali functions. A comprehensive accreditation, such as that of JCI, needed to be implemented across all departments, with the involvement of all the employees who take part in the patient's journey from admission to discharge.

In JCI, there are 565 standards divided into 197 core standards that must be met to achieve accreditation and 368 other standards that lead organisations to best practice levels. These standards are further divided into 1033 measurable parameters, which focus on aspects such as patient safety, patient rights, facilities, and physicians' credentials besides policies and procedures of the organisation. To get accredited, a hospital has to fully meet these parameters and Fortis Hospital Mohali has passed this litmus test with distinction.

References

ALPHA Agenda, International Society for Quality in Health Care, Vol. 1:2, May, 2000.

Anrudh K. Jain, Managing quality of care in population programs, Kumarian press. QA Brief. *The Quality Assurance Project's Information,* Outlet. Vol. 8, No. 1.

Baker R, Fraser RC. Development of review criteria: linking guidelines and assessment of quality. *Br Med J* 1995; 311:370-373

Bero LA, Grilli R., Grimshaw JM, *et al.* Getting research findings into practice: Closing the gap between research and practice: an overview of systematic reviews of interventions to promote the implementation of research findings. *Br Med J* 1998; 317:465-8.

Buttery Y., Walshe, K., Coles J, Bennett J. The development of audit: findings of a national survey of health care provider units in England. London: CASPE Research, 1994.

Department of Health. A first class service: quality in the new NHS. 1998. http://www.open.gov.uk/

Donabedian A. The criteria and standards of quality. In explorations in quality assessment and monitoring. Vol II, Ann Arbor: Health Administration Press; 1982.

Eliasson G, et al. Facilitating quality improvement in primary health care by practice visiting. Quality in Health Care 1998; 7: 48-54

Ellis R, Dorothy Wittington. Quality Assurance in Health Care, a handbook. Edward Arnold.

Enhancing the role of Civil Society. The International Council on the Management of population programs, 1999. 2007-08-28 16:47:09. *Source*: Moneycontrol.com

ExPeRT website: www.caspe.co.uk

External evaluation of health care, *International Journal for Quality in Health Care*, Vol. 12:3, Special issue, June 2000.

Gill Walt 1986. Paying for the health sector, Evaluation and Planning Centre for health Care, London School of hygiene and Tropical Medicine

Hearnshaw H, Reddish S, Peddie D, *et al.* Introducing a quality improvement programme to primary health care teams. *Quality in Health Care* 1998; 7:200-8.

http://www.achs.org.au/-ACHS—Australian Council on Health Care Accreditation.

http://www.agpal.com.au/-Generak Paractice Accreditation.

http://www.cchsa.ca/-Canadian Council on Health Services Accreditation.

http://www.chapinc.org/-Community Health Accreditation Program—CHAP.

http://www.efqm.org-EFQM—The European Foundation for Quality Management.

http://www.hqs.org.uk/-The Health Quality Service.

http://www.isqua.org.au/-ISQua—International Society for Quality in Health Care

http://www.jcaho.org/-JCAHO—Joint Commission on Health Care Organisations (USA) http://www.kingsfund.org.uk/-HQS—Health Quality Service (formerly King's Fund UK)

http://www.nhsetrent.gov.uk/noticeboard/tas.htm-Trent Acceditation Scheme (UK)

http://www.quality-foundation.co.uk/-British Quality Foundation.

http://www.qualityhealth.org.nz/-Quality Health New Zealand.

http://www.urac.org/-URAC—American Acccreditation Health Care Commission.

ISQua International Indicators Initiative Melbourne; 1999. http://www.isqua.org.au/ISQUAPAGES/ProgramsEvents.html#ALPHA

Joint Commission on Accreditation of Health Care Organisations in the USA. National Library of Health Indicators. www.jcaho.org/perfmeas/mlhi/appendc.htm

Lawrence M, Olesen F, for the EQuiP working party on indicators. Indicators of quality in health care. *Eu J Gen Pract*, September 1997; 3: 103-108

Lawrence M, Packwood T. Adapting total quality management for general practice: evaluation of a programme. *Quality in Health Care* 1996; 5:151-158

Maxwell RJ, Quality assessment in health. *BMJ* 1984; 288:1470-2.

nerenz DR. Accountability for health outcomes and the proper unit of analysis: what do the experts think? *International journal for quality in health care* 1998; 10(6): 539-46.

O'Connor P, Spann S, Woolf S. Care of adults with type 2 diabetes mellitus: a review of the evidence. *J Fam Pract* 1998; 47(suppl):S13-S22.

O'Leary DS, O'Leary MR, From quality assurance to quality improvement. The Joint Commission on Accreditation of Health Care Organisations and Emergency Care. *Emerg Med Clin North Am* 1992 Aug; 10(3): 477-492.

Ovreitveit J. Health Service Quality: an introduction to quality methods for health services. Oxford: Blackwell Science Ltd., 1992.

P, Campion-Smith C. Editorial. Never mind the quality, feel the improvement. *Quality in Health Care*. 1998; 7:181.

Practice Standards Pilot, Summary. Report to the Health Funding Authority; 1999

Reason J. Human error: models and management. *Br Med J* 2000; 320: 768-70.

Schyve P. Models for relating performance measurement and accreditation. International journal of health planning and management, 1995; 10: 231-41.

Shaw C. Health service quality assessment: external assessment of health service standards. *Health Care Review*, Online TM 4(6); June 2000. http://www.enigma.co.nz/hcro_articles/0006/vol4no6_001.htm

Shaw CD. External quality mechanisms for health care: results of the ExPeRT project on visitatie, accreditation, EFQM and ISO assessment in European Union countries. *Int J Quality in Health Care*. June 2000. (in press)

Strategies for medical technology assessment, September 1982. Washington DC.

Strengthening of secondary level hospital services in West Bengal, Dept. of Health and Family Welfare, 1995.

Tregloan, M.L. Health service quality assessment: defining and assessing health care standards; an international picture. Health Care Review—Online TM. 4(6); June 2000. http://www.enigma.co.nz/hcro_articles/0006/vol4no6_002.htm

Using Quality improvement tools in a health care setting. Joint Commission on Accreditation of Health Care Organisations, 1992.

Wellingham J. Health service quality assessment: a common framework for accreditation—what is possible? A New Zealand general practice perspective.

APPENDIX

BANGKOK INTERNATIONAL HOSPITAL, THAILAND

(observed by the authors and from the brochures supplied by the management)

Asian countries have excelled in providing international medical services, despite serious difficulty of language. Two groups of hospitals viz., Bangkok hospitals group and Bumrungrad International Group have proved to be shining stars in offering world class international medical services with a smile. The authors had the opportunity to visit the Bangkok hospital with the courtesy of Mr. Veerachat Petpisit, Marketing Director and Mr. Tawhid Iqbal, Marketing Executive.

WELCOME TO THAILAND

Welcome to the Kingdom of Thailand. This amazing country never fails to amuse the foreign eyes. Ranked as one of the most popular tourist destinations in the world, Thailand leads you to an adventure of fascinating destinations and experiences that can be explored throughout the whole year.

BANGKOK INTERNATIONAL HOSPITAL—THE HUB OF HEALTH TOURISM

Bangkok International Hospital (BIH) is the newest addition to the Bangkok Hospital Group. Recognized as the leader in private medical health care in Thailand and the SE Asian Region, our outstanding facilities, leading expertise and latest advancements in medical technology place us amongst the world's premier global health care providers.

Started in 1972, Bangkok Hospital has grown from a small private hospital to a campus for Bangkok Hospital, Bangkok Heart Hospital, Wattanosoth Hospital and more importantly Bangkok International Hospital.

At Bangkok International Hospital, our world renowned physicians, cutting edge technology and excellent nursing staff provide all of our patients with the utmost level of medical care. With overseas training and experience, we can assure that all of your needs and expectations will be met.

BIH is the medical hub for an increasing number of global patients seeking treatment in Bangkok. Each patient is granted the privacy of their own room, ensuring complete consideration and respect is received.

Bangkok International Hospital's vision, to create a comfortable ambience for all cultures from over 140 nationalities is reached by our dedicated international team, giving full provision to the understanding and needs of each individual patient. We "speak your language" to ensure your time with Bangkok International Hospital is a pleasant one.

There's basically no disease the Bangkok Hospital Campus can't treat. Its hospitals have successfully treated thousands and thousands of patients. In 2001, the group established the Bangkok Hospital Office in Phnom Penh as a one-stop liaison center to facilitate direct patient enquiries from Cambodia. Soon afterwards it opened a clinic in Siern Reap, Cambodia and then offices in Bangladesh, Vietnam and Myanmar. Today, Bangkok Hospital is taking care of international patients traveling from Europe, US and Australia for cost effective medical treatment.

Wherever you go in Thailand, the Bangkok Hospital Group is available to assist you with any medical requirements.

A network of nine branch hospitals throughout the country is able to deal with all the routine medical problems at the following locations:

- Bangkok—Bangkok Hospital
- Prapadang—Bangkok Prapadang Hospital
- Pattaya—Bangkok Pattaya Hospital
- Rayong—Bangkok Rayon Hospital
- Chantaburi—Bangkok Taksin Chantaburi Hospital
- Trat—Bangkok Trat Hospital
- Phuket—Bangkok Phuket Hospital
- Hatyai, Songkla—Bangkok Hatyai Hospital
- Koh Chang—Koh Chang International Clinic
- Koh Samui—Bangkok Samui Hospital.

An experienced Medevac team is also available, at all times, to rapidly transfer patients from regional hospitals, by helicopter, to the Bangkok Hospital.

Medical assistance companies, from neighbouring countries, choose to evacuate their patients and transfer them to Bangkok Hospital, knowing that they will receive the very best treatment available.

In Bangkok, a fleet of ambulances and motorlance vehicles is on 24-hour stand-by to transfer patients rapidly and effectively.

VACCINES AND VACCINATIONS

Chickenpox
Cholera
Hepatitis A
Hepatitis B
Meningitis
Typhoid
Polio
Tetanus
Yellow Fever

- Vaccination are used as a stimulus for the body to create antibodies for a specific disease. Vaccination, if successful, results in immunization.

- Vaccines are generally very safe and adverse reactions are uncommon. Routine immunization programs protect most of the world's children from a number of infectious diseases, which previously claimed million of lives each year. For travelers, vaccinations offer the possibility of avoiding a number of dangerous infections that may be encountered abroad. However, vaccines have not yet been developed against several of the most life-threatening diseases including malaria and HIV/AIDS.
- The vaccinated traveler should not assume that there is no risk of catching the disease against which they have been vaccinated. All additional precautions against infection should be followed carefully, regardless of any vaccines or other medication that have been administered.

TETANUS (Lockjaw) AND DIPHTHERIA

Tetanus, a bacterial disease, is one of the leading cause of death in the tropical countries. The bacterial spores are everywhere and are indestructible, but pose no threat except in the presence of wounds. Once contracted, symptoms arise 7-14 days later. Diphtheria is a bacillus that lives in people's throats; it most common manifestation is in the throat and as skin ulcers. A toxin produced by the bacillus can cause paralysis, which is very serious. These diseases are easily prevented through immunization and following careful hygiene. To also prevent getting these diseases, wash out small wounds with hydrogen peroxide and in case of deep, dirty wounds or animal bites, you should immediately go and get an immunization booster shot. Beware of and stay away from tattooing, ear piercing, chronic ulcers and ear infections, all of which can cause tetanus. Avoid coughing strangers and staying clean will usually prevent diphtheria.

TYPHOID FEVER

High fever, spots, and abdominal pains characterize this acute infectious disease. A bacillus ingested by eating food or drinking water causes the disease. Anyone with these symptoms should seek immediate medical help.

MALARIA

Malaria is a parasite that is spread by Anopheles mosquitoe. Many of the popular jungle trekking areas and rural islands, in Thailand, are places where you are in risk of being bitten by a malaria-infested mosquito. In Bangkok and most popular tourist centers in Thailand, the risk of being bitten by a malaria infested mosquito is low.

The best way to prevent getting bitten would be to use good mosquito repellent, avoid perfumes and scented aftershaves, wear light coloured long-sleeved shirts, long pants, and hoes. At night, sleep with your air-conditioning or a ceiling fan on. Symptoms of malaria are fever, chills, sweating, severe headache, and abdominal pains. Treatment for malaria are very effective and the recovery is very rapid, but not treating malaria could be fatal. So if you have these symptoms you should see a physician immediately.

TYPHUS

All four types of typhus cause fever, headache, and skin rash, but the intensity of symptoms vary according to type. Mountain trekkers are at higher risk of getting this disease. Biting mites that cling to scrub and vegetation in secondary forests spreads this disease. To prevent getting bitten, trekkers should wear long thick pants and use mite repellent, such as diethyl phthalate, and rub it into their skin every four hours. Effective treatment is available but only if it is started early into the illness; there is no vaccination.

DENGUE FEVER

Dengue fever is caused by a virus transmitted to humans through the bite of an infected mosquito. The disease has spread rapidly throughout tropical areas of the world. These infected mosquitoes are much less common in rural areas. This means that bites can occur both in Bangkok and outside the city, 24 hours a day!

People who carry dengue fever have symptom that appear suddenly such as a fever, chills, headache, nausea and vomiting, eye pain and joint and muscle pain, especially in the lower back. This is followed by fatigue, a change in taste and pain when touching the skin. Respiratory and abdominal symptoms may also appear, as with the flu. Sometimes the fever appears to settle after a few days, only to reappear.

It is extremely important to drink plenty of water in order to prevent dehydration. A blood test can help to diagnose dengue fever, which is the best action to take if any symptoms occur. The treatment of dengue fever is primarily aimed at the relief of pain through the use of paracetamols and drinking sufficient amounts of fluid.

Currently there isn't a vaccine for the disease. The only way to avoid dengue fever is to prevent getting bitten by mosquitoes. Using a good mosquito repellant and wearing clothes that cover the entire body can help to prevent this from occurring.

Insects spread many serious, life-threatening diseases. The careful traveler should always keep a good insect repellent nearby. Those of you who experienced reactions to familiar over-the-counter preparations, should seek medical help, and so should those of you entering areas known to be hazardous.

RABIES

The time interval between being bitten and having symptoms is usually about two months, but can vary from a few days to years. The initial symptom of rabies is itching, tingling, or pain at the site of the healed bite. Then the symptoms turn to headache, fever, spreading paralysis with episodes of confusion, aggression, hallucination, and hydrophobia, or an inability to drink water. After these symptoms the infection is fatal. Fortunately the incubation period allows time to get treatment. So if an animal or a stranger bites you, seek medical advice immediately. To prevent getting rabies avoid stray dogs and look for unusually tame behaviour in wild animals, because this is one of the early signs of the disease. Pre-and post-exposure vaccinations are available for this disease.

OTHER THINGS TO CONSIDER

Aside from the preceding list, there are a number of other precautions to bear in mind while visiting Thailand:

(1) Excessive sun exposure can cause skin damage, and or skin cancer. So please, always wear sunscreen lotion while in the sun.
(2) Anyone visiting the tropics with a fever is a serious matter. If you or anyone near you comes down with fever, please remember that it may not be a brief, mild, elf-limited illness. For any persistent or severe fever, especially one associated with persistent diarrhea, vomiting, or jaundice, to seek medical attention immediately.
(3) Those of you affected by motion sickness can minimize this by gazing at a stable external orientation reference. Such as the horizon, if you are on a boat, or straight down the road, if you are in a car. You can also minimize it by holding yourself rigidly to the thing that is moving, instead of allowing yourself to be tossed back and forth within it.
(4) Pregnant women should always remember that most miscarriages occur during the first three months of pregnancy. This is therefore the most dangerous time to travel. In the last three months of pregnancy, women should avoid unnecessary medications, except for vaccinations and anti-malarial drugs, which should be taken where needed and under a doctor's advice. Also, remember to stay within the vicinity of a good hospital during the last wee months of pregnancy.
(5) Vaccinations—it is recommended that people traveling to Thailand should have up-to-date vaccinations against Tetanus, Polio, and Hepatitis A. All children must be vaccinated and must also have proof to say they have been vaccinated.
(6) Post-tropical check-up persons that have experienced illnesses during their trips through the tropical areas, such as diarrhea and fever, or have been exposed to a high-risk disease for even a short time should undergo a specific screening procedure before or after returning borne. Long-term traveler and expatriates living in the tropics should consider undergoing the same procedures from time to time, because examinations often reveal lurking, unsuspecting diseases.

Finally, aircraft passengers with chronically stuffy sinuses should bring along, with them, a decongestant or else they may experience severe sinus pains during the descent. Swollen feet and ankles after a long flight are normal, and there is no need to be alarmed.

Here are some Thai words and phrases to help you on your way:

Medical Problem	*How to say it in Thai*
Abscess/boil	Fee
Aches	Puad
Allergic/sensitive to	Phae
Backache	Puad-lung
Broken bone	Kra-duke-hak
Broken leg	Kha hak
Burns	Mai
Cancer	Ma-reng
Cholera	A-hi-wa
Cut	Bat
Cuts/wounds	Phlae
Dengue Fever	Khai luat auk
Dizzy	Wian hua
Drown	Jom nam
Faint	Pen lom
Fever	Khai
Flu	Khai wad yai
Headache	Puad-hua
Heart Disease	Rok-hua-jai
Help	Chuay duay
I can't breathe	Hai-jai mai awk
I have a cold	Chan pen wad
I have a cough	Chan ai
I have constipation	Chan thong phook
I have Diarrhea	Chan thong-sia
Illness	Puay
Infected	Ak-sayp
Itches	Kun
My eye stings	Seab ta
My hand hurts	Jep-meu
Pains	Jep; puad
Shake/tremble	Sun
Sore Throat	Jep-khaw
Stomachache	Puad-thong
Sunburn	Phiu mai/daet phao
Swollen/inflamed	Buam
Toothache	Puad-fun
Unconscious	Sa-lop/mot sa-ti
Vomit	Uak/a-jian
Weak	Awn plea

HEART HOSPITAL

WHAT IS CARDIOVASCULAR MAGNETIC RESONANCE IMAGING (MRI)?

Magnetic resonance imaging (MRI) uses powerful magnets that cause hydrogen nuclei in the body's molecules to vibrate or resonate and emitting radiofrequency energy. The MRI machine detects these energy emissions and converts them into images, which allows clinicians to see and evaluate many cardiac conditions. Importantly, some diseases and conditions were previously difficult to determine but this technology improves the diagnostic capabilities.

Since the introduction of MRI technology in late 1970's, it has been used as diagnostic tools mainly in neurology and orthopedics. However, the utilities of the machine for heart imaging were limited due to inability to capture a clear image of a beating heart. With the recent development and advancement in hardware and software, MRI can be utilized to image the heart in real time. Cardiovascular MRI offers significant advantages over other imaging methods because it produces excellently clear, complete and detailed three dimensional images of cardiac anatomy without interference from adjacent bone or air. Importantly, patients do not expose to the potential harmful radiation unlike most other non-invasive cardiac tests.

Comprehensive cardiovascular examination now is possible with this powerful technology. Several common heart diseases are benefit from cardiovascular MRI examinations which are:

1. Assessment of coronary artery disease

Coronary artery disease is the condition of reducing the blood flow or oxygen to the heart muscle due to coronary arterial luminal narrowing. MRI can be utilized to assess coronary artery disease patients in many ways.

These include:

- determining whether significant coronary artery stenosis by evaluating myocardial function and perfusion during stress testing,
- providing the most accurate measurement of cardiac volume and function (especially left ventricular ejection fraction) which are the important predictors for coronary artery disease patients,
- evaluating heart muscle damage due to myocardial infarction and determining how much available of viable heart muscle,
- examining structures around the heart which can cause the symptoms of chest pain including aortic dissection, pulmonary embolism, pericardial effusion, etc., and
- detecting significant atherosclerosis of the thoracic aorta which may be important for coronary bypass graft surgery planning.

2. Assessment of congestive heart failure

Heart failure is the condition which can be caused from several etiologies. The most important task is to differentiate between ischemic and non-ischemic heart disease which MRI can be useful in this scenario. Other important information needed for managing other heart patients can be obtained from MRI exam.

- providing the structural and functional status of cardiac chambers,
- evaluating the presence of significant valvular heart disease,
- excluding concurrent conditions with reducing heart function including clot in the left ventricle or pericardial effusion,
- following the effects of medications treating heart failure, and
- examining the functional properties of the aorta which is correlated with the exercise capacity in these patients.

3. Assessment of valvular heart disease

MRI can be used to evaluate the severity of the valvular lesions and follow several parameters to guide the need for either medical or surgical treatments.

These parameters can be provided with MRI examination:

- cardiac chamber size and volume,
- cardiac function,
- the degree of the stenosisor regurgitation of the valve lesions, and
- valve and perivalvular structures evaluation which is important for planning intervention or surgery.

4. Assessment of congenital heart disease

Because there is no limitation on image plane acquisition, complex congenital heart diseases can be assessed with MRI. Functional and structure information can be obtained.

5. Assessment of pericardial disease

Disease of the sac and soft tissue around the heart (pericardium) can cause symptoms including shortness of breath, extremities swelling, hypotension, etc. MRI can be used to examine whether there is significant amount of fluid in the pericardial sac, how thick of the pericardium, and how the heart responses to those abnormalities.

6. Assessment of cardiac tumors

MRI can cover the large examining area; the surrounding structures can be as well evaluated. This provides information of the extension of the mass and the involvement of surrounding structures.

7. Assessment of great vessels and peripheral arteries

MRI can be used to visualize and evaluate the diseases of the aorta and peripheral arteries using gadolinium-based contrast, which is different from the contrast used in conventional angiography. The dose of contrast using during routine MR angiography examination is not nephrotoxic.

Cardiovascular MRI at Bangkok Heart Hospital

Bangkok Heart Institute has been a leader in using innovative tools in diagnosis treatments and prevention of heart disease. The Bangkok Heart Cardiovascular Magnetic Resonance Center develops cardiovascular applications for MRI and utilizes them to benefit of patients with heart disease. Our equipment which include Philips MRI 3.0 Tesla. Intera Achieva, specialized coils with very fast imaging acquisition method. and cardiovascular image software is the most advanced and sophisticated available in the world. Information obtained from cardiovascular MRI examination will help in diagnosis, treatments and planning for interventional procedures or surgery. Center members have been well trained in this highly specialized field.

How to prepare for a MRI study

Please notify your physician or MRI technician, if you have had any brain, eye, ear or other surgeries such as:

- Pacemoker
- Metal implants
- Aneurysm clips
- Surgical clips
- Neuro-stimulater
- Foreign metal objects in the eye
- Bullet
- Inter-uterine devices

If you have gone through the MRI screening procedure with the study representative: and they determine that it is safe for you to have MRI study, the preparation is then simple

"You may eat or drink, sleep and behave as you normally would before your MRI study, unless instructed otherwise by our representative."

Follow these guidelines:

- Do not wear clothing with metal components if you have contact lens, wear these instead of glasses.
- Remove body piercing and other jewelry if possible.
- You may be asked to remove dentures or removable dental bridges, retainers, etc.
- If you have tattoos that may contain metal dye, notify the study representative.

- Do not wear eye shadow or any makeup that may contain metal speckles.
- If you are pregnant. please notify your physician.

What should you expect?

The procedure typically will take anywhere from 30 to 60 minutes, depending on the type of information required by your physician. You just need to be as still as possible during the exam. Sometimes you will be asked to hold your breathing 5-10 seconds during scanning. A technician will be able to see you all the time and there is a built-in intercom system, which you can communicate with us at anytime. A contrast agent or medication given during the study, will give important information to the requested physician.

The newest addition to the Bangkok Hospital Group

Recognised as the leader in private medical health care in Thailand and the South East Asian region, our outstanding facilities, leading expertise and latest advancements in medical technology place us among the world's premier global health care providers.

Bangkok International Hospital's vision is to create a comfortable ambience for people of all cultures. Our dedicated international team gives full attention to the understanding and needs of each individual patient. With 26 languages spoken, we ensure a welcoming experience for everyone and ensure your time spent with Bangkok International Hospital is a pleasant one.

The finest physicians over a range of specialties

Our sixteen specialized centres, ranging from pediatrics to geriatrics, neurology to cardiology, bring together some of the finest internationally trained and qualified physicians, complemented by state-of-the-art medical technology. All centres offer the latest diagnostic and treatment methods, integrated into a comprehensive care programme, within a welcoming, friendly environment.

A world of attention

Our policy of attentive service stretches beyond the simply medical. We are well equipped to make every facet of your stay in Thailand a comfortable one. Scheduling of travel arrangements as well as assistance with preferential room rates at local hotels and apartments mean that patients and their loved ones will be taken care of at every moment of their stay. Other services include airport pickup, round the clock contact for medical assessments, advice on treatment options and doctor's appointments, ambulance services, liaison with embassies and international organisations, claims liaison with insurance companies, and 24-hour medical evacuation and repatriation.

Catering to your particular needs

Our outpatient clinics are designed around the requirements of our patients. Cultural and personal needs are taken into account with unique facilities for International Medical Services, Japanese Medical Services, and Arabic Medical Services

A comfortable stay

Inpatients will find that their every need—cultural, personal and religious—is taken care of while at Bangkok International Hospital. Dietary requirements are strictly respected and adhered to. To help the time pass quickly, each room is equipped with 32 inch LCD television, satellite TV, internet access, microwave oven, refrigerator and telephone as well as a safety deposit box for peace of mind.

Unparalleled Technology

Our medical team are second to none, and the caring nature of our Thai staff is legendary. This would not be complete without the equipment we use being at the forefront of medical technology.

Da Vinci Robotic Cardiac Surgery

The most advanced cardiac technology, providing minimally invasive cardiac treatment.

PET-CT (Positron Emission Tomography)

PET scanning and CT imaging, for faster and more accurate diagnosis of cancer and heart problems.

IMRT (Intensity Modulated Radiotherapy)

BrainLAB is dedicated system for non-invasive surgery or stereotactic radiotherapy to treat cancer (radiation administered in a series of treatment sessions): SRS/SRT.

Leksell Gamma Knife

Neurosurgical Gamma Knife Treatment for brain tumors, AVM, Epilepsy, Parkinsonism.

MRI (Intra Achiva 3.0T MRI)

The latest MRI with 3.0 Tesla. Reduced MRI time, providing clearer imagery with less exposure.

64-slice Multi-Detector CT Scan

High Speed CT SCAN with today's modern technology.

GAMMA KNIFE CENTRE

Once a patient and a doctor have decided on a GAMMA KNIFE procedure, the patient should be admitted into the hospital a night prior to the treatment to have a health check-up and to wash the hair (no shaving is necessary). The next morning, a neurosurgeon applies a head frame to the patient's head and then a CT or MRI scanning procedure is performed. The scanned images produced are entered into a computer system operated by the neurosurgeon to identify the exact location of the lesion and to measure the amount of radiation to be used. When the radiation therapy is completed, the frame is removed. The patient might be asked to stay overnight for observation. The patient is released the next day and can resume his/her normal activities immediately. Follow-up appointments are to be made for every three to six months.

TREATMENT PROTOCOL: FOUR EASY STEPS

1. Frame Fixation

The neurosurgeon places the Leksell Stereotactic frame to the patient's head. The frame is attached to the head with adjustable pins. The frame is used to pinpoint the exact position of the target brain tissue.

2. Diagnosis Imaging

After the Leksell Stereotactic frame is fixed to the head, the technician will scan the image of the brain with CT or MRI or Angiography scanner. The images produced are used for treatment planning and for measurement of the size of the target lesion.

3. Computerized Treatment Planning

Scanned images are sent to the planning center and entered into the computer system to create a three dimensional image. The doctor and the medical physicist can then calculate the amount of radiation to cover the tumor or the lesion.

4. Treatment

The patient is sent to the Gamma Knife room and the helmet is placed on the patient's head. The Stereotactic frame holds the head in place to make sure that the head lies absolutely still so that the target tumor is positioned at the radiation beam. The finely focused beams are emitted continuously in a 1-2 hour time frame. During that time, the patient experiences no pain or discomfort. After the treatment is complete, the patient is escorted to a patient room and may be discharged the following day.

ABOUT THE GAMMA KNIFE

GAMMA KNIFE treatment has been researched and studied for over 30 years with continuous follow-up and development. Since the beginning of 2003, several medical institutes across America, Europe and Asia have used GAMMA KNIFE to treat more than 230,000 patients with brain disorders.

In Thailand, Bangkok Hospital has offered GAMMA KNIFE treatment for Thai patients since 1996. Since the center is an open institution, doctors from any medical establishments are welcome to send their patients to be treated here at Bangkok Neurosurgical Gamma Center or to join the treatment with the center's neurologist. The center helps reduce the patient's cost and time travelling abroad for the treatment. Meanwhile the patient can feel comfortable at home with the support of family and friends.

What is the Gamma Knife?

Leksell Gamma Knife is a radiosurgery tool to treat patients with brain disorders. The instrument emits the proper amount of radiation to the target such as tumors or AVM.

How does the Gamma Knife Work?

Leksell Gamam Knife contains 201 radioactive cobalt-60 sources. The intense-dose radiation beams are delivered through holes in the helmet to the target lesion in the brain with minimal effect to the surrounding tissue. The Gamma Knife instrument is highly accurate; therefore, it gives a very successful result.

Why use the Gamma Knife?

In the past, to cure some brain diseases we needed an open-brain surgery to expose the lesion or to cure the illness. Thanks to Bangkok Hospital, the hospital responsible for bringing the technology of radiology to Thailand eight years ago, Thai people now have more choices and opportunities to be treated for brain diseases.

Comparison between the Gamma Knife Treatment and the Open-Brain Surgery

Gamma Knife is a safe alternative treatment compared to open brain surgery. The Gamma Knife treatment minimizes the risk of surgical complication. There are also fewer side effects and lower risk of post-surgical disability. Meanwhile, the patient saves time and expense of rehabilitation.

GAMMA KNIFE: The Technology Trusted All Over the World For Treating

- Vascular disorders such as arteriovenous malformation (AVM).
- Brain tumours
- Brain cancer, cancer from somewhere else to the brain.
- Certain brain dysfunction such as Parkinson's disease and Epilepsy.

	Comparison Chart	*Gamma Knife*	*Open-Brain Surgery*
1.	The risk of discomfort and pain	None	High
2.	The risk of bleeding	None	High
3.	The risk of infection	None	High
4.	Anesthesia	No	Yes
5.	Convalescent time at the hospital	1-2 days	30-60 days
6.	Incision scar	No	Yes
7.	The efficiency to expose the lesions	High	Deep or inaccessible lesions might remain
8.	The risk of a patient over 50 years of age	Low	High
9.	Operation time	1-2 hours	3-18 hours or more
10.	Head shaving	No	Yes

UROLOGICAL CENTRE

Bangkok Urological Center was established in 1995. The center has gone through great improvement and new development to increase its effectiveness in medical service especially for the diagnosis and treatment of patients with urinary tract diseases. We are equipped with carefully selected high-technology and state-of-art equipment to perform proper medical treatment including:

- Urological investigations including cystoscopy, ureterorenoscopy and nephrosopic examination.
- Uroflowmetry and urodynamic study
- Ultrasonography and Transrectal ultrasound
- Endourological investigation and surgery
- Extracorporeal Shockwave Lithotripsy (ESWL)
- Brachytherapy for prostate cancer
- Advance urological surgeries including Microwave and Laser surgery (VLAP)
- Sex diagnosis and sex reassignment surgery
- Kidney Transplantation
- We also offer counselling and treatment on sexual dysfunction, genital abnormality and aging male by experiences urologists with high standard technology.

The center provides a complete one-stop medical service with experienced staff who work as team. The complete urological investigations as one-stop service at Bangkok Urological Center:

Urinary Tract Tumour Clinic

The center provides the diagnosis with ultrasound scanner, X-ray, computer scan, endoscopic examination and surgical biopsy if necessitate. The treatment including medication, surgical intervention and radical surgery for tumour. The chemotherapy or radiation therapy are available as conventional needed.

Prostate Gland Clinic

The complete investigations for prostate problems are available at all time. This is including the prostate examination, uroflowmetry, urodynamic study, transrectal ultrasound, cystoscopic examination and needle biopsy. The blood test for prostatic cancer are routinely done. The treatment for prostate gland are conventionally available either medical treatment and surgical treatments. The Laser and Microwave prostatic surgeries are frequently used. The Brachytherapy for non-invasive carcinoma of prostate is our experienced procedure.

Stone Diseases Clinic

The urinary tract stones are one of the most common daily diseases. The complete investigation and treatment can be done as one stop occasion. The management can be immediately treated by medication, cystoscopic lithotripsy, URS lithotripsy, Percutaneous nephrolithotripsy (PCNL) and Shockwave lithotripsy (ESWL). This is depending to the size and location of stones.

The Incontinence Clinic

The clinic specialized in treatment of patients with problem related to urinary incontinence (urine leakage) and pelvic floor relaxation disorder especially in women, patients with spinal cord or brain injury and pediatric incontinence. Patients will be served for neuropathic bladder test by uroflowmetry or urodynamics study.

Aging Male Health Clinic

Is specialized in aging male. The male with the hormone or mental health imbalance. The symptoms of sexual disorder, erectile dysfunction. The clinic will provides physical, psychology couselling, alternative medical, hormonal and surgical treatments. Those including viagra, apomorphine medications, intracavenous injection, vacuum devices and surgical prosthesis. The implantation of artificial device, depending on the doctor's psychological and medical guidance.

Kidney Transplantation Clinic

We have the team of nephrologist, immunologist and transplant surgeons. The clinic is able to provide excellent medical service to patient with chronic renal disease and kidney transplantation in order to provide the better quality of life.

Sex Reassignment Clinic

The clinic offer counselling on sexual disorder in children, men and women. We also provide the sex recorrection surgery as well as a sex reassignment surgery especially for a man to woman by experienced surgeons.

LIVER CANCER CENTRE

The liver is the largest organ in the body, and extremely important organ that has many functions. This includes producing proteins that circulate in the blood. Some of these help the blood to clot and prevent excessive bleeding, while others are essential for maintaining the balance of fluid in the body. Hepatoma, or hepatocellular carcinoma is the most common primary liver cancer and related to chronic viral hepatitis B and C. This section gives more information about this kind of liver cancer.

- What is liver cancer?
- What causes liver cancer?
- What are the symptoms?
- How is it diagnosed?
- Treatment?

What is Liver Cancer?

There are two different types of liver cancer. The commoner kind is called hepatoma or hepatocellular carcinoma (HCC), and arises from the main cells of the liver. This type is usually confined to the liver, and occurs mostly in people with a liver disease called cirrhosis. There is also a rarer sub-type of hepatoma called Fibrolamellar hepatoma, which may occur in younger people and is not related to previous liver diseases. The less common type of primary liver cancer is called cholangiocarcinoma or bile duct cancer, because it starts in the cells lining the bile ducts.

What causes liver cancer?

Most people who develop hepatoma usually also have a condition called cirrhosis of the liver. This is a fine scarring throughout the liver which is due to a variety of causes including infection and heavy alcohol drinking over long period of time. Infection with either the hepatitis B or hepatitis C virus can lead to liver cancer, and can also be the cause of cirrhosis which increases the risk of developing hepatoma. In Asia a poison called Aflatoxin, found in mouldy peanuts and grain, is an important cause of hepatoma. In the western world, cancer of the liver usually occurs in middle-aged and elderly people, although rarely it can also affect children and young adults.

What are the common symptoms?

In the early stages of liver cancer there are often no symptoms. Sometimes people notice a vague discomfort in the upper abdomen that may become painful. This is due to enlargement of the liver. Loss of appetite, weight loss, jaundice, ascites, nausea, and weakness and tiredness are common symptoms.

Whatever the cause of these symptoms will always indicate a condition that needs medical attention and would not be ignored and should be checked by your doctor.

How to diagnose?

Usually you begin by seeing your doctor who will examine you and arrange for any tests or x-rays that may be necessary. Your primary physician will refer you to a hospital specialist for appropriate tests and for expert advice and treatment.

You will have a physical examination and blood tests such as liver function tests and AFP: liver cancer screening.

Your doctor may arrange for you to have a liver ultrasound, an abdominal CT scan, a magnetic resonance imaging (MRI) scan, or a liver biopsy.

Types of treatment

Surgery is the most effective treatment for primary liver cancer, but this is not always possible due to the size or position of the tumor. It is also not possible to operate if the cancer has spread beyond the liver. Liquids such as alcohol may be injected into the tumour to destroy it (known as tumour ablation). Chemotherapy may also sometimes be used.

BACK PAIN CENTRE

Back Pain is a common problem among people of just about any age, most of it can be treated with bed rest or in conjunction with medication. Some of it is bad enough or chronic that may disturb working and routine daily activities.

Most back pain comes from the muscles, ligaments and joints in the back when they are not moving the way they should. Many different factors can work together to cause back pain.

Causes of back pain can be categorized into 2 groups

1. Musculoskeletal system disorder occur by abnormal development of the back bone, excessive stress on the back, injury, or anyone of a number of physical disorders that affect the bones or the discs in the spine. The cause of pain may be differentiated by character of pain such as—

a. Back pain alone may be caused by

- Inflammation of back muscle and joint from working in poor posture or back injury.
- Infection of back bone or in spinal column.
- Spinal tumor.
- Degenerative process of facet joint and intervertebral disc.

b. Back pain with radiating pain to other places

Such as hip, either leg or both legs. These symptoms are due to the compression of the spinal nerve root. The degeneration of the back bone, joint and disc may be the cause of compression. The patient may experience weakness and numbness of the legs with more severe compression. This leg pain, which may be accompanied by numbing or tingling sensation, and weakness may affect the thigh, the calf and also the foot.

2. Diseases from other organ that can create back pain such as flu, gastritis, kidney disease, gynaecologic disease, intrapelvic tumor.

Treatment

Aim of treatment is to make the patient return to their normal activities as soon as possible and prevention of severe back pain.

Treatment according to the causes

1. In case of musculoskeletal system disorder, doctors generally prescribe one or more of the following treatments:

- Medication
- Physical therapy such as heat, rest, exercise, postural training, weight loss
- Back support
- Local injection such as epidural injection, selective nerve root block, facet joint injection
- Surgery if indicated

2. Disease from other organs

- Diagnose and treat that cause

A guide to prevent low back pain

Changing posture in routine daily life will prevent and lessen back pain.

Sleeping Sleep on a firm mattresses. If the mattresses is to soft, your back would be overbending and that make your back hurt.

SLEEPING POSTURE

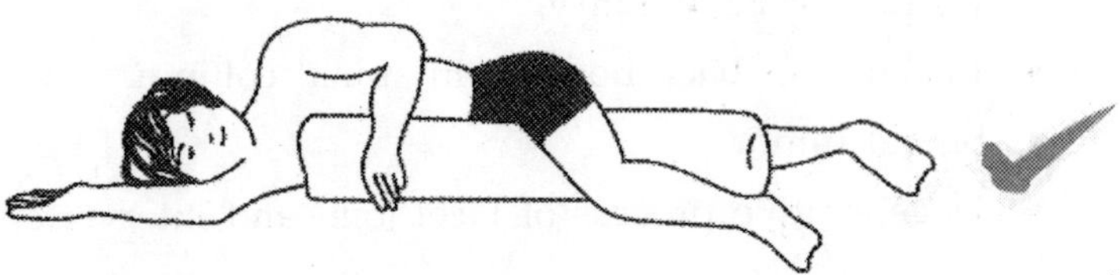

If you sleep on side, place a pillow between your knees.

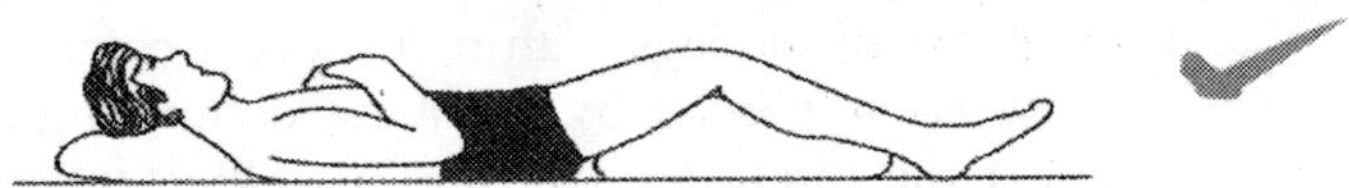

If you sleep on back, place a pillow between your knees.

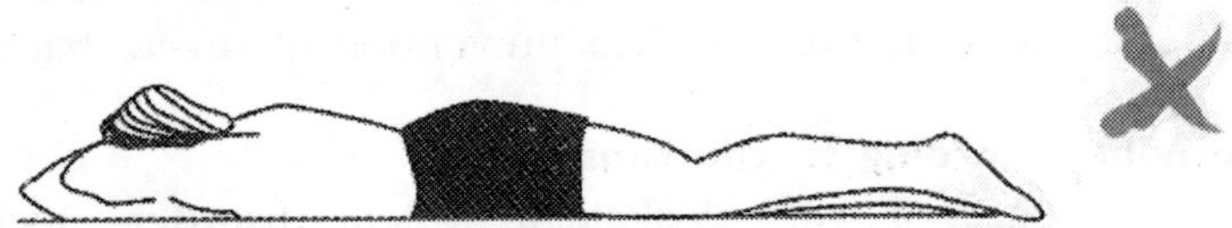

Sleeping on your stomach is not good. That arch your back too much and make your back hurt.

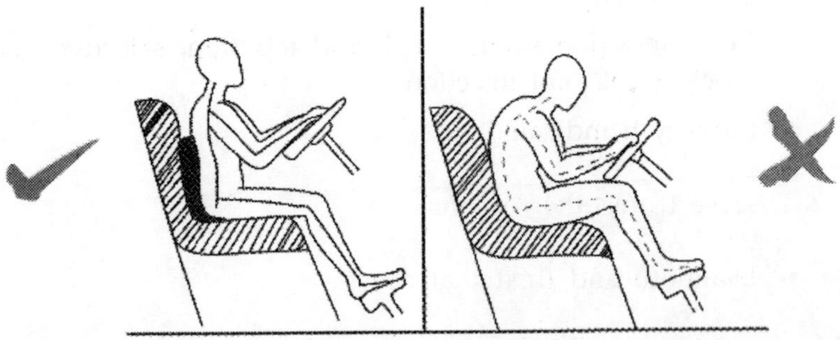

When driving, keep your back in a normal, slightly arched positino. Place a small pillow to support your low back.

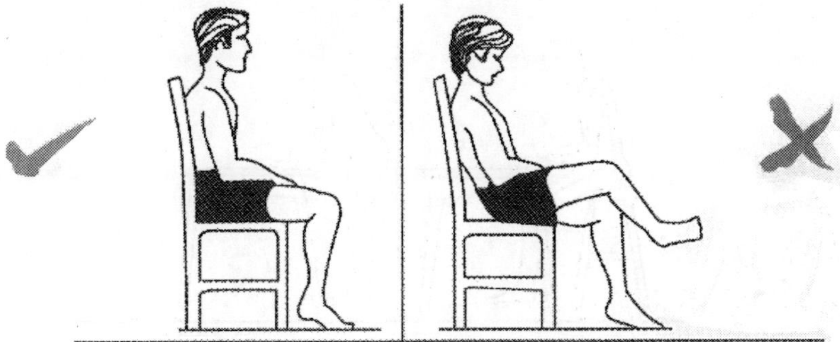

When sitting, keep your back in a normal, slightly arched position. Make sure your chair supports your lower back, keep your head and shoulder erect.

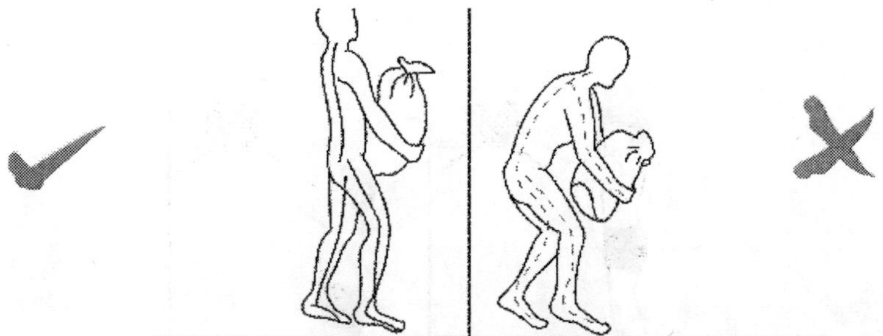

When lifting loads, do not bend at your waist. Bend at the knees and lift with your leg, maintain a straight back with your head up. Don't try to ilft by yourself an object that is too heavy or an awkward shape. Get help.

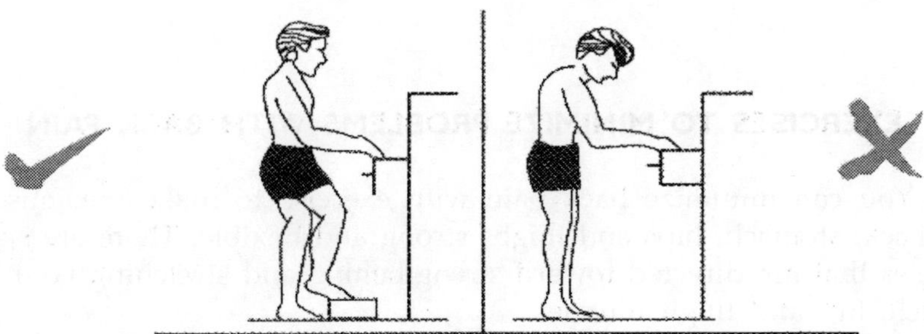

When standing for a long time, rest oen foot on a stip to lessen arching of the back.

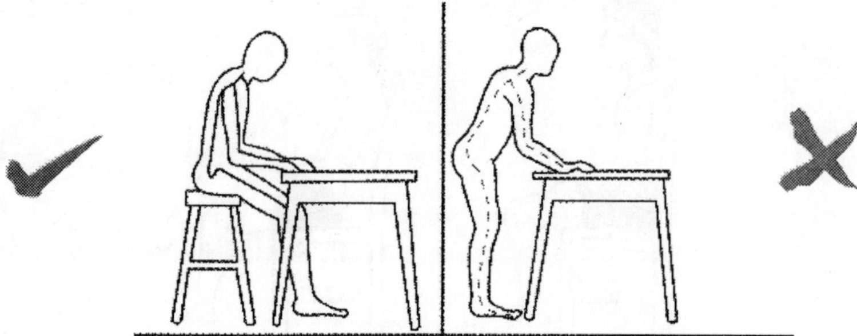

When working on table, make sure your working surface is at the proper height so you dno't have to lean forward.

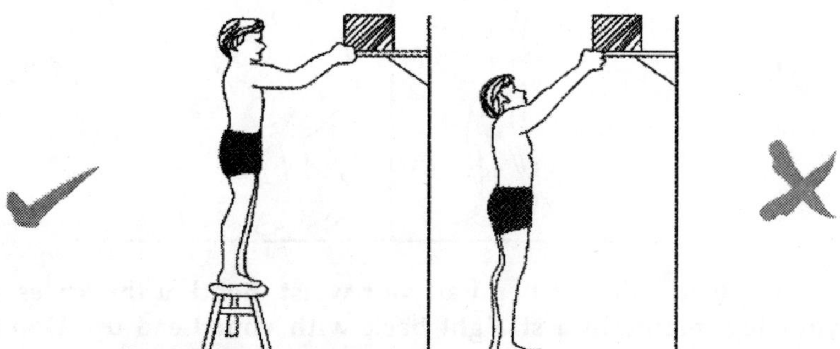

If the shelf is chest high, move close to the shelf. Use steps if the object is over chest high.

EXERCISES TO MINIMIZE PROBLEMS WITH BACK PAIN

You can minimize back pain with exercise to make the muscle in your back, stomach, hips and thighs strong and flexible. There are specific exercises that are directed toward strengthening and stretching your back, stomach, hip and thigh muscles.

It is important to exercise regularly, every other day. A little exercise every day can make a huge difference. If your back hurts during exercise, stop doing immediately.

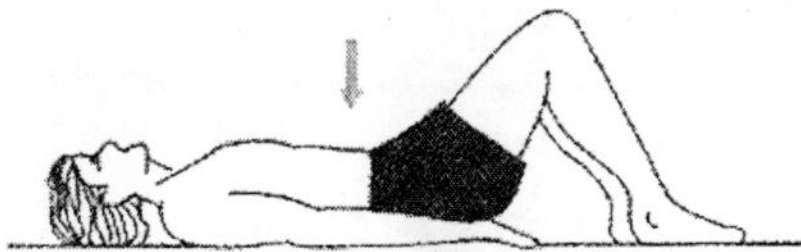

Act. 1

Lie on your back with your arms at your sides and knee bent.
Step 1 tighten your stomach muscle to push your back against the floor. Count to 3.
Step 2 relax your stomach muscle, repeat five times.

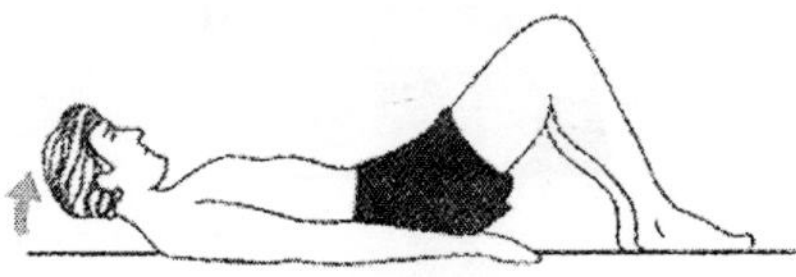

Act. 2

Lie on your back with knee bent and feet flat on the floor.
Slowly raise your head off the floor. Count to 2. Repeat 10 times.

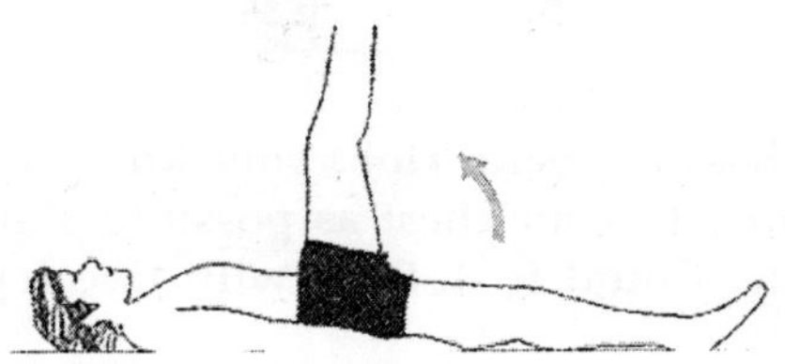

Act. 3

Lie on your back with your arms at your sides. Lift one leg off the floor, hold your lege up for a count of 0 and return it to the floor. Do the same with the other leg. Repeat five times with each leg.

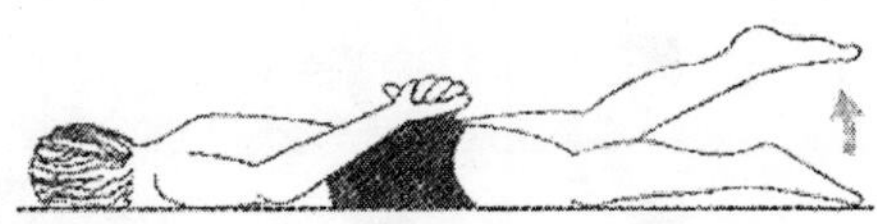

Act. 4

Lie on your stomach. Tighten the muscles in one leg and raise it from the floor. Hold your leg up for a count of 10 and return it to the floor. Do the same with the other leg. Repeat five times with each leg.

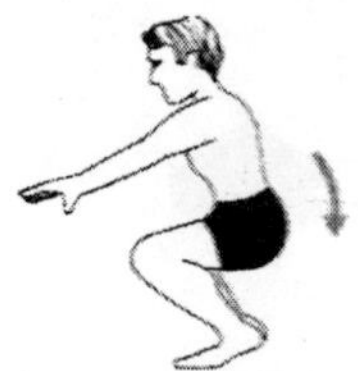

Act. 5

Stand with your feet slightly apart. Slide down into a crouch with knees bent to about 90 degrees. Keep the back straight. Count to give and silde back up. Repeat five times.

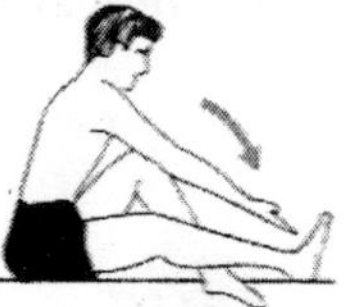

Act. 6

Sit upright with one leg straight and the other knee bent. Reach with both hands toward your feet. Count to 3. Repeat five times.

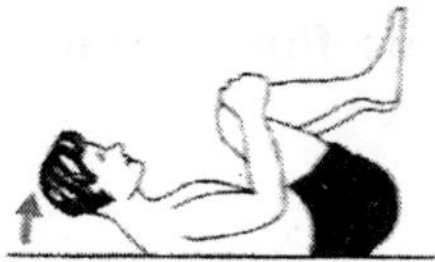

Act. 7

Lie on your back with knees bent. Hold your knees with both hands and pull your knees as close to your chest as possible. Raise the hand-off the floor at the same time. Count to 3. Start with five repetitions.

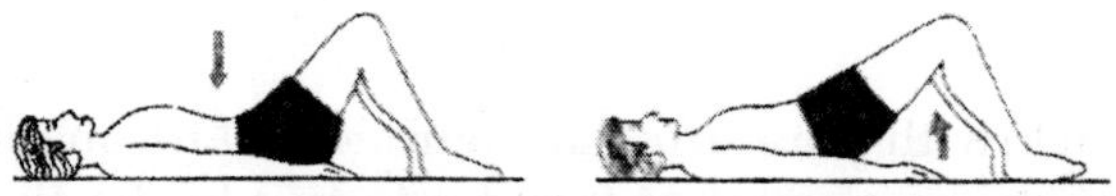

Act. 8

Lie on your back with arms at your sides and knees bent. Step 1 tighten your stomach muscle to push your back against the floor. Step 2 raise your buttock off the floor. Count to 3 and return it to the floor.

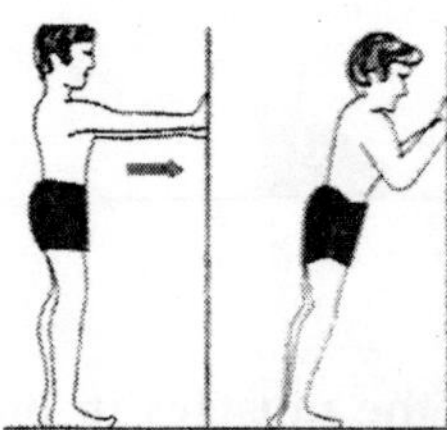

Act. 9

Stand with your feet slightly apart and about 1/2 meter away from the wall. Stretch your arm and push your hands against the wall. Lean forward and Count to 3. Return to standing positino.

DENTAL CARE

BANGKOK DENTAL AND MAXILLOFACIAL CENTER

It will help our team to make preliminary plan, if you can provide us in advance with the panoramic and periapical x-rays of your teeth. Contact Bangkok Dental and Maxillofacial Center: e-mail dental@bangkokhospital.com

Some of Dental and Maxillofacial Services that we offer: March 2005

Esthetic and Operative Dentistry

1. Laser Tooth Whitening — 14000 bahts/mouth
   Treatment Time : approx. 1 visit

   Customized Home Used Tray — 4000 bahts/set
   Home Used Set

2. **Anterior Porcelain Full Veneer** — 9,000 bahts/mouth
   [to correct brown/grey colored tooth]
   Treatment Time approx. 2-3 visits (1-2 weeks total)

3. Posterior Tooth Colored Restoration [price varies per surface of tooth]
   - With Composite Filling — 1,000-3000 bahts/tooth
   - With Composite Inlay or Onlay — 4,000-5,500 bahts/tooth
   - With Porcelain Inlay or Onlay — 9,000-10,000 bahts/tooth

   Treatment Time approx. 2-3 visits (1-2 weeks total)

Full Mouth Tooth Cleaning

Full Mouth Tooth Cleaning — 900-1,500 bahts/mouth
Stain Removal with Air-flow — 900 bahts/mouth
Treatment Time: approx. 1 visit.

Periodontal Treatment and Surgery

Treatment for Periodontitis — 5,200-8,000 bahts/mouth
Treatment Time : approx. 2-3 visits (2-3 weeks total)

Periodontal Surgery — 5,500-12,000 bahts/procedure
Treatment Time : approx. 2-3 visits (1-2 weeks total)

Root Canal Treatment

RCT for anterior and posterior tooth — 5,500-10,500 bahts/tooth
Retreat of old root canal — +2,000 bahts/tooth

Treatment Time: approx. 1-3 visits (1-2 weeks total)

Fixed Crown and Bridge

Diagnostic model, radiograph, consultation and treatment plan	2,460	bahts
All Ceramic crown	15.400	bahts/crown
Full Precious Crown	13,200-15,400	bahts/crown
Porcelain Fused to Precious Crown	13,200-15,400	bahts/crown
Pin [for root canal treated tooth]	3,300-4,400	bahts/pin

Treatment Time: approx. 2-3 visits (1-2 weeks total)

Removable Denture

Diagnostic model, radiographs, consultation and treatment plan	2.460	bahts
Full Denture [with metal or acrylic high impact base]	11,000 15,400	bahts/arch

Treatment Time: approx. 5-6 visits (3 weeks total)

Partial Denture [price varies per number of teeth]	9.000-5,400	bahts/arch

Treatment Time: approx. 4 visits (2-3 weeks total)

Dental Implant

Diagnostic model, radiographs, consultation and treatment plan	2,000-3,000	bahts
Dental Implant (Replace Implant System)	80,000	bahts/Implant
Dental Implant (Branemark Implant System)	88,000	bahts/Implant

Treatment Time : approx. 4 visits

[first 2 visits and last 2 visits about 3-6 months apart]
1st visit Consultation, Radiographs and Treatment Plan
2nd visit Implant Surgical Part
(wait 3-6 months for bone attaches to Implant)
3rd visit Take Impression for Prosthetic Pant
4th visit Insert Prosthetic Part

Please visit our Website: www.bangkokhospital.com
for more dental information about Implant in Dentistry, Laser Tooth Whitening, Air Flow Stain Removal, etc.

HEALTH CHECK UPS

Health Check-up at Bangkok International Hospital

As long as we are feeling healthy we see little need to go to the doctor, however, yearly check-ups can be very beneficial and sometimes life saving. Yearly check-ups help to detect minor problems before they become major problems. At Bangkok Hospital we have a full range of standard check-up packages as well as tailor making health check-ups to your needs.

The following guidelines are to assist you in gaining the most from your check-up:

- Please do not eat or drink for at least 8 hours before taking any tests as this can effect the results (a small amount of water is acceptable)

Selecting the right check-up package:

We want you to select the package option which best suits your needs and is most relevant to your health (please see overleaf for standard packages)

- The packages are divided into age and sex groups with additional options.
- Each package has a fixed price, unless you include extra checks.
- You can select the package by yourself or consult with the doctor for advice—please inform our staff if you would like to visit the doctor first.

Your check-up

- Firstly you will be asked to fill out a form about your lifestyle, medical history and family history
- The nurse will then check your height, weight and sight.
- You will then be given some pyjamas to change into and a container for your urine sample.
- Please change your clothes and keep your belongings in the locker provided.
- Please place your urine sample container in the basket located outside the bathroom.
- Our nurse will now guide you through the program until all tests are done.
- Usually your blood will be taken first as these results take the longest to develop.

Most check-up results are received within an hour after finishing, however some checks can take up to 3 hours.

- Once your results have been processed, you will receive a booklet from the checkup department analysing all your test results.
- You should then visit the doctor for the final diagnosis and overview of your check-up test results.

Payment

Please ensure that you pay for your health check-up package before leaving the hospital. Payment can be made at any of the cashier counters located around the hospital. Please have your appointment slip or hospital number for reference.

Health Check-up Packages

Items Please keep fasting (no food and drink) at least 8-10 hours before coming for checkup	Vital Age Age range	14-30 yrs.	Supreme 30-45 yrs.	Ultimate Male 45 yrs. up	Ultimate Female 45 yrs. up
Examination by doctor	Physical Examination	√	√	√	√
Eye Screening	Eye Exam Screening			√	√
Dental Screening	Dental Screening			√	√
Hearing Screening	Hearing Screening		√	√	√
complete blood count	CBC	√	√	√	√
Blood sugar	FBS	√	√	√	√
	SGPT	√	√	√	√
	SGOT	√	√	√	√
Liver function test	Alkaline phosphatase		√	√	√
	GGT			√	√
Bilirubin (Total Bilirubin, Direct	Bilirubin, (Total Bilirubin,			√	√
	Direct Bilirubin			√	√
	Total Protein (Albumin Globulin)			√	√
Kidney function test	BUN			√	√
	Creatinine	√	√	√	√
Thyroid screening	TSH			√	√
	Free T4			√	√
Gout screening	Uric Acid		√	√	√
	Cholesterol	√	√	√	√
Lipid screening	Triglyceride	√	√	√	√
	HDL	√	√	√	√
	LDL	√	√	√	√
Tumor marker for liver cancer	AFP			√	√
Tumor marker for colon cancer	CEA			√	√
Tumor marker for prostate cancer	PSA			√	√
Urine analysis	Urine Exam	√	√	√	√
Stool exam for occult blood	Stool Exam			√	√
Chest x-ray	Chest x-ray	√	√	√	√
Rest EKG	EKG		√	√	√
Heart screening	Exercise Stress Test		√	√	√
Ultrasound abdomen	Ultrasound Whole Abdomen		√	√	√
Osteoporosis screening	Bone Densitometry				√
Peripheral vascular blockage screening	ABI			√	√
Cervix cancer screening	Thin prep pap test				√
Breast cancer screening	Digital Mammogram				√
Ultrasound Breast	Ultrasound Breast				√
	Regular Price (THB.)	4,830	24,830	23,180	32,295
	Special Price (THB.)	2,600	8,100	12,700	17,770

POSITRON EMISSION TOMOGRAPHY AND CT

Bangkok PET/CT Center is very proud to present the latest generation of the PET/CT scanning technology to serve patients in Thailand and from other countries in the Asia-Pacific region. The combination PET/CT is a major advance in imaging technology and patient care. The our PET/CT scanner (GEMINI, Philips) is the first to be installed for medical services in Thailand.

What is PET?

PET (Positron Emission Tomography) is a functional imaging technology using radioisotopes. The medical application of PET primarily includes early detection of cancers, assessment of heart muscle viability in heart diseases and evaluation of functional brain anatomy in dementia, epilepsy and stroke. Across various applications to cancers, the average sensitivity and specificity of 18F-FDG PET were estimated at 84% and 99% respectively. The accuracy ranged from 87% to 90%.

How is PET different from CT or MRI?

By labelling foci of metabolically active cells or tissues in the body, PET provides functional information, which is not available from structural images such as CT (Computed Tomography) and MRI (Magnetic Resonance Imaging). However, the spatial resolution of PET is intrinsically limited, that is, it does not generate as detailed a pictorial representation of an organ structure as CT or MRI.

What is PET/CT Scanning?

PET/CT scanning is a combination of PET and CT that generates precisely co-registered functional and structural images. This can be achieved by performing both PET and CT studies on the same scanner with no necessity to move the patient. The integrated PET/CT images provide functional information on detailed organ structures in the body.

How does PET work?

PET images are produced by the emission of radiation by an injected or inhaled isotope in tissue. By using different substances of biology interest labelled with positron emitting radionuclide (PET radiopharmaceutical). The PET systems have the advantage of using physiologically important isotopes, such as 11-Carbon, 13-Nitrogen, 15-Oxygen, and I8-Fluorine (18F). A cyclotron is needed in generating these positron-emitting isotopes that have short half-lives.

18F-FDG (2-[18F]fluoro-2-deoxy-D-glucose) PET is able to measure different rates of glucose metabolism in various tissues or organs that use glucose to obtain energy. The radiation during PET/CT scanning is equal to the amount of radiation exposure during two chest x-rays.

Applications of 18F-FDG PET in cancer scanning

- Early detection of cancers of various organs, such as lung cancer, head and neck cancer, colourectal cancer, melanoma, lymphoma, breast cancer, ovarian cancer, and pancreatic cancer.
- Staging of cancers.
- Monitoring the response to therapy.
- Assessment of the effectiveness of treatments.
- Detection of the metastasis and recurrence.

18F-FDG PET by means of providing information on the metabolic activity of tissues, is able to detect small foci of early cancer, especially in case it has spread to other organs of the body (metastases). In contrast, with CT or MRI the cancer must reach a significant size enough to distort the surrounding structures before the effect will show up on the scans.

PET/CT in Heart System

PET/CT can be used for assessment of heart muscle viability in heart diseases and myocardial perfusion. The sensitivity is more than 90%.

PET/CT in Brain System

- Brain tumor: diagnostic and follow up after treatment.
- Diagnostic and high accuracy of localization of seizure in the brain results in very effective surgery treatment.
- Dementia: diagnostic pathology and the cause of dementia for an efficient and accurate treatment (especially in elder persons).

What are the procedures involved in PET/CT scanning?

- Fasting for a period of at least 6 hours prior to scanning.
- Measuring fasting blood glucose.
- Injecting the radioisotope agent via the patient's cubital vein.
- Resting for a short period of time.
- Positioning on the scanning bed and keeping till during scanning.
- Scanning times vary with the procedure, generally about 20-60 minutes.
- After the scanning, the radiologist will interpret the images and report to the referring physician who will then discuss the findings with the patient.

NON-INVASIVE STEREOLACTIC RADIOSURGERY (NOVALIS)

What is Novalis®?

Novalis®, BrainLAB's dedicated system for non-invasive stereotactic radiosurgery (a high dose of radiation applied in a single session) or stereotactic radiotherapy (radiation administered in a series of treatment sessions) (SRS/SRT).

Novalis® is the optimal tool to effectively and safely perform the advanced techniques of 3-D CRT, high resolution Intensity Modulated RadioSurgery (IMRS) and Intensity Modulated RadioTherapy (IMRT) on tumors throughout the body.

IMRS: IMRT combined with accurate target positioning. Only the combination of IMRT with precise target positioning will allow to tailor the IMRT dose as tight as possible around target volume.

Novalis® shapes the radiation beams to match the exact shape of the tumor or lesion by using micromultileaf collimator (mMLC). Even the irregularly shaped tumors or lesions receive doses of radiation totally consistent with what the physician prescribes. The result is the tumor or lesion receives its prescribed dose of radiation while avoiding critical tissues and organs. The mechanical accuracy of the Novalis' system, as well as its precise localization and positioning technology, allows for the patient to reduce the total number of fractions for the treatment of certain indications, thus minimizing the cost per patient.

What cancers and illnesses can Novalis® treat?

- Primary brain tumors
- Gliomas (astrocytomas, glioblastomas, oligodendrogliomas, ependymomas)
- Acoustic neuromas/acoustic schwannomas
- Pituitary tumors
- Meningiomas
- Chordomas and chondrosarcomas
- Brain metastasis
- Hepatocellular carcinoma
- Cholangiocarcinoma
- Liver metastasis
- Lung cancer

Non-cancerous conditions

- Arteriovenous malformations (AVMs)
- Cavernous malformations
- Trigeminal neuralgia
- Intractable seizures
- Parkinson's disease
- Extracranial disorders

Why would I like to choose Novalis® for Treatment?

The primary advantages of stereotactic radiosurgery are its precision and minimal risk. Equipped with highly sophisticated computer-based imaging techniques, Novalis® delivers the radiation beam with a high precision and produces a sharp radiation dose gradient at the tumor and normal tissue boundary.

It may therefore be the treatment of choice for patients whose doctors cannot perform traditional surgery due to the increased risk of harming critical structures inside the brain. Tumors located deep in the brain or in other inoperable areas may be treated with Novalis®. Novalis® is also increasingly a treatment of choice for patients with multiple tumors in different areas of the brain or tumors throughout body. Novalis® has an exceptionally high dose rate of 800 cGy/min. resulting in a total treatment time much shorter than that obtained with conventional linac or cobalt-based radiosurgery units.

Novalls® Basic Principle

Novalis® device is a high precision LINAC (linear accelerator) unit, which generates single energy x-ray (6 MV photon beam) and is equipped with an m3 High-Resolution Multileaf Collimator (52 leaves) with its fine 3 mm leaves width at isocenter. Novalis= has revolutionized radiosurgery by introducing conformal treatments that precisely tailor the dose to the shape of the tumor. The shape of treatment field ranges from 3 x 3 mm^2 to 100x 100 mm^2.

The system is capable of performing dynamic a· segmented IMRT or IMRS. BrainSCAN is the software for the inverse IMRT treatment plans. The m3 enables the delivery of superior homogeneous dose distributions with a steep dose gradient-an essential requirement for SRS treatments.

The leaves of the m^3 are automatically placed around the target for all beam angles with the desired margin. Risk organs may be automatically protected by the leaves, with manual adjustments possible at any time.

EXACTRAC PATIENT POSITIONING PLATFORM is an infared-based patient positioning platform, which relates the patient's current position to the planned position. The integrated real-time verification of the patient's positioning during treatment results in greater patient set-up accuracy compared to conventional skin markers. Furthermore, the automatic table movement provides greater efficiency during clinical routines and is suited for conformal and IMRS/IMRT treatments. Moreover, by using Image-guided technology (IGRT), Novalis=has an x-ray image verification system (EXACTRAC X-RAY 6D) in order to assure the accuracy and reproducibility of pre-defined treatment set-up.

ExacTrac X-ray Adaptive Gating

Respiration induced motion of lung and liver tumors make the accurate delivery of radiation to these lesions particularly challenging. ExacTrac X-Ray Adaptive Gating of BrainLAB is a new tumor tracking and targeting system. Due to Respiratory Gating, the system increases the treatment accuracy.

Novalis® Treatment Procedure

Step 1: Fitting of the Headframe/Mask Attachment/Custom body support system.

The doctor will select the immobilizing device best suited for the patient's therapy.

The headring works to hold reference markers in a fixed position in relation to your head during imaging and treatment for SRS. If you are undergoing fractionated stereotactic radiotherapy (SRT), a face mask will be used instead of the metal head ring. Its use is painless. For a lesion outside the brain, a custom body support system may be used instead.

Step 2: Diagnostic Imaging

After the immobilizing device is secured, you will undergo a series of diagnostic scans in order to precisely define the size and shape of the lesion and its relationship to other structures. During the diagnostic imaging the metal head ring I the face mask I custom body support system will be worn.

Step 3: Image Transfer and Planning

The radiosurgery team gathers information from the scans and enters it into the Novalis® computer program to determine the precise target position, dosage and configuration of radiation beams. While the treatment is being planned, the patient will be free to move. Once the customized treatment plan has been completed, the patient will be positioned comfortably on a specially designed couch. Next, a series of carefully controlled quality checks using Novalis® instruments are performed prior to treatment in order to assure that the radiation beams will be guided precisely to the chosen target position.

Case Study

Hepatocellular carcinoma (HCC) 3-D conformal radiation therapy (CRT) is very useful for the unresectable and medical inoperable disease in liver cancer patients. the patients were treated with 3-D CRT which reduced the symptoms and resulted in a better quality of life after treatment.

Step 4: Treatment

The actual treatment session typically takes less than 30 minutes. This involves the movement of the Novalis® machine around your head or your body as the focused beams converge on the target. Multiple radiation beams radiate the tumor from different angles. The invisible radiation is not felt at all.

2

Health Tourism: Definition, Nature and Scope

Health tourism can be broadly defined as provision of 'cost effective' private medical care in collaboration with the tourism industry for patients needing surgical and other forms of specialized health care. This process is being facilitated by the corporate sector involved in medical care as well as the tourism industry—both private and public. It entails patients going to a different country for either urgent or elective medical procedures—is fast becoming a worldwide, multibillion-dollar industry. The reasons patients travel for treatment vary. Many medical tourists from the United States are seeking treatment at a quarter or sometimes even a 10th of the cost at home. From Canada, it is often people who are frustrated by long waiting times. From Great Britain, the patient can't wait for treatment by the National Health Service (NHS) but also can't afford to see a physician in private practice. For others, becoming a medical tourist is a chance to combine a tropical vacation with elective or plastic surgery. And many more patients are coming from poorer countries e.g. Bangladesh, Nepal, Pakistan, Bhutan, etc. where treatment may not be available.

MEDICAL TOURISM IS NOT NEW

Medical tourism is actually thousands of years old. In ancient Greece, pilgrims and patients came from all over the Mediterranean to the sanctuary of the healing god, Asklepios, at Epidaurus. In Roman Britain, patients took the waters at a shrine to bathe, a practice that continued for 2,000 years. From the 18th century wealthy Europeans traveled to spas from Germany to the Nile. In the 21st century, relatively low-cost jet travel has taken the industry beyond the wealthy and desperate. The most recent trend in privatisation of health services is medical tourism, which is gaining prominence in developing countries. Globalisation has promoted a consumerist culture, thereby promoting goods and services that can feed the aspirations arising from this culture. This has had its effect in the health sector too, with the emergence of a private sector that thrives by servicing a small percentage of the population that has the ability to "buy" medical care at the rates at which the "high end" of the private medical sector provides such care. This has changed the character of the medical care sector, with the entry of the corporate sector. Corporate run institutions are seized with the necessity to maximise profits and expand their coverage. These objectives face a constraint in the form of the relatively small size of the population in developing countries that can afford services offered by such institutions. In this background, corporate interests in the Medical Care sector are looking for opportunities that go beyond the limited domestic "market" for high cost medical care. This is the genesis of the "medical tourism" industry. With global revenues of an estimated $2.8 trillion, the health care industry is the world's largest industry. The Indian health care industry has the potential to show the same exponential growth that the software and pharmaceutical industries have shown in the past decade. Countries that actively promote medical tourism include Cuba, Costa Rica, Hungary, India, Israel, Jordan, Lithuania, Malaysia and Thailand. Belgium, Poland and Singapore are now entering the field. South Africa specializes in medical safaris—visit the country for a safari, with a stopover for plastic surgery, a nose job and a chance to see lions and elephants.

Need for Medical Tourism

Medical tourism has become a common form of vacationing, and covers a broad spectrum of medical services. It mixes leisure, fun and relaxation together with wellness and health care. The idea of the health holiday is to offer you an opportunity to get away from your daily routine and come into a different relaxing surrounding. Here you can enjoy being close to the beach and the mountains. At the same time you are able to receive an orientation that will help you improve your life in terms of your health and general well-being. It is like rejuvenation and clean up process on all levels—physical, mental and emotional. Many people from the developed world come to India for the rejuvenation promised by yoga and Ayurvedic massage, but only a few consider it a destination for hip replacement or brain surgery. However, a nice blend of top-class medical expertise at attractive prices is helping a growing number of Indian corporate hospitals lure foreign patients, including a few from developed nations such as the UK and the US.

As more and more patients from affluent nations with high Medicare costs look for effective options, India is pitted against Thailand, Singapore, Malaysia and some other Asian countries, which have good hospitals, salubrious climate and tourist destinations. While Thailand and Singapore with their advanced medical facilities and built-in medical tourism options have been drawing foreign patients of the order of several lakhs per annum, the rapidly expanding Indian corporate hospital sector has been able to get a few thousands for treatment. But, things are going to change drastically in favour of India, especially in view of the high quality expertise of medical professionals, backed by the fast improving equipment and nursing facilities, and above all, the cost-effectiveness of the package. As Indian corporate hospitals are on par, if not better than the best hospitals in Thailand, Singapore, etc there is scope for improvement.

Scope of health tourism

With internationally recognized health care professionals, holistic medicinal services and low cost of treatment, India has the potential to attract over one million health tourists every year, according to confederation of Indian industry (CII). The country offers a unique mix of systems such as yoga, ayurveda and meditation and modern medical system. This, along with world-class experts and the cost advantage, can help earn $5 billion every year, a CII release said. While a heart surgery costs $30,000 in the US, it costs $6,000 in India. Similarly, a bone marrow transplant costs $26,000 here compared to $250,000 in the US. If a liver transplant costs in the range of Rs. 60 lakhs-70 lakhs in Europe and double that in the US, a few Indian hospitals, such as Global in Hyderabad, have the wherewithal to do it in around Rs. 15 lakh-20 lakhs. Similarly, if a heart surgery in the US costs about Rs. 20 lakhs, the Chennai-headquartered Apollo Hospitals Group does it in roughly Rs. 2 lakhs. Knee surgery (on both knees) costs 350,000 rupees ($7,700) in India; in Britain this costs £10,000 ($16,950), more than twice as much. Dental, eye and cosmetic surgeries in Western countries cost three to four times as much as in India. Take the rising popularity of "preventive health screening". At one private clinic in London a thorough men's health check-up that includes blood tests, electro-cardiogram tests, chest x-rays, lung tests and abdominal ultrasound costs £345 ($574, €500). By comparison, a comparable check-up at a clinic operated by Delhi-based health care company Max Health Care costs $84. The Indian government predicts that India's $17-billion-a-year health care industry could grow 13 per cent in each of the next six years, boosted by medical tourism, which industry watchers say is growing at 30 per cent annually. Price advantage is, of course, a major selling point. The cost differential across the board is huge: only a tenth and sometimes even a sixteenth of the cost in the West.

Citing the example of Thailand, CII said India should aggressively publicize its traditional medicinal system and surgical services in association with the tourism authorities. Indians, NRIs and tourists from around the world are beginning to realize the potential of modern and traditional Indian medicine. Indian hospitals and medical establishments have also realized the potential of this niche market and have begun to tailor their services for foreign visitors. At a regional level, this nascent industry came to limelight with the arrival of 'Naby Noor' from Pakistan, who came by the Indo-Pak bus service and got a red-carpet treatment at a hospital in Bangalore. Several Indian state governments have realized the potential of this 'industry' and have been actively promoting it. Visitors, especially from the west and the middle-east find Indian hospitals affordable and viable option to grappling with insurance and National medical systems in their native lands. Many prefer to combine their treatments with a visit to the 'exotic east' with their families, however, the country would have to improve its health care infrastructure, connectivity between major cities and streamline immigration procedure for medical visitors. Accreditation of Indian hospitals is also essential for attracting such tourists, it added.

Government as well as corporate sector is promoting health tourism

Close on the heels of introducing a medical visa, the Government has started overseas marketing of India as a medical tourism destination. According to senior Government officials, they hope to complete the process of price-banding of hospitals in various cities. By marketing India as a global medical tourism destination, the Government hopes to capitalize on the low-cost, high-quality medical care available in the country. Medical tourism focuses on treatment of acute illness, elective surgeries such as cardiology and cancer, among others. Statistics suggest that the medical tourism industry in India is worth $333 million (Rs. 1,450 crore) while a study by CII-McKinsey estimates that the country could earn Rs. 5,000-10,000 crore by 2012. Probably realising the potential, major corporates such as the Apollo, the Tatas, Fortis, Max, Wockhardt, Piramal, and the Escorts group have made significant investments in setting up modern hospitals in major cities. Many have also designed special packages for patients, including airport pickups, visa assistance and board and lodging, health care industry officials said. While the trickle of foreigners coming to India for treatment has started, officials are hopeful that this will become a flood once the various initiatives being taken by the Government take-off. Apart from receiving patients from those parts of the globe that have poor medical facilities, India has also been getting some medical visitors from the West for a variety of reasons including the long waiting period there for treatment in Government hospitals there. Indian Government has introduced the following policy measures to encourage medical tourism.

National Health Policy recognizes the treatment of international patients as an export, which allows private hospitals treating such patients to enjoy benefits such as lower import duties, increase in the rate of depreciation (from 25 per cent to 40 per cent) for life-saving medical equipment, and several other tax sops.

- India's relatively developing medical tourism segment has been anointed by health care and tourism industry pundits as the next 'best' thing for the country.
- There are plenty of challenges that need to be addressed for India to become the world's preferred health care destination.

- Prominent among them being the need for proper accreditation and requisite standardization systems in place, a tripartite synergy between hospitals, tour operators and respective state governments.
- They spoke about the various challenges impeding the growth of the medical tourism industry and emphasized the need for a synergy between hospitals, state government and international tour operators.
- India will have to project itself as being a holistic medical destination to get an edge over other countries.
- We need to club together a couple of 'pathies' because we have a very strong base of alternative healing therapies like yoga, naturopathy, ayurveda, etc.
- Creating awareness about India's facilities is a must to establish credibility in foreign markets.
- Standardization of a price band for graded hospitals and a quality assurance model should be taken up immediately to take medical tourism ahead.
- The private health care industry is quietly facilitating a revolution to enable India to emerge as a health destination.
- STARK contrasts are no surprise in urban India, and in the health care sector, the difference between what is available (world-class techniques and service, at a price) and what the common denominator urgently needs is no less so.
- private sector health care centres are gleaming "islands of excellence", as the industry calls them, all too often surrounded by seas of medical neglect.
- When the mix is just right (support from the government in the form of incentives and tax breaks, international health care accreditation standards in place, breakthroughs in insurance coverage for overseas patients, and savvy promotion of India as a tourism-plus-medical tech destination) the sector is certain the numbers will fall into place.
- What's more, the beneficiary of such growth will be the country's desperately overburdened public health system, say industry associations such as the Confederation of Indian Industry (CII) and the Federation of Indian Chambers of Commerce and Industry (FICCI), which see medical tourism a mirror of the early years of India's info-tech growth.
- Look at the possibility of the public hospitals being technologically upgraded to world-class standards with this source of income.
- Such optimism apart, India's three-tier public health system --- primary health centres (PHC) in villages, district hospitals, and tertiary care hospitals ---is increasingly unable to attend to the medical needs of the population.

- There is no doubt that a technology-centric approach to health care, such as that promoted by the major private hospitals, will inevitably affect the cost of care to the common man.

India moving ahead

India is considered one of the leading country promoting medical tourism—and now it is moving into a new area of "medical outsourcing," where subcontractors provide services to the overburdened medical care systems in western countries. India's top-rated education system is not only churning out computer programmers and engineers, but an estimated 20,000 to 30,000 doctors and nurses each year. The largest of the estimated half-dozen medical corporations in India serving medical tourists is Apollo Hospital. Dr. Prathap C. Reddy, the chairman of the company, began negotiations in the spring of 2004 with Britain's National Health Service to work as a subcontractor, to do operations and medical tests for patients at a fraction of the cost in Britain. Apollo now has 37 hospitals, with about 7,000 beds. The company is in partnership in hospitals in Kuwait, Sri Lanka and Nigeria. Apollo has also reacted to criticism by Indian politicians by expanding its services to India's millions of poor.

India will be happy to provide fixed-price treatment packages, integrating all transport, medical and living costs into one price. Plus a vacation at any of India'·s fabulous destinations. India is hoping to expand its tourist industry—to include visitors with heart conditions and cataracts. The sight of the country's overcrowded public hospitals, open sewers and garbage-littered streets would unsettle most visitors' confidence about public sanitation standards in India. Though the quality of health care for the poor in countries like India is undeniably low, private facilities offer advanced technology and procedures on par with hospitals in developed nations.

Vishal Bali, of Wockhardt Hospitals, points out as proof of quality that the US private health insurers Blue Cross and Blue Shield insure patients treated at his group's hospitals. The British health insurer Bupa also insures the costs of treatment at Wockhardt hospitals. Mr. Bali adds that Wockhardt is in talks with Britain's National Health Service about outsourcing the treatment of British patients to India. Early this year Rosemarie—who is into tourism business—encountered a leg ailment which curtailed her active life. She made extensive enquiries with the Turkish hospitals. She wanted to know what exactly was wrong with her leg, what are the corrective procedures available, what are the latest advances in the field, what is the success rate and how long will it take her to bounce back to her active life. Around this time, she happened to read "Stern," a popular German magazine, which had a special feature on India. It featured India's advancement in medical field. She will have to undergo special hip resurfacing surgery, she landed in Mumbai. Rosemarie speaking from Workhardt Hospital, Mumbai where she is undergoing post surgery physiotherapy told that her entire medical experience in India was wonderful.

IndUS health

If you or a loved one have a health problem that is causing concern about the cost and quality of available care, IndUShealth suggests you consider the excellent, high-quality treatment options available to you in India at a fraction of the cost in a U.S. hospital.IndUShealth's case managers and alliance of physicians in North America are ready to work with you to evaluate your needs and provide the necessary guidance that will help you take advantage of the exceptional care options available to you at one of our partner super-specialty hospitals in India.

At IndUShealth, we strive to make each patient's experience nothing short of an outstanding success. Any patient seeking affordable, high quality medical care can benefit from the IndUShealth system. However, those who may benefit the most are uninsured individuals who may face staggering medical bills for serious procedures. It's notable that half of U.S. bankruptcies are a direct result of catastrophic medical events and their associated costs.

- Patients seeking treatments that are routinely performed in India, but not approved in the U.S. (robot assisted joint replacement as an example).
- Patients that want to take personal accountability for their health care decisions, and make the best choice from global, rather than local options.
- Wait-listed patients with chronic pain or disability e.g. Canada.

Advent Medical Services

Advent Medical Services group is a leading medical service provider based in India with accomplished and distinguished physicians and surgeons with a vast experience in variety of disciplines including cardiothoracic surgery cosmetic and plastic surgery, laparoscopic surgery, endoscopic surgery, microsurgery, joint replacements and highly advanced form of ophthalmic and ear surgery. Advent is closely affiliated with world-class medical laboratory and research facilities. The group offers the best of class and personalized medical care in a cost-effective manner. It provides a risk-free concept of medical evaluation. After completing the registration, he/she can complete the medical history form which is securely transmitted to expert team of Board Certified physicians and surgeons in India. Team evaluates the patient's medical history and provides a professional opinion and an estimated cost for the treatment.

Every year 1 billion dollars are spent by Nigerians, on Medical Care in US and Europe. This expenditure can be reduced as much as 50% or more, through quality service available in India. The package offers free Preventive Health Care Program (PHP) for one person accompanying the patient. This package includes Echocardiography; CT scan; Ultrasonography; Treadmill testing; X-ray Hormonal levels, Liver, Kidney and Pulmonary function tests, Blood Urine and Stool investigations or any other relevant investigation.

India's Health Care Tourism

The health care sector in India has witnessed an enormous growth in infrastructure in the private and voluntary sector. The private sector which was very modest in the early stages has now become a flourishing industry equipped with the most modern state-of-the-art technology at its disposal. It is estimated that 75-80% of health care services and investments in India are now provided by the private sector. An added plus had been that India has one of the largest pharmaceutical industries in the world. It is self-sufficient in drug production and exports drugs to more than 180 countries.

- Bone Marrow Transplant
- Brain Surgery
- Cancer Procedures (Oncology)
- Cardiac Care
- Cosmetic Surgery
- Dialysis and Kidney Transplant
- Drug Rehabilitation
- Gynaecology and Obstetrics
- Health Checkups
- Internal/Digestive Procedures
- Joint Replacement Surgery
- Nuclear Medicine
- Neurosurgery and Trauma Surgery
- Preventive Health Care
- Refractive Surgery
- Osteoporosis
- Spine Related
- Urology
- Vascular Surgery
- Dental jobs

A typical package will consist of:

- Assessment of medical history.
- Patient received at the airport/Package inclusive of accompanying person.
- Transfer to a hotel.
- Escorted to the specialty hospital as per appointments for admission.
- Treatment administered.
- Rejuvenation holiday begins.
- Post treatment check-up.
- Transfer to airport and departure.

Dental care Packages

Following are some of the procedures offered under Dental care packages:

- Veneers
- Filling and Aesthetic reconstruction
- Dental Implants
- Bleaching
- Crowns and Bridges
- Cast partial dentures
- Periodontal Surgery
- Oral Surgery
- Pedodontics

Eye Care

India's ophthalmologists offer you custom made solutions for all your eye care problems. From corrective eye disorders to Diabetic retinopathy, Glaucoma, Cornea and Refractive Surgery to Low-stress cataract surgery. The eye surgery techniques have now become so advanced that the cataract surgery can be done in a day. LASIK (Laser Assisted Stromal *In-situ* Keratomileusis), a method of re-shaping the external surface of the eye to correct low, moderate and high degrees of nearsightedness, astigmatism and far-sightedness is also offered. The cost of such treatment in the UK is Pound 4000 and in the USA $ 5000 as against $ 1200 or less in India for the same treatment with highly experienced Indian doctors. A cataract surgery in the UK costs about Pounds 3000 and in the USA about $11000. In India in one of the best eye hospitals the cost is about Pound 400 or $ 700. This includes all investigations including the A scan on the IOL Master, the best intraocular lenses (Alcon Acrysof and the Allergan Sensar from USA, Pharmacia Tecnis Wavefront IOL from Sweden and also the Acritec from France) hospital stay, surgeon's fee, pre and post-operative treatment as well as follow ups. Chandigarh has a centre of excellence in eye care at Advanced eye centre, PGI. Several private clinics also offer world class services.

A worldwide market

While, India has attracted patients from Europe, the Middle East and Canada, Thailand has been the goal for Americans. India mainy attracted people who had left the country for the West; Thailand treated western expatriates across Southeast Asia. Many of them worked for western companies and had the advantage of flexible, worldwide medical insurance plans geared specifically at the expatriate and overseas corporate markets. With the growth of medical-related travel and aggressive marketing, Bangkok became a centre for medical tourism. Bangkok's International Medical Centre offers services in 26 languages, recognizes cultural and religious dietary restrictions and has a special wing for Japanese patients. The medical tour companies that serve Thailand often put emphasis on the vacation aspects, offering post-recovery resort stays.

Cuba, for example, first aimed its services at well-off patients from Central and South America and now attracts patients from Canada, Germany and Italy. Malaysia attracts patients from surrounding Southeast Asian countries; Jordan serves patients from the Middle East. Israel caters to both Jewish patients and people from some nearby countries. One Israeli hospital advertises worldwide services, specializing in both male and female infertility, in-vitro fertilization and high-risk pregnancies. South Africa offers package medical holiday deals with stays at either luxury hotels or safaris.

The newest and fastest-growing area of medical tourism is a visit to the dentist, where costs are often not covered by basic insurance and by only some extended insurance policies. India, Thailand and Hungary attract patients who want to combine a filling, extraction or root canal with a vacation.

Procedure Charges in India and US (US $)

Procedure	*Cost (US$)*	
	United States	*India*
Bone Marrow Transplant	2,50,000	69,000
Liver Transplant	3,00,000	69,000
Heart Surgery	30,000	8,000
Orthopedic Surgery	20,000	6,000
Cataract Surgery	2,000	1,250

Here's a brief comparison of the cost of few of the Dental treatment procedures between USA and India.

Dental procedure	*Cost in US ($)*	*Cost in India ($)*	
	General Dentist	*Top End Dentist*	*Top End Dentist*
Smile designing	-	8,000	1,000
Metal Free Bridge	-	5,500	500
Dental Implants	-	3,500	800
Porcelain Metal Bridge	1,800	3,000	300
Porcelain Metal Crown	600	1,000	80
Tooth impactions	500	2,000	100
Root canal Treatment	600	1,000	100
Tooth whitening	350	800	110
Tooth coloured composite fillings	200	500	25
Tooth cleaning	100	300	75

Facilities Available in India

Indian corporate hospitals excel in cardiology and cardiothoracic surgery, joint replacement, orthopedic surgery, gastroenterology, ophthalmology, transplants and urology to name a few. The various specialties covered are Neurology, Neurosurgery, Oncology, Ophthalmology, Rheumatology, Endocrinology, ENT, Pediatrics, Pediatric Surgery, Pediatric Neurology, Urology, Nephrology, Dermatology, Dentistry, Plastic Surgery, Gynecology, Pulmonology, Psychiatry, General Medicine and General Surgery

The various facilities in India include full body pathology, comprehensive physical and gynecological examinations, dental checkup, eye checkup, diet consultation, audiometry, spirometry, stress and lifestyle management, pap smear, digital Chest X-ray, 12 lead ECG, 2D echo colour doppler, gold standard DXA bone densitometry, body fat analysis, coronary risk markers, cancer risk markers, carotid colour doppler, spiral CT scan and high strength MRI. Each test is carried out by professional M.D. physicians, and is comprehensive yet pain-free.

There is also a gamut of services ranging from General Radiography, Ultra Sonography, Mammography to high end services like Magnetic Resonance Imaging, Digital Subtraction Angiography along with intervention procedures, Nuclear Imaging. The diagnostic facilities offered in India are comprehensive to include Laboratory services, Imaging, Cardiology, Neurology and Pulmonology. The Laboratory services include biochemistry, hematology, microbiology, serology, histopathology, transfusion medicine and RIA.

QUESTIONS AND ANSWERS ON HEALTH TOURISM

Que.: Is India really a better place to get medical treatment?

Ans.: Yes, Currently India receives patients from over 50 countries across the world. Here are some reasons behind its emergence as the preferred health care destination: India has a vast reservoir of skilled doctors. Many of them have proved their mettle in the US and UK and returned to India to work in hospitals here. The caliber of other doctors practicing in India is also of a very high order.

Que.: Why should patients come from USA for treatment to India?

A recent film 'Sicko' has indicted the American health care system; the insurance and pharma companies are exploiting the American citizens. Those who are not insured cannot afford treatment at home and hence come to India for world class health care at a fraction of cost.

Que.: I always thought India was a poor nation of snake charmers and rope tricks. How then can it offer world-class health care, that too at minimal costs?

Ans.: India has all along been a knowledge-oriented nation. However, it never had a chance to showcase its expertise. The revolution in Information Technology changed the rules of the game. And India made complete use of the knowledge base built by its English-speaking engineers to come out and display its immense capabilities.

And now for the costs. India is a diverse economy where a family of four can live comfortably, without debt, on a monthly income of just $300. As a result, the costs of services and products too have stayed at extremely low levels.

Now, thanks to the world becoming inter-connected and people being more willing to explore other nations, India has emerged as a preferred source of low cost health care. An extremely welcome alternative to the prohibitive costs prevalent in the western countries.

Que.: I don't know anyone in India. I'm already ill. Then how am I to cope with travel, stay and surgery in India?

Ans.: It's ok if you don't know anybody in India. After all, Mediescapes India brings you comprehensive, custom-built schemes for health care. This includes:

++Getting second opinions from well-known board certified doctors in India

Offering all support information on:

++Your ailment
++Recommended mode of surgery
++The hospital that will perform the surgery
++Costs involved
++Mediescapes India has entered into exclusive affiliate arrangements with a leading hospital in India. This means that you can count on special and personalized attention when you come to India for medical treatment through Mediescapes India.

Que.: I just need a second opinion. I don't intend to come to India. Is it possible to get an opinion alone from one of your affiliated hospitals?

Ans.: Yes, of course. Just pay $ 50 and get a second opinion from one of our affiliate hospitals. You are not obligated to have your surgery in India through Mediescapes India just because you have asked for a second opinion.

Que.: Do I have to pay any fees or commissions for your services?

Ans.: We do not charge any fees or commissions from people who want to use the services of our health care partners.

Que.: How do I pay the costs of surgery?

Ans.: You pay the costs of surgery directly to the hospital. The benefits of such a payment are:

Your money is paid directly to the service provider, i.e., the hospital and not to any intermediary

Our health care partner have been rich expertise in treating patients from almost all parts of the world. Hence, the Payment systems are well in place in the partner hospital to accept payments from almost any part of the world.

Que.: What are the surgeries offered by your partner hospital and what are the rates?

Ans.: Click here to find the spectrum of hospitals as well as surgeries/treatments our partner hospitals/clinics offer.

Costs exclude travel, visa and any other incidental costs. Cost only include cost of surgery, boarding and lodging for the package period for the patient and the boarding and lodging expenses of ONE accompanying person.

Que.: I want to get my surgery/medical treatment done in India. How should I go about it?

Ans.: Here's suggested step-by-step process:

Ist step—With your initial medical enquiry sent to us, submit your name, e-mail address, postal address and contact phone numbers.

IInd step—Complete the second opinion questionnaire (Medical Quote Request Form) that we send to you by email. Basically this Medical Quote Request Form covers current nature of your ailment/your need for second medical opinion/various types of Diagnostic reports available with you and other medical records such as CT Scan/MRI Scans/back home hospital or clinic or your personal doctor's conducted test reports/X-Rays, etc. All these past or current medical history of a patients' information's helps our board certified medical specialists in answering your medical query with full details.

IIIrd step—If further asked by our attending medical specialists/ doctors for better understanding your medical conditions then send scanned copies of all your diagnostic reports/pathological reports/MRI/ CT-Scans/OPG Images/Dental, Moulds/X-Rays/Angiograms, etc. to facilitate out specialists second opinion. You can also use our postal address to send CD's or Xerox copies of all reports or use our Telefax or can also use postal mail or courier to send these.

IVth step—Based on all above receive full information from our board certified attending specialist doctor's/medical consultants advice on your medical treatment approximate cost for rough planning purposes and total duration of your stay required at the hospital with pre-operative and post operative extra stay requirement, etc. based on your posted surgery/medical treatment in India medical enquiry.

Vth step—Also receive full details about cost of your stay at respective treatment city using a hotel or service apartment or guest house from us. Also receive full details about your treating institution/hospital in India with profile of attending doctor's/specialist and respective department at the Hospital where your medical treatment is suggested for your approval/ consent and for planning purposes.

VIth step—Acquire consent of your local physician to fly down to India. Inform us about consent/medical trip making condition.

VIIth step—Enter into the required agreements (Pre-Registration/ Indemnity or Consent Bond or Agreement) with the hospital in India for your firm medical treatment with them.

VIIIth step—Enter into similar agreements (Indemnity Bond) with chosen hotel/service apartment/guest house in India for pre-operative and post-operative stay duration.

IXth step—Pay the surgery/medical treatment full cost/full fees to the hospital directly via us to book OT/doctors' appointment/ward or room category chosen by you booking, etc.

Xth step—Receive details of your date of surgery/medical treatment via email support from us.

XIth step—Proceed for India Medical Visa (given for special medical emergencies). Here you have to carry confirm appointment with your Indian medical specialist/India hospital booking, etc. papers given by us for speedy India Visa clearance (we can issue you medial visa recommendation letter)

XIIth step—Book tickets to fly to India. Inform us about your international arrival/departure flight timings and flight number, etc.

XIIIth step—Fly down to India receive by our representative. Orientation of your treatment city/hotel or service apartment or guest house stay, etc. are undertaken by us for your familiarization.

XIVth step—Meet the attending specialist/treating doctor at the hospital/treating Institution where you will undergo surgery/your medical treatment and proceed on your specific treatment/medical surgery there.

XVth step—On completion of treatment/medical procedure/discharge from the hospital with final medical bill clearance and as per post-operative stay requirement suggested by your attending Indian medical specialist/ doctor stay at the pre-booked hotel or service apartment or guest house and ones full clearance received from attending medical specialist/doctor is received either fly back home or enjoy a recuperative holidays in India for few weeks or as per opted choice.

XVIth step—Carry medications or prescriptions for generic medicines/ drugs recommended by your attending medical specialist/doctor to carry home. Afterwards continue your post treatment follow-up if any, through email with attending medical specialist/doctor.

Health tourism promotion in India

The scope and concept of Medical Tourism (MT) has today transgressed and evolved from healing by mineral and hot spring in the Neolithic and Bronze Age to today's health farms. India should provide the best of Eastern and Westerm health care systems. Ayurveda, Yoga and

Siddha can be India's gift to the world. "Ayurveda is recognised as an official health care system in Hungary. Doctors in the West are increasingly prescribing Indian Systems of Medicine. More than 70 per cent of the American population prefer a natural approach to health," Dr. Bhaskar Shah, said. Americans are said to spend around USD 25 bn on non-traditional medical therapies and products. Addressing the same conference organized by INDIAN EXPRESS, Anil Maini, said, "MT has gained prominence with the advent of cutting edge technologies in India in specialties like cardiology, oncology, neurology, molecular and receptor imaging, which have improved sensitivity and specificity, early diagnosis, accurate and precise staging in oncology, significant input in decision-making, evaluation of treatment outcome and improved morbidity and mortality." The main deterrents to MT are poor airports and infrastructure, non-medical people getting into the business, unnecessary investigation and treatment, no replies to follow-ups and Indian doctors not providing sufficient information to patients. The threats to India are the practice of Indian hospitals raising their prices every now and then, while treatment in Eastern European countries like Poland and Hungary are good and cheap, with France being just around 25 per cent costlier.

The key "selling points" of the medical tourism

"Cost effectiveness, world class treatment" and its combination with the attractions of tourism are the key selling points. The latter also uses the ploy of selling the "exotica" of packaging of health care with traditional therapies and treatment methods. For example open-heart surgery could cost up to $70,000 in Britain and up to $150,000 in the US; in India's best hospitals it could cost between $3,000 and $10,000. The outcome of such a surgery in Indian hospitals matches with the best in the world. India is now moving into a new area of "medical outsourcing," where sub-contractors provide services to the overburdened medical care systems in western countries. India's Policy declares that treatment of foreign patients is legally an "export" and deemed "eligible for all fiscal incentives extended to export earnings. Anil Kamath, pointed out that good news about India is that medical tourism is growing at a rate of 7.5 per cent to 8.0 per cent with health care growing at a rate of 20 per cent. MT has also received a boost with corporatisation of the hospitals sector and interest of international players with reference to investment and foreign direct investment. The medical tourism market is estimated to grow by USD 2.2 bn with a corresponding increase in the health care market by USD 60 bn by 2012. The growing international competition is another attribute with India facing a stiff competition with the East Europe having approximately half of US tariffs, Thailand having approximately 1/8th of US tariffs and India having 1/10th US tariffs.

National Health Policy

National Health Policy recognizes the treatment of international patients as an export, which allows private hospitals treating such patients to enjoy benefits such as lower import duties, increase in the rate of depreciation (from 25 per cent to 40 per cent) for life-saving medical equipment, and several other tax sops. Medical corporations in India serving medical tourists led by Apollo Hospital Enterprises are aggressively moving into medical outsourcing.

The following points merit attention:

- We need to club together 'pathies' because we have a very strong base of alternative healing therapies like yoga, naturopathy, ayurveda, etc.
- Creating awareness about India's facilities abroad is a must to establish credibility in foreign markets.
- Standardization of a price band for graded hospitals and a quality assurance model should be taken up immediately to take medical tourism ahead.
- India's relatively developing medical tourism segment has been anointed by health care and tourism industry pundits as the next 'best' thing for the country.
- There are plenty of challenges that need to be addressed for India to become the world's preferred health care destination.
- There is a need for a synergy between hospitals, state government and international tour operators. India will have to project itself as being a holistic medical destination to get an edge over other countries
- The private health care industry is quietly facilitating a revolution to enable India to emerge as a health destination.
- STARK contrasts are no surprise in urban India, and in the health care sector, the difference between what is available (world-class techniques and service, at a price) and what the common denominator urgently needs is no less so.
- Private sector health care centres are gleaming "islands of excellence", as the industry calls them, all too•often surrounded by seas of medical neglect.
- When the mix is just right (support from the government in the form of incentives and tax breaks, international health care accreditation standards in place, breakthroughs in insurance coverage for overseas patients, and savvy promotion of India as a tourism-plus-medical tech destination) the sector is certain the numbers will fall into place.
- The beneficiary of such growth will be the country's desperately overburdened public health system, say industry associations such as the Confederation of Indian Industry (CII) and the Federation of Indian Chambers of Commerce and Industry (FICCI).
- Look at the possibility of the public hospitals being

technologically upgraded to world-class standards with this source of income.

- India's three-tier public health system ---primary health centres (PHC) in villages, district hospitals, and tertiary care hospitals ---is increasingly unable to attend to the medical needs of the population.
- Technology-centric approach to health care, such as that promoted by the private hospitals, will affect the cost of care to the common man.
- "If we can build our brand, there will be no stopping us," says Dr. Prathap Reddy, chairman of the Apollo Group.
- Price-banding exercise by a cii-affiliated industry body, the Indian Health Care Federation, completed late last year, indicates fair prices for standard treatments in a good hospital. This was preceded by complaints of wide variation in prices and indiscriminate fee-hikes.
- Imminent launch of campaign using brochures and advertorials by the tourism ministry to project Indian health care, will disseminate case-studies and the new pricing information. Targeting GP practices in western countries, especially those run by Indian doctors.
- Growing interest by foreign governments and public health care bodies in checking out Indian health care. Side-trip to hospitals being included in official itineraries, like the now-mandatory visit to Infosys.
- Satisfied customers and free publicity in the western media for top Indian hospitals for delivering on price and quality.
- A newly-created autonomous Indian accreditation board to set standards in safety and patient care. Expects to accredit 50 hospitals this year. Simultaneously, a drive for American accreditation by leading hospitals.

What's not happening?

- Industry and government not working in a coordinated manner. Progress so far driven mainly by individual players and ministries. Inter-ministerial taskforce on medical tourism, with representatives from six ministries and the private sector, set-up two years ago, has little to show.
- The much-touted new 'medical visa' is a disaster, say facilitators, more expensive and cumbersome than a regular visa, and requiring an array of documents.
- Medical tourists still negotiate snake-like immigration queues at airports, despite promises of a fast-track for the last two years. Recently, a Pakistani child needing a liver transplant took an hour and a half to clear at Delhi airport.

- Government failing to deliver on quality of airports, roads and infrastructure which don't make India look like a destination for "world class" medical treatment.
- Much more needs to be done to enforce norms, standards and ethical practices in a notoriously unregulated health care sector.
- Big breakthroughs depend on insurance companies, corporations and public health care bodies like Britain's nhs picking up the tab for medical treatment in India. Such deals have so far proved elusive, but the industry maintains they will happen.
- Handful of top doctors' names crop up in testimonials by medical tourists. Hospitals will have to maintain quality as numbers increase. It takes thousands of testimonials to build a brand, but just a few brickbats can destroy one.

Noises from a global health care bazaar

"We have no health insurance. My wife suffers constantly with her back pain. We cannot even begin to think about treatment here in the US because of the extremely high cost. After seeing your operations on 60 Minutes, we both have new hope. Please contact us. "Shortly after it was featured in the American TV programme 60 Minutes, e-mails began hitting the inbox of Delhi's Indraprastha Apollo Hospital, seconds apart from each other. From Illinois, Florida, Washington, Texas, New Mexico, California, Oregon, Oklahoma, Tennessee, Virginia, from British Columbia and Alberta, Canada. Curious, hopeful or frankly desperate, they were all looking for deals, asking prices, checking out packages: what will a new hip cost, by itself, and with bigger breasts thrown in? What about a package for two—a facelift for me, Lasik eye surgery for my companion? How much for a bridge, a root canal, IVF, angioplasty, gastric bypass surgery. This is my budget, what can I get for it?

It might sound discordant, this price-tagging of body parts, but for Indian private hospitals, nothing is more musical than these noises from a global health care bazaar. They demonstrate that an idea that seemed absurd at the start of this decade has entered the realm of reality: that people from the West will travel thousands of miles, to so-called cholera country, for medical treatment—if the price is right, and the quality is right. It's an idea with big money attached to it: medical tourism is forecast to become a $2.3 billion business for India by 2012. Some analysts predict it could be the next major driver of the Indian economy after information technology—if the industry and the government play their cards right.

Western TV crews accompanied often elderly people to India, filmed them hobbling out of Third World airports, with bhangra on the soundtrack, and driving into First World tertiary hospitals with the best technology money could buy. They showed them being "swamped by staff" and "feeling like kings", as one delighted patient described it, and seen by western-qualified senior consultants within an hour of arrival—which could be 2 a.m.

The crews tracked the pilgrims' progress, finding their way into an operating theatre where a surgeon obligingly delivered a tribute to the British system that trained him. But the main message came through loud and clear: white people getting knees replaced, hips resurfaced, and dental work done at bargain-basement prices by experienced doctors who knew their job. British tabloids went to town on teenager Elliot Knott who successfully underwent spine surgery here last August after being told to wait a year for an operation by the National Health Service U.K. Most private hospitals saw a marked upward trend in western arrivals last year, most of them from the UK, US and Canada.

The Apollo Group saw an overall five per cent increase in the number of western medical tourists, according to executive director (finance) Sunita Reddy, despite no special effort to market to them. But at Apollo's flagship Delhi hospital, which gets more medical tourists than its other hospitals, the arrivals from some countries seem to have doubled. For example, it got around 80 American patients from April to November 05, more than the entire number in the previous financial year. Any international marketing executive—and every upmarket private hospital now has one—can recite the numbers in her sleep: 8,50,000 waiting for a hospital bed in the UK, 47-million plus uninsured in the US. Medical value-travellers, as hospitals like to call them, are also people looking for body shapes that insurance companies won't pay for and dreams that even efficient public health care systems won't deliver, like those of the 5 feet 4 tall Frenchman who recently came to India for a leg-lengthening operation. Many are also in quest of treatments not available at home, like hip resurfacing, less radical than hip replacement, but yet to be approved by the US Food and Drug Administration.

Foreign medical tourists

Agonizing pain kept his wife in bed for 16 to 20 hours a day, and the wait for an appointment with the right kind of doctorwas no less painful. Google took Smith to India. "Much of Marlene's pre-operative pain has gone. We're 100 per cent satisfied. We paid $19,000, including airfare. In the US, the metal alone would have cost $40,000."

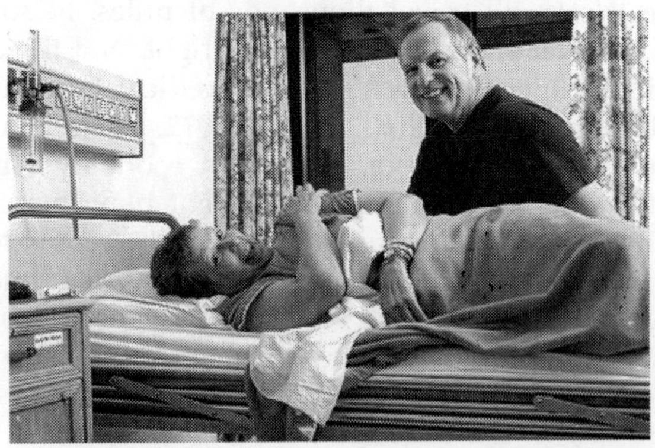

Marlene and Paul Smith; Canadians

Treatment: Spinal fusion surgery

Contrary to the popular stereotype, not every medical tourist is dying to see the Taj. He could be someone for whom a hospital room is the only piece of India he can handle. In a month's stay at Apollo Hospital for complicated surgery to correct his wife Marlene's curved spine, Paul Smith, from Barrie, a small picture-postcard town in Ontario, left the hospital only once, on a trip to the airport to sort out ticketing. "With Marlene in bed, why would I want to sightsee?" he said. In December, however, thanks to Elliot, and other high-profile visits arranged by their start-up, Taj Medical Group, they were able to send 27. They are going home in a few hours and they won't be returning. One giant leap into the unknown was probably enough. And yet, they couldn't be more grateful, raving about their doctor, dreaming about a better life for Marlene, determined to spread the word about India. Fortunately for the tourism ministry not all medical tourists confine themselves to hospital rooms.

Dr. Trehan says American citizens not covered by insurance—or those in countries such as the United Kingdom where there are long waiting lists for many National Health services—prefer to receive treatment in a country like India where top-tier institutions can provide high-quality health care at a fraction of the cost. Trehan recently operated on an 83-year old Canadian cardiac patient who needed a valve replacement with a bypass, but had been turned down by doctors back home. "No doctor was willing to do it for him. It's my specialization, patients with 10 or 20 per cent heart function. I told him the risk was less than five per cent," said Trehan.

Language is another big advantage in India, says Howard Staab, who spent more than three weeks in Escorts Hospital and at a resort, recuperating after surgery: "Doctors and nurses were all Indians, and many of the doctors were trained in the United States and Britain and most of them spoke very good English. I did not have any trouble understanding them." Howard Staab's partner Maggie Grace, who accompanied him on his medical trip to India, is writing a book about their experience. "We want to help people in the United States know they have choices," says Mr. Staab. "There will be our book coming out very soon. My partner Maggie Grace is writing it. The book title is "Patient Pilgrimage: A True Story of the First Americans Travel to India for Heart Surgery" and the website is www.howardsheart.com."Howard Staab says one key to his trip's success was that it combined a high degree of medical excellence with a human touch.

Amitabh Kant, the bureaucrat who led 'Incredible India' and helped successfully reinvent Kerala as God's own Ayurvedic paradise, is leading the ministry's initiative to promote India as a "global health care destination". So, after incredible temples, incredible tigers and incredible yoga, it's now going to be incredible doctors backed by incredible technology. Glossy brochures, prepared with the help of ad agency Ogilvy and Mather, feature men and women in spotless white coats bending over patients against backdrops of sleek medical hardware. The patients in the brochure seem mostly white and middle-aged, for a reason: Kant is aiming way beyond the harried middle classes from SAARC countries, Afghanistan and poorer African countries who have been flocking to India for specialised medical care which their countries lack. They, too, are coming in rising numbers, especially from Afghanistan and Africa, and sure, hospitals want their custom. But for reasons of both prestige and money, what really excites both government and industry is the fatter wallets in western countries with ageing populations and rising health care costs—and the Gulf, where seekers are finding it harder to access medical treatment in the West, post 9/11.

It's definitely not the titled rich that are showing up here. Cosmetic surgeon Mohan Thomas's upcoming patients include a pair of London cabbies, husband and wife, coming for facelifts. But even a school teacher from Bognor Regis can book a nice room when a hip replacement costs less than half of what it does back home. If they like the main course, western patients will also splurge on side dishes. Like Briton Barry Peters, who came to get a hip replaced, and got his teeth done as well, paying less for the whole treatment, including airfares, than just the dental would have cost him in London. Or Serena Taylor from California, who came to look after her friend seeking plastic surgery, and decided to buy an eyelift. It must be like eyeing a pricey handbag for several weeks and suddenly finding it at 80 per cent off. What else can you say but, "I'll have that"?

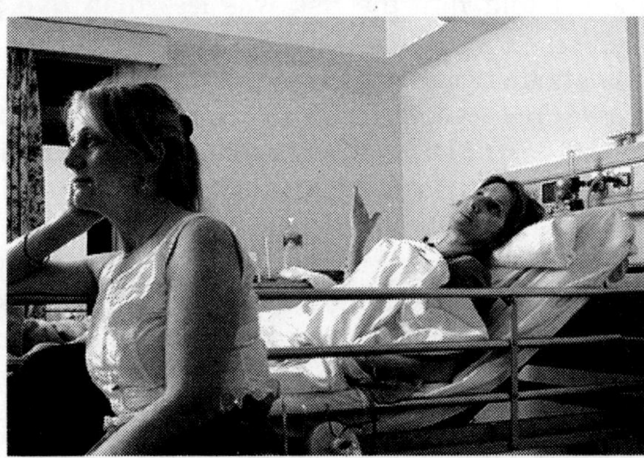

"A hospital cannot replace a hotel. We should not keep these patients in hospital a minute more than required, we must send them to a place where they can recuperate," says Apollo group chairman Dr. Prathap Reddy. In Bangalore, patients can check out of leading private hospitals, and convalesce in places like Soukya, a sprawling health farm on the outskirts of the city. With an in-house team of ayurvedic physicians and allopathic doctors on call, when needed, its medical director, homeopath Dr. Isaac Mathai, claims to have the "lowest doctor-patient ratio in the world". It's the detox destination for Indian software and media tycoons, and its international guests.

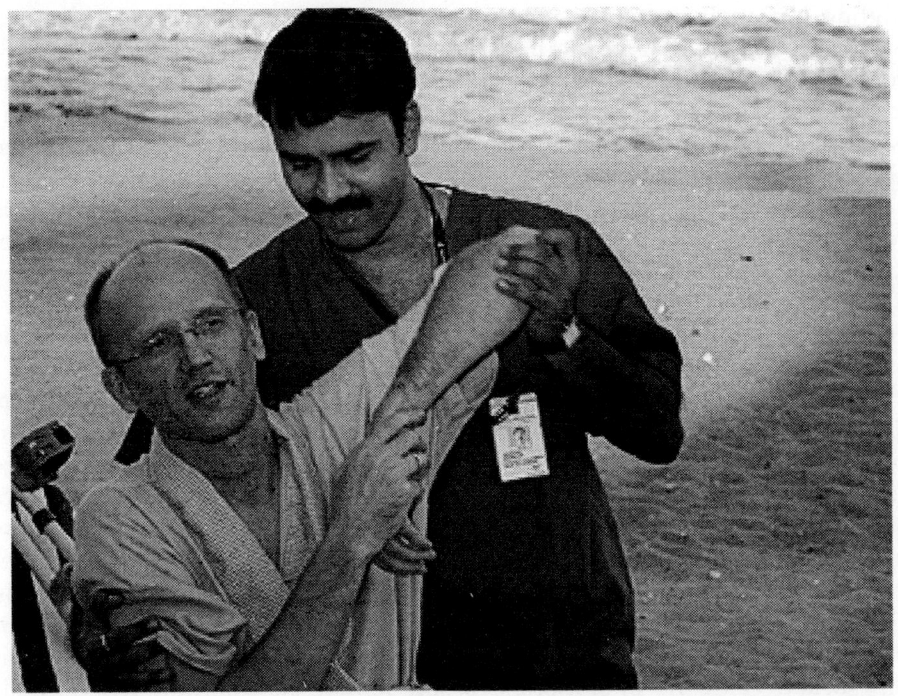

Scot Johnson; American

Treatment: Cervical disc replacement

"I heard about medical treatment in India from the TV show 60 Minutes. Big American hospitals are full of Indian doctors, that's how I knew they'd be good."

Howard looked into state-of-the-art cardiac facilities in India, Argentina and Texas, where top U.S.-trained doctors do the same procedures for a fraction of the cost. Of course, Howard would prefer to stay in the Triangle to be near his son and wide circle of friends. But who could resist these other options? After much deliberation Howard and his partner, Maggi, will fly to India for the surgery as soon as they can obtain the appropriate visas. Indian Hospitals Lure Foreigners with $6,700 Heart Surgery.

Dhanyavaad

Staab was rolled into Escorts' operating room on Sept. 28. Grace, who'd picked up a smattering of Hindi, wrote "dhanyavaad," for "thank you," on his bare chest with purple marker. The surgeons first decided to repair Staab's mitral valve. A day later, the valve walls thickened and obstructed blood flow. Staab went in for a second operation on Sept. 30, and doctors replaced the valve. He was ready to leave on Oct. 8 when blurry vision from suspected blood clots kept him for another two days to thin his blood. Staab and Grace returned to the U.S. on Oct. 24. Grace says finding out about India was the tough part. If not for Srivastava, she and Staab never would have figured out where to look, let alone gather the courage to make the trip. Back in North Carolina, Staab had an opportunity to compare health care in the U.S. with his treatment in India. An early November checkup found that his blood was still too thick, and he entered Durham Regional Hospital.

Grace says she had to ask for sheets to make Staab's bed and get him water herself. The bathroom wasn't cleaned, and they had to ask twice for the intravenous bag containing blood-thinning heparin to be changed when it became empty, she says. Carol Clayton, senior public relations specialist at Durham Regional, says the hospital addresses patient concerns as soon as they are brought to the staff's attention.

In April, Ian Stuart Crombie, 64, couldn't finish his round of golf at the Bonny Island course in Rivers State, Nigeria, because of pain in his right hip. Doctors gave him two choices: live on painkillers or undergo surgery. Crombie opted for a route that more Europeans and Americans are taking. He looked beyond a decrepit airport and teeming streets and chose India for medical care. In September, the British citizen flew 5,159 miles (8,303 kilometers) from his home in Winchester to Apollo Hospital in Chennai. Doctors performed a hip resurfacing, which involved shaving his thighbone and fitting it with a metal head that was then anchored in his hip socket. With the operation, Crombie joined the international clientele flocking to India for cut-rate services that include telephone call centers, software design and financial analysis. Indian hospitals are a very cheap option where patients get the same quality they're used to back home," says Sanjay Dongre, who manages the equivalent of $237 million of shares at UTI Asset Management Co. in Mumbai, which owns Apollo stock.

For Crombie, who was working as a human resources manager in Africa, Apollo presented a low-cost option. He says his medical plan didn't cover the hip operation. He didn't bother with the U.K. National Health Service because of its waiting list and decided not to pursue treatment in Nigeria. A private hospital back home would charge 15,000 pounds ($27,965), he says. Instead, Crombie paid a total of 5,000 pounds for his India trip, including the operation, airfare and a stay at the $130-a-night Park Hotel in Chennai. Crombie was familiar with India, where his job had taken him to recruit workers in Cochin, Mumbai and New Delhi. He found Bose on the Internet and checked his credentials with doctors Bose had worked within the U.K. He decided on India after e-mail exchanges persuaded him that hip resurfacing rather than hip replacement would give him a better shot at playing golf again. "I can imagine someone who's not been to India before may find it intimidating," Crombie says.

On vacation in India in September, Brown experienced chest pain again and was rushed to Wockhardt Hospital in Bangalore. Wockhardt performed an angioplasty the next day, inserting a wire mesh tube called a stent to prop open an artery. "The hospital could have been in London," Brown recalls. "It was immaculately clean and had good standards." Back in England, Brown says, he got a letter from the National Health Service in November asking him to come in for his initial test --two months after he'd had the surgery in India.

Some Middle Eastern patients began choosing India after the Sept. 11, 2001, attacks on New York and Washington, says Suneeta Reddy, 45, director of finance at Apollo Hospitals and daughter of founder and Executive Chairman Prathap Reddy, 71. In November, Waleed Khalid Al-Zadjali, 40, a doctor in Oman, picked Apollo for his father's angioplasty and his mother's knee replacement. Oman hospitals often refer patients to India for complicated procedures because the country is familiar, closer than the U.S. or Europe and cheap, he says. "After 9/11, people were scared to go to the U.S.," he says.

Healthy competition in health care

Top private hospitals are also vying with each other in other ways to attract an international clientele. As in an accelerated race for the latest hardware—you can't miss the giant boards advertising the latest scanner-and for that prized certificate by the Joint Commission International (JCI) in the United States, a non-governmental body that accredits international hospitals meeting exacting American standards. The early birds who have it, such as Apollo in Delhi and Wockhardt in Mumbai, display it big, and other hospitals are in the queue. "The fact that we are JCI-accredited is a symbol of quality assurance for patients in the western world. The hospital room is changing too, with globalisation clearly the spur, though all CEOs maintain that demanding Indian patients are driving the changes, too. John Connell, a primary school teacher from Southampton in the UK, who came to Wockhardt in Mumbai earlier this month for a new minimally invasive procedure to treat a hole in his heart, had the following in his hospital room: a computer, internet, a DVD player with regional compatibility that could play British DVDs, a mini-bar, a coffee-maker, a cellphone. The hospital also offered him and wife Amanda "virtual family visits"—that is, a video of them shot in the room and uploaded for their families back home. A hospital car was made available for them to move around in the neighbourhood. John's room still managed to look like a hospital room, but at new hospitals like the Max Devki Devi Heart and Vascular Institute in Delhi, it's all blonde wood, expensive blinds, and leather sofas, the work of a British designer hired by the company to get the look right. And prices? Ashmeena Ghei, international marketing head, who is already facilitating visits by a stream of international patients, quotes them in dollars: $150 for a room, $300 for a suite.

But the 2.3 billion dollar question is: Will the stream turn into a flood?

Judging by the talk on the hospital circuit, it won't be long before every upmarket private hospital offers ayurvedic massages, aromatherapy, mudbaths, pranic healing, yoga, the works. And full-fledged departments of alternative medicine, with homeopaths, naturopaths, and unani medicine specialists on board to deliver that authentic dose of India. The BPO sector, in comparison, earned $5.2 billion last year. (Source: CII-McKinsey report) The government hopes to encourage a budding trade in medical tourism, selling foreigners the idea of travelling to India for low-cost but world-class medical treatment. Naresh Trehan, executive director of Escorts Heart Institute and Research Centre, a leading private health care provider, says India has established world-class expertise in practices such as cardiac care, cosmetic surgery, joint replacements and dentistry. Merging medical expertise and tourism became government policy when finance minister Jaswant Singh, in this year's budget, called for India to become a "global health destination". If foreigners respond, a new medical tourism industry could be generating revenues of Rs. 100bn ($2.1bn, €1.9bn, £1.3bn) by 2012, according to a report by McKinsey Consultants and the Confederation of Indian Industry, a business group.

Take the rising popularity of "preventive health screening". At one private clinic in London a thorough men's health check-up that includes blood tests, electro-cardiogram tests, chest x-rays, lung tests and abdominal ultrasound costs £345 ($574, €500). By comparison, a comparable check-up at a clinic operated by Delhi-based health care company Max Health Care costs $84.

According to Hari Prasad, vice-president of Apollo Hospitals in Hyderabad, foreigners should have confidence in India's medical system because many Britons and Americans are accustomed to being treated by expatriate Indian doctors. In any case, most private health care providers hold modest ambitions about which foreign patients would come to India seeking treatment. For instance, of the 5,200 hospital beds run by the Apollo hospital group, about 100 beds are usually occupied by foreign patients, mostly from the Middle East, Africa and countries of South Asia. Indeed, demand for medical tourism is most likely to come from among the 25m-strong Indian diaspora, says Deep Kalra, chief executive officer of travel agency makemytrip.com. Mr. Kalra says wealthy first-and second-generation expatriate Indians are aware of the rise of India's high quality, low-cost hospitals. He estimates there is a potential market of some 12m expatriate Indians who would combine regular visits to India and save time and money by undergoing non-emergency procedures such as eye operations, dental work, cosmetic surgery and knee surgery. Mr. Kalra's agency plans to launch a medical tourism package later this year. Still, some remain sceptical about medical tourism's potential. Sumanjit Chaudhry, an executive at India's Max Health Care group, says: "I imagine if someone is sick and ill they won't want to have a holiday. You'll hardly see a guy who comes here for heart surgery leaping off and going to the beach."

Maharashtra Medical Tourism Council (MTC)

Initially the MTC plans to woo foreign patients who pay for private health care in their own countries. But it also plans to work with state-run systems. For instance, Anapum Verma, the council's honorary secretary, believes Britain has a "huge potential" for medical tourism owing to its long waiting lists for surgery. He has already had exploratory conversations with some British National Health Service managers about the possibility of sending patients to India. For the MTC, its plans are the next chapter in globalization and the outsourcing of work to India. As Sanjay Agarwala, the Hinduja's chief neurosurgeon, says: "Wherever you can offer better services at a more competitive price, that is the place that is going to win in the end." Contrary to the claims of the council, Dr. Baru believes there will be no trickle down of money to the impoverished public health system, which currently receives just 0.9% of India's gross domestic product. The MTC's plans may well benefit the doctors and patients involved, but it is currently unclear how a country that still suffers from malaria and TB will reap the rewards of a new wave of medical tourists coming to India.

In recent years Indian Medical Tourism Sector has exhibited tremendous potential. Studies reveal that the Sector is growing at an exaggerated rate of 15% for last five years. It is expected that with the current growth rate the Industry will reach Rs. 270,000 crores by 2012. Statistics show that the medical tourism industry in India is worth $333 million at present (Rs. 1,450 crore), while a study by CII-McKinsey estimates that the country could earn Rs. 5,000-10,000 crore by 2012. Probably realizing the potential, major corporates such as the Tatas, Fortis, Max, Wockhardt, Piramal, and the Escorts group have made significant investments in setting up modern hospitals in major cities. Many have also designed special packages for patients, including airport pickups, visa assistance and board and lodging, health care industry officials said. Foreigners have already started trickling into India for medical treatment thus officials are hopeful that this will become a flood once the various initiatives being taken by the Government take off. With world-class medical care, equipment and facilities now available in India, patients from the United States and other developed countries are going there for treatment. A number of private hospitals in India offer packages designed to attract foreign patients, with airport-to-hospital bed transfer service, Internet access, and other facilities. Some packages include add-ons, such as a yoga holiday or a trip to the world-famous Taj Mahal.

RELIGIOUS TOURISM; AS AN ENGINE OF GROWTH OF MEDICAL TOURISM IN INDIA

Synergy of religious tourism and medical tourism can work. It can improve health care for the countrymen and earn dollars from foreign medical tourists. It will not put any burden on the state exchequer or burden the country with debts. It will be self financing as well as fulfilling to the community. This is in consonance with Indian tradition to help the people in pain and disability. If the donations from all over the country are channelised to health care, it will not only lead to health care for all in India, but also make it attractive for the medical tourists from abroad. Various religious sects and their heads have to come forward to further a common cause that is good for the humanity. See appendix on the list of religious places in India.

Agra moving forward

While the states of Karnatka, Maharashtra, Gujarat, Tamil Nadu, Andhra Pardesh are quite ahead in tourism promotion, other states are also making efforts to march ahead. Agra is definitely moving in the direction of a well developed medical tourism centre. With the new international airport coming up soon, and competent city doctors working abroad, this process will start soon enough. "Medical facilities in Agra have expanded immensely. Earlier we referred our patients to hospitals in Delhi, now with the latest gadgetry and facilities available locally, patients take advantage and save both money and time."

Apollo Hospitals has also entered into partnership with Pankaj Mahendru's medical outfit. The new venture is called Apollo Pankaj. Said Apollo Pankaj director Pankaj Mahendru: "Earlier during the British and Mughal empires also, Agra was the main centre of health services. Now embassies and corporate houses are referring patients to hospitals here which have a fairly competent base of manpower and facilities." An American company Mefcom Agro Ind has acquired stakes in Kamayani Patients Care India, a multi-specialty hospital, providing specialty cancer treatment. Metro, Heritage, Pushpanjali, Shanti Ved, Pareek's, Nawal Kishore's, GG Nursing Home and Sarkar's, the oldest nursing home in Agra, are some of the other hospitals that have broken new ground in Agra by modernizing their infrastructure and facilities. To support the fast growing medical tourism industry, at least a dozen training institutes for paramedic staff as well as research centres have come up. The Agra Mental Hospital is conducting several programmes to train personnel for this specialised sector. Even the 150-year-old S N Medical College now presents a new profile in a bid to attract patients from the rest of India and even abroad.

Rajasthan enterprise

For this, land would be provided at special prices to all new private medical institutions, including medical and dental colleges, diagnosis centres, blood banks, and nursing and paramedical training institutes. The policy will also boost other medical streams like ayurveda, homoeopathy and naturopathy. A "land bank" will be created to give land to medical institutions that are promoting and practicing alternative medical therapies.

To benefit from the policy, nursing and paramedical institutions will have to make an investment of at least Rs. 50 million. Similarly, nursing homes and 15-bed hospitals planning a facility within 50 km from regional headquarters or 20 km from district headquarters or in a village or town with a population of less than 50,000 will have to invest at least Rs. 5 million. Investors will also have to abide by environment protection rules for hospital waste disposal and follow the rules and regulations set by the committee of standards.

Obesity treatment looks attractive

In a development that could bring patients from US and Europe to the country, a private hospital today launched a world class bariatric surgery clinic in Gujarat to treat people suffering from severe obesity, a disease that is fast attaining epidemic proportions in India.

The star-studded launch of the clinic at Apollo Gleneagles Hospitals here saw at least 25 people queuing up for surgery to get rid of excessive body weight and in turn associated diseases like high blood pressure, diabetes and cardiac ailments. The new facility, first of its kind in India after sporadic attempts elsewhere in the country, is also eyeing patients from the west, where the cost of treatment is more and the waiting time enormous. "The facility, being backed by a support group for obese people, is a comprehensive unit, which will benefit not only domestic patients but also thousands of patients in the Americas and Europe, who are showing interest in flying down to get operated," says laparoscopic and bariatric surgeon, who heads the clinic. Quoting the WHO, he says 17 per cent of men and 15 per cent women in India were confirmed to be obese and the numbers were growing by leaps with changing lifestyles and eating habits. "Globally, over 1.7 billion people are affected by the disease. In the US, over 300,000 people die of obesity while in Europe around 250,000 people are killed by the scourge," he warned.

3

Asian Hospitals take a Leap Forward in Health Tourism

The birth of new technologies, has transformed the globe's vast population into a boundary-less "Global village Community." From a 'consumer' point of view, it is now possible to take advantage of both cheap airfares and often higher standards or more affordable medical treatment in foreign countries, than those available in their own countries. From a patient perspective, the benefits of global health care are numerous. Though cost is the over-riding factor, the wait for surgeries in some developed nations can also be annoying. USA, Canada and Great Britain have reported a surge in the number of people traveling outside the country to avoid long queues in the National Health Service, which can often be for a year or more for some surgical procedures. The South East Asian countries such as Thailand, Malaysia, Singapore, Korea and Philippines are the popular destinations for medical treatment. India is positioning itself as the primary destination for advanced medical procedures in the world. Some of Indian hospitals are also competing with their Asian peers to get a slice of the cake in the booming health tourism market for international patients.

ASIA LEADING

Health tourism is a promising new industry in Asia, offering prospects for private hospitals facing saturation in patient growth. It is with a clearer view of the addressable market potential, internal strengths and limitations, as well as the level of external competition, that health care providers may best move forward to realize this potential. Health Care providers may now consider the medical quality of their services, how non-medical services are key to encouraging patient access, and the various marketing options available to them. Thailand's Bumrungrad Hospital was among the first in the region to focus on attracting foreign patients. Thailand's Bangkok Medical centre is also excelling in health tourism (see appendices at the end). The Malaysian Government has successfully exerted its leadership to facilitate and encourage hospital industry development, with the formation of National Committee for the Promotion of Health Tourism. The Hong Kong Government is starting to consider to possibility of marketing its Traditional Chinese Medicine (TCM) capabilities to the region, while concerted efforts have similarly been launched by government agencies in Singapore to market its world-class medical capabilities. In countries such as Thailand, the onus remains on the private sector to analyze available opportunities, spearhead sectoral development, and formulate strategies to improve their competitiveness.

With the tightening of immigration rules and security checks, the US has seen a decline in the number of foreign patient visits. More patients, especially those in the Middle-East, are moving towards alternatives like Thailand. Over 100,000 foreign medical tourists visit Malaysia annually, while Singapore and India are also starting to experience positive growth in patient visits as a result of their aggressive marketing initiatives to source countries like Indonesia. However, Thailand leads the Asia-Pacific region. Thailand is able to attract a large volume of patients as it has a variety of existing tourist attractions for recuperating patients, a relatively low cost of living, expat-friendly locals, and a respectable quality of health care, in cosmetic surgery.

Industry's best practices for International patients

Medical tourists expect the highest possible quality of care, having traveled great distances to seek world-class doctors and hospitals. Many leading hospitals have expounded on this by branching their medical expertise into super-specialization. For instance, some Australian hospitals focus not only on cancer, but perhaps on specific variations of skin cancer. This also builds credibility and buy-in, when the referring doctors are trained in the post-procedural stage to provide a continuum of patient care. Even nursing teams are trained to specialize as oncology nurses, while the cross-fertilization of medical teams such as with dermatologists, radiologists and oncologists ensures that all complications are completely accounted for. Medical quality is also supported by hardware and software investments. Hardware investments include the purchase of cutting-edge technology such as MRI or Gamma Knife machines. Software refers to the intellectual output of the hospitals as demonstrated by the latest medical research.

Non-medical services

Many hospitals offer airport pick-up services for patient convenience. Hospital reception areas are fitted as luxuriously as five-star hotels; Bumrungrad Hospital in Thailand for instance even features a Starbucks café and McDonald's outlet. Bangkok's Piyavate Hospital may even feature spa facilities that offer a holistic wellness experience. Western-style hospitals such as in the US, UK or Australia feature their own on-site accommodation, both for patients in the aftercare stage, as well as for their relatives. Similarly, many Asian hospitals that do not manage their own accommodations also offer link-ups with different hotels, hostels, etc. Apart from bedside manners, hospital staff members are also being recruited to accommodate to their religious, dietary and cultural needs.

Hospitals that are successfully attracting foreign patients enlarge their geographical footprints with representative offices or agencies in other countries. For example, Cromwell Hospital in the UK has representatives in India and Pakistan, while hospitals in Singapore are also setting up offices such as in Indonesia or the Middle-East. These agents help establish and maintain relationships such as with local hospitals, doctors, embassies, sponsor corporations, or insurers. Participating in different events also facilitates such relationships. For instance, trade shows, exhibitions or training seminars allow health care providers to share their medical expertise.

With budget air travel and the Internet providing access to information about cheap or specialist treatment overseas, medical centers across Asia are vying with each other to become regional or even global hubs for health care. Singapore is aiming to attract one million foreign patients per year by 2010 while India is gunning to be a top medical tourist destination, benefiting from its huge base of medical professionals and low costs. Pioneering stem or embryonic cell work is attracting patients to South Korea and China to undergo treatment that is not available, or legally permissible, in many other countries. The work may be controversial but it is providing new hope to paralyzed patients.

Medical tourism as an engine of economic growth

In the past 30 years or so, the costs of health care have soared in developed countries, especially the United States. Americans and, to some extent, the British, Canadians, Australians began to look for ways to reduce these expenses. Certain services and procedures in American hospitals are now being contracted out to Third World countries, from transcriptions of medical records to the reading of X-rays. Medical tourism presents an opportunity for hospitals to fuel economic growth by tapping the potential of the international patient market. To attract foreign patients, health care providers may consider leveraging on both business and clinical considerations. The advancement in medical technologies, increased patient mobility and demand for immediate quality health care is arousing interest among health care providers globally. To set-up world class medical tourism centers, massive investment in health sector is called for. This will not only improve health care for the countrymen, but also attract patients from all over the world on the strength of quality, promptness and economy.

However needs can vary widely between the 'essential' health care seekers—traveling by necessity, because treatment is not available or unaffordable locally—and the 'premium' medical tourists, who are typically looking for wellness or cosmetic procedures and may want first-class flights and exclusive add-ons. Pacific Health Care Holdings Patient Relations Manager Alison Lim says, our International Patient Liaison Centre has seen an increase in these "premium" medical tourists seeking high end elective treatments like titanium dental implants, complex cosmetic procedures as well as deluxe health screening. An emerging trend is the bundling of five-star health care services with unconventional post-operation treatment. India is providing traditional recuperation forms such as yoga and naturopathy, while Thailand is promoting its ancient Thai herbal remedies to the West, Middle East and Far East. To create awareness and market their medical services, Singapore's Raffles Hospital works with 50 agents in 12 countries. Parkway Group Health care has marketing offices in 15 countries including China, India, Bangladesh, Sri Lanka, Vietnam, Brunei, UAE, Brittan, Russia, Canada, Indonesia and Malaysia, which last year helped attract over 17,000 indoor patients and 140,000 outpatients.

Top 10 in medical tourism

- Bumrungrad International Hospital in Bangkok
- Buchinger Clinic in Germany
- All India Institute of Medical Sciences in Delhi
- The Fyodorov Clinics in Russia
- A Technology Prescription: Denver Health
- Brigham and Women's Hospital
- Sourasky Medical Center in Tel Aviv
- Hôpital Edouard Herriot in Lyons
- Hospital for Tropical Diseases in London
- Mount Sinai Medical Center

The medical tourism policy can draw strength from recommendations that the corporate sector has been making in India, and specifically from the "Policy Framework for Reforms in Health Care", drafted by the Indian prime minister's Advisory Council on Trade and Industry, headed by Mukesh Ambani and Kumaramangalam Birla. Certain other Asian countries have taken Giant strides in promoting medical tourism in their respective countries. However, the current market for medical tourism in India is mainly limited to patients from the Middle East and South Asian economies, besides the NRIs from all over the globe. Analysts say that as many as 150,000 medical tourists came to India in the year 2005 and over 200,000 in the year 2006. Afro-Asian people spend as much as $20 billion a year on health care outside their countries—Nigerians alone spend an estimated $1 billion a year. Most of this money is spent in Europe and America, but it is hoped that this would now be increasingly directed to developing countries like India.

The foreign patients come from SAARC region, Afghanistan, Ethiopia, Nigeria, Tanzania, other parts of Africa, CIS countries and the Middle East, especially Oman and Yemen As per New trends from 2003, patients from the US, UK and Canada, escaping high costs and waiting lists are coming to India. Also from Europe, Australia and New Zealand for procedures not covered by insurance such as cosmetic surgery, obesity treatment, and new techniques like hip resurfacing Around 30 private tertiary hospitals, mainly in Delhi, Mumbai and Bangalore; but also Chennai, Calcutta Thiruvananthapuram, Coimbatore and Hyderabad. It Includes hospital groups like Apollo, Wockhardt, Fortis, Max, Escorts. At an Indian medical tourism expo in the UK last year, 25 per cent of visitors were seeking medical treatment in India. India's Apollo is setting up hospitals in joint ventures in Dhaka and Colombo; and clinics in Yemen and Saudi Arabia Parkway Holdings of Singapore in tie-up with Apollo in Calcutta; with Asian Heart Institute and Research Centre in Mumbai; International chain Columbia Asia has a 75-bed multi-speciality hospital in Bangalore.

Indian corporate hospitals have a large pool of doctors, nurses, and paramedics ensuring individual, personalized care for all. The highly skilled personnel, with wide experience and international exposure excel in cardiology and cardio thoracic surgery, joint replacement, orthopedic surgery, gastroenterology, ophthalmology, transplants and urology to name a few. The various specialties covered are Neurology, Neurosurgery, Oncology, Ophthalmology, Rheumatology, Endocrinology, ENT, Pediatrics, Pediatric Surgery, Pediatric Neurology, Urology, Nephrology, Dermatology, Dentistry, Plastic Surgery, Gynecology, Pulmonology, Psychiatry, General Medicine and General Surgery.

Bangkok; the hub of medical tourism

Catch some sun, take in a few golden temples, and get a new hip- a new slogan coined by the Thailand Tourism, to promote medical tourism. It's an increasingly popular itinerary for foreign visitors who are flying into Thailand in ever greater numbers to get quality hospital care at bargain prices, part of a 'medical tourism' boom that is turning into a multi-billion dollar industry in Asia. The kingdom is one of several countries in the region cashing in on its ability to use cheap but highly skilled labor, affordable hospital accommodation and offer specialist treatments. Of a total of one million patients each year at Bumrungrad, nearly 50 percent are foreigners with Americans making up the biggest group, followed by patients from the United Arab Emirates, Bangladesh, Oman, Britain, Japan, Australia, Cambodia and Myanmar. Among Americans, back surgery and hip and knee replacements are the most popular procedures at Bumrungrad, while many Australians seek plastic surgery. Bumrungrad International Hospital offers a full spectrum of services from executive health tests to cardiac packages, cancer therapy, eye surgery, liposuction and other cosmetic options. Bumrungrad has more than 700 internationally-trained and board-certified doctors, and a complete range of health care services and facilities.

Which Thai Hospital is Best: Bumrungrad vs. Bangkok Hospital

Charles Runckel writes about two leading hospitals in Bangkok, Thailand. Thailand is the world leader for medical tourism, but which hospital within Thailand is best for you? This article, part three of a series on Medical Tourism, explores the top two choices. While there are many hospitals in Thailand that cater to medical tourists, these are two full-service facilities that have strong reputations for quality and experience with foreigners. The aspiring medical tourist should consider these two before any other Thai hospitals, even ones with a slightly lower cost, as they are the gold standard for medical tourism not only in Thailand but worldwide.

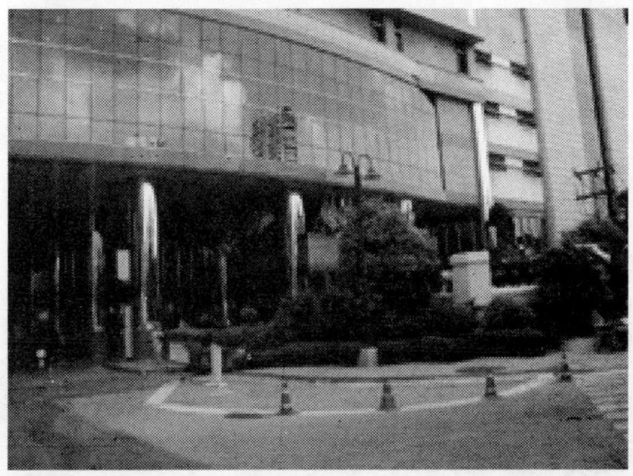

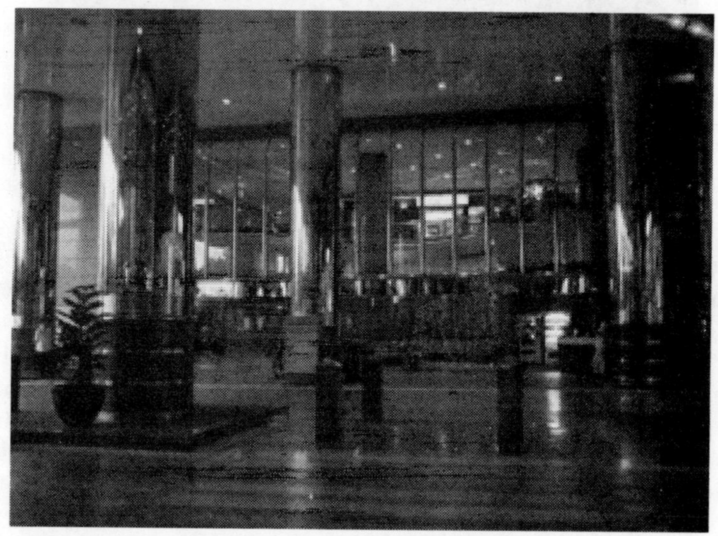

Pictures (top) Bumrungrad Hospital's main Building and Entrance

Pictures (below) Bangkok Hospital's Buildings and one of their Entrance

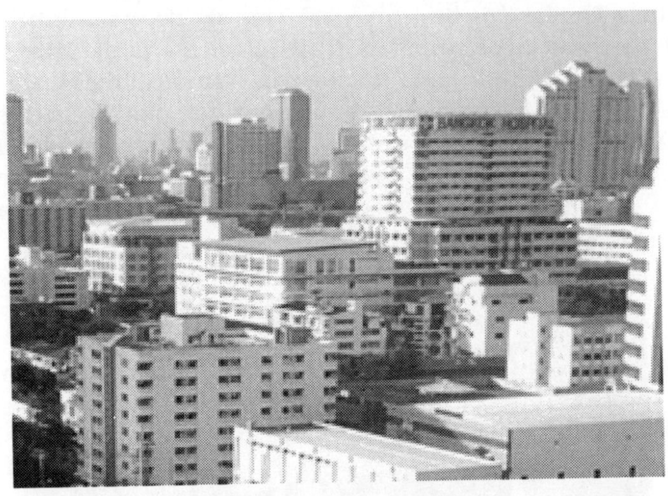

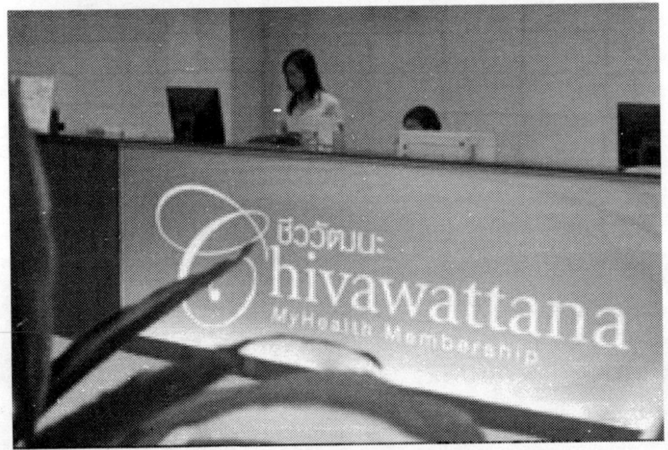

Background and Location

Bumrungrad Hospital treats over 400,000 foreign patients every year and has made medical tourism its major focus. The monolithic hospital consists of a large tower and several associated buildings adjoining, all conveniently located in downtown Bangkok. The hospital is within walking distance of Bangkok's Skytrain (light rail system) but only barely, and given the heat usual in Thailand most patients are strongly advised to take a taxi. International patients are so much a part of Bumrungrad's focus that they recently broke from their single tower architecture and built a separate International Tower that caters specially to foreigners with a brand new Physical Exam wing and upgraded VIP rooms.

Bangkok Hospital Group is a network of Thai hospitals focused on Bangkok and sprawling into the provinces and even Cambodia, though the portion of this that is most important to foreigners is their Bangkok Hospital Medical Center (BMC) complex. This campus consists of their International Hospital as well as their main General Hospital and a collection of specialty hospitals, including their Heart Hospital, Rehabilitation Center and Dental Clinic. The BMC is a series of adjacent buildings connected by skywalks and, apart from the main General Hospital building, are new having been built in the past five years. The BMC is located near, but not walking distance from, several Sky-train and sub-ways stations, so a taxi is in order in this case as well. While BMC and Bumrungrad treat about the same number of total patients each, a lower proportion of BMC's patients are from overseas and total only 150,000 annually, though these are often for more serious treatments.

Layout and Impressions

Bumrungrad Hospital is, as previously mentioned, monolithic. Visitors enter into the lobby of the main tower at the ground floor, but this and the next floor contain mostly restaurants, coffee shops and the cafeteria. The Hospital portion does not begin until the third floor, where the patient is greeted with a larger lobby and registration area. Elegantly uniformed staff register new patients with digital cameras—both Bumrungrad and BMC are very tech savvy hospitals with test results updated and delivered electronically and pictures of each patient checked at every stage to avoid foul-ups. This registration area is both the point of entry and exit, and next to registration are desks for checkout and a pharmacy.

On every floor of Bumrungrad runs a long, wide hallway with specialty clinics and divisions branching off, generally four to six per floor. Each has its own lobby, which looks out onto the hall. The older main tower and new international tower are quite different, with the older tower very much feeling like a mature hospital, with traditional waiting areas and layout, while the new wing is decidedly more modern and up-to-date, from the lobbies and hallways to furnishings in patient rooms.

Upon walking into BMC's main building, one is immediately greeted with the registration staff. They are far more eager to register you than those at Bumrungrad, though this has a strong basis in necessity. Upon registration, a patient's schedule will likely initially take them to another building, or several buildings if they have multiple appointments. The BMC staff then ensure that you are taken to the right building or floor of the main structure. There are enclosed walkways between the buildings, however most patients are initially led to the shuttles, which are over-sized gold carts or minivans that scoot patients around the campus.

Each division, clinic or specialty hospital at BMC has its own modular area with it's own independent registration and cashier services (so you don't have to go through the main lobby at all, if you know where you're going). These lobbies, especially in the newer buildings, are considerably more aesthetically appealing and pleasant to wait in than many of Bumrungrad's specialty clinic lobbies, mostly due to their smaller size, more updated furnishings and clever architectural design. Like Bumrungrad, there is a clear difference in ambiance between their older General Hospital building and the new, adjoining specialty centers.

The famed, or infamous, Bangkok Hospital Phuket is renowned as a world leader in sex-change operations, but is also a state-of-the-art hospital for more mundane purposes and nothing beats Phuket's beaches for physical therapy and recuperation after a surgery in Bangkok, which the Phuket Hospital supervises and coordinates.

One of many MRI scanners at the Bangkok Hospital

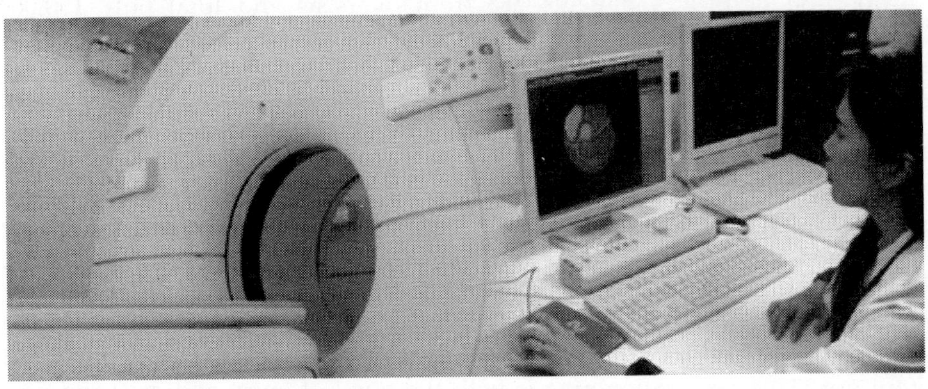

Unlike many other aspects of a hospital experience, the sheer technical capabilities of a hospital are somewhat easily quantified, and it is in this aspect that Bangkok Hospital most outshines its competitor. BMC has focused a tremendous amount of resources to being on the cutting edge of medical technology, and while Bumrungrad is certainly not unsophisticated, there is general agreement that Bumrungrad is a solid step behind BMC technologically. BMC's hi-tech drive falls into two general areas: advanced imaging and non-invasive surgery. Their advanced imaging options include at least seven MRI scanners in their main campus alone. Each department receives its own specialized diagnostic equipment, unlike many hospitals which must pool resources, including Digital Mammography and a brand new 128-slice CT scanner currently being installed. It is peerless in South-East Asia, and BMC boasts one of Thailand's only two clinical PET-CT scanners. The non-invasive offerings include state-of-the-art radiation systems such as the Novalis device for brain tumors and robotic laparoscopic surgery for both heart and joint operations (with different robots, of course). Bumrungrad simply does not compete in this field, which gives BMC a decisive advantage in the specific operations these advanced machines enable; reducing risk, discomfort and hospital stay time.

Reputation and Marketing

Bumrungrad is probably the best-marketed hospital in the world. Their fame is well deserved, but their marketing staff and management have put a tremendous effort in being "The" medical tourist hospital that potential patients in the Western world have heard of, specifically through news reports on ABC and CBS as well as multiple appearances in Newsweek. BMC, in contrast, is more famous within Thailand and elsewhere in Asia and the Middle East. Both hospitals treat approximately the same total number of patients—about 1 million a year—however Bumrungrad began courting foreign patients much earlier than BMC and now draws 400,000 foreign patients a year to BMC's 150,000-250,000. It is worth noting that different hospitals use different metrics to calculate these numbers (visits vs. patients) so these comparisons must be taken with a grain of salt, however it is commonly accepted that Bumrungrad's proportion is higher than BMC's, though not by as much as the disclosed numbers suggest. While BMC's focus for the future includes increasing the proportion of foreign patients, the target countries of both hospitals will likely remain the same with Bumrungrad focusing on the US and BMC focusing on the Middle-East and Asia, affecting the level of marketing in each area.

Part of Bumrungrad's early marketing included aggressive pursuit of international certification, and as a result Bumrungrad correctly claims a number of regional "Firsts" with various international credentialing organisations. In many ways, Bumrungrad was a trendsetter and these certifications were necessary when no one had even heard the term "medical tourism" and there were serious doubts about the quality of a Thai hospital. Today, the first and second tier of Thai hospitals are firmly within international standards and rising acceptance of medical tourism make this less necessary. BMC has, itself, a slew of acronyms attesting to its quality, many of which overlap Bumrungrad's, and comparing certifications should be less important to the potential medical tourist than other aspects of reputation, but for a nervous first time medical tourist Bumrungrad's list of "firsts" can be welcome reassurance.

The savings on one 'major tooth repair' can pay for an economy level 2 week vacation including air:

- Root canal and cap front tooth 14,000 thb US $354. AUD $481. EU284.
- Significant dental work (2 teeth) would result saved money in your bank account + the vacation!
- Very simple but necessary dental procedures from cleaning to cosmetic .. available at significant savings..
- Diagnostics, imaging, lab analysis, physical rehabilitation, cosmetic surgery, dental .. all 80% off US pricing.

Anonymous violent crime/robbery, common in the West, is all but unknown in Thailand:

- Most "Thailand Citizen US Educated Doctors" return to Thailand after graduation from their US Medical School.
- Plus, access to top Thai specialists within 24 hours is pretty reassuring
  - .. no waiting, ever, for anything! + a free tasty lunch!
- The Dell computer system at Bumrungrad is equal to any in the world.
  - Orthopedic images, blood work, diagnostics, specialist notes .. all are available across the network.
  - No carrying film/records to a specialist .. it's in the system and instantly available.
  - Doc suggests additional imaging: .. OK, he orders it, the test is completed and you are back in his office getting his interpretation within 24-48 hours.
  - Doc orders a CAT scan and it's completed the next morning and immediately it's in the computer system! .. !!
- Appointments are coordinated system wide .. smooth patient flow .. no bottle necks .. no waits, respect .. professional! + smiling happy Health Care team and bilingual clerical staffing.

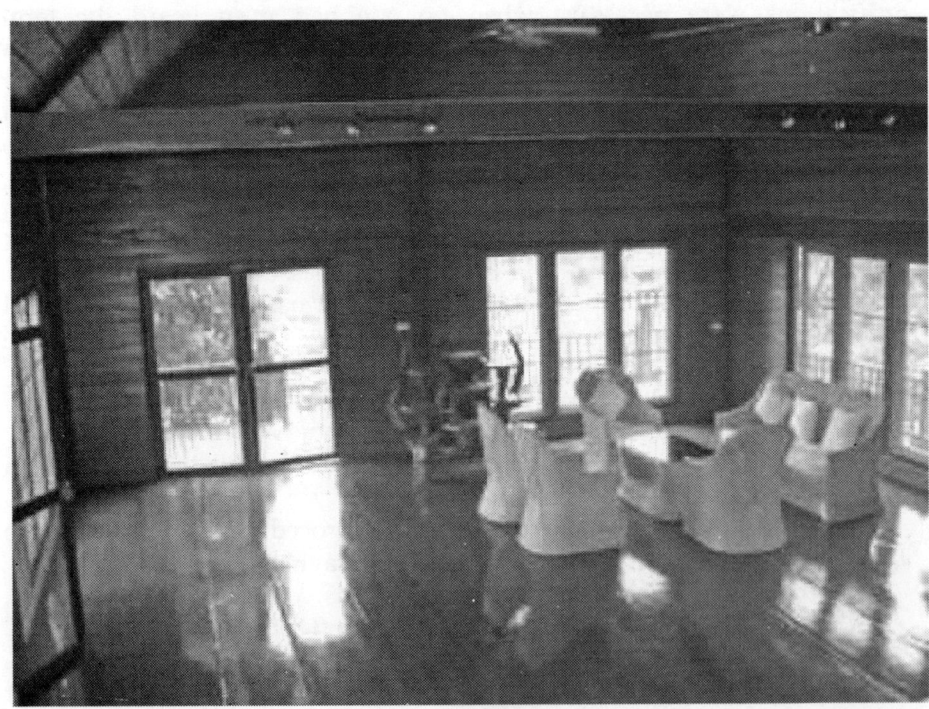

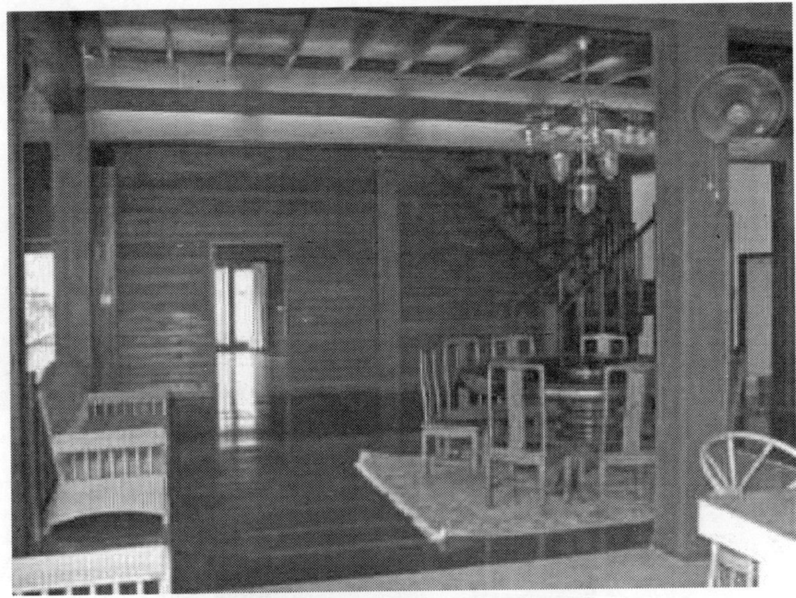

In the Chiang Mai/Chiang Rai area some incredible Lanni Thai style house are available for short term rental .. quite marvelous houses built from 100% teak. The house above rents for 17,000 Thb (US $400, Euro 325 per month)

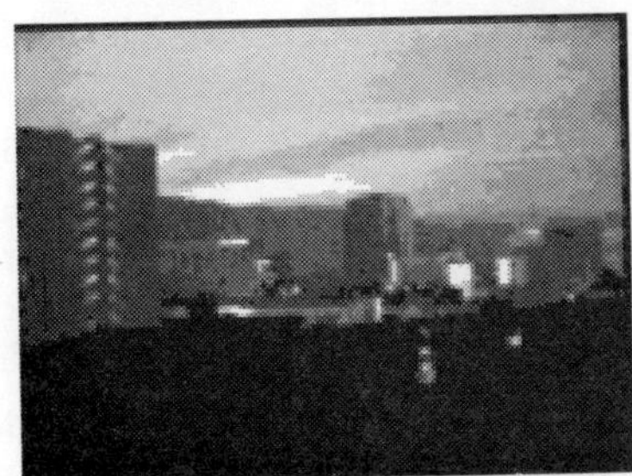

Golden Triangle

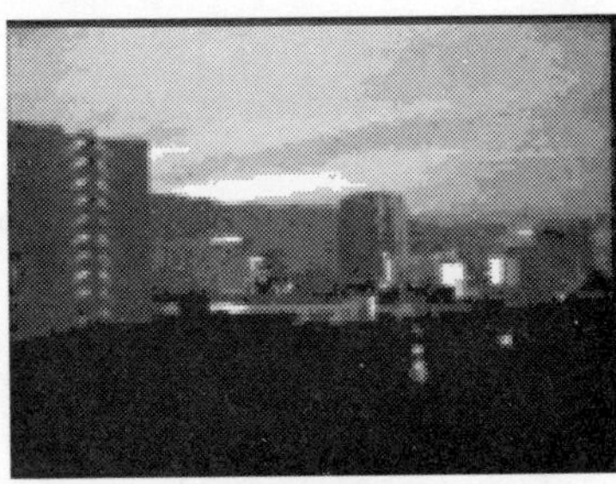

Beaches

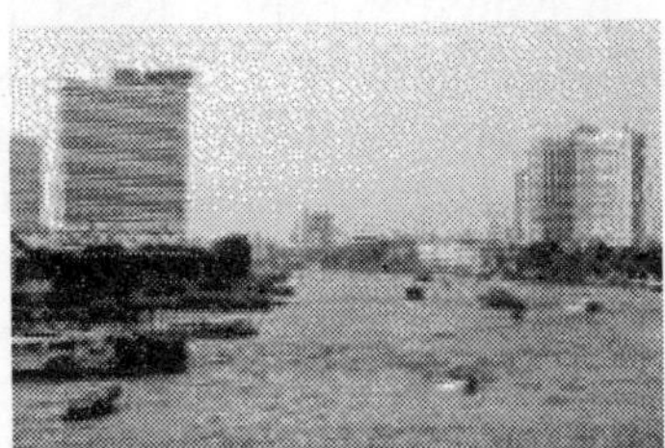

Bangkok

Bangkok is a wonderful mix of Ancient Far East and Ultra Modern West

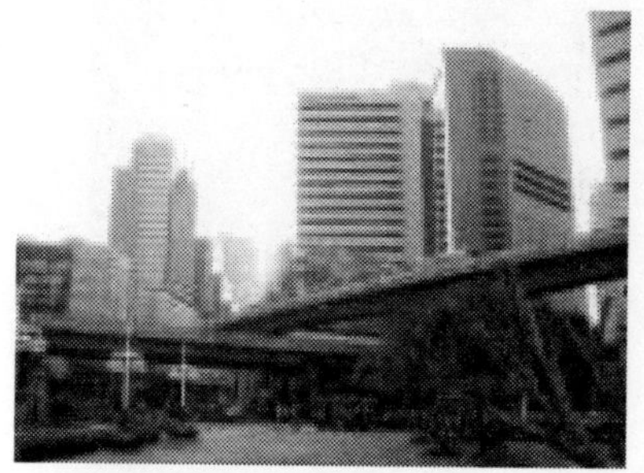

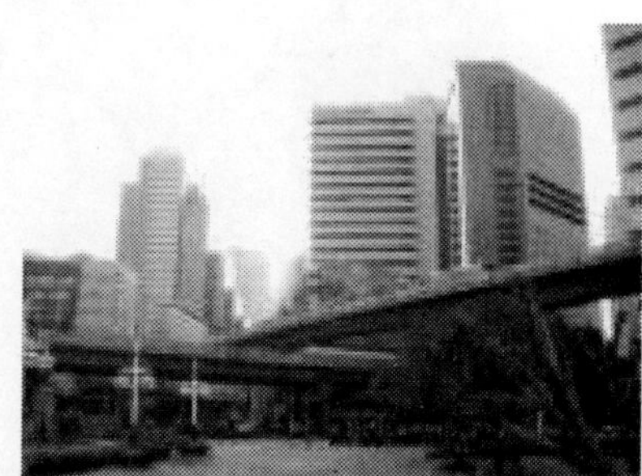

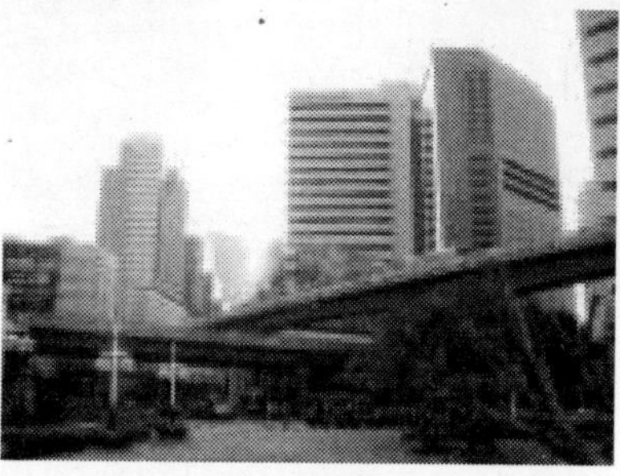

Thailand can provide an "extremely cost effective" Health Vacation.

- Grand Imperial Travel of Bangkok offers Executive Medical Tourism Packages!
- They assist with appointments and suggest hotels/apartments near your medical provider.
- They pick you up at the airport, provide a cell phone for your stay, provide a personal guide for both tourist outings and medical appointments .. all for a flat fee.
- Bumrungrad and Bangkok Hospital compare well to US Med Center Hospitals .. and far better than rural US hospitals.

Bumrungrad Hospital, is very foreigner friendly. Said to be #1 in Asia! Bangkok Hospital, off New Petchaburi Road, is foreigner friendly and comparable to most western hospitals. Private hospital room is $60. per day. A few extra days in the hospital, no problem. Many Japanese companies send their employees to Thailand for annual physicals as well as long-term medial care modalities. The savings on medical fees and the high quality medical care makes the air fare inconsequential. See attached appendix to this chapter for more details on Bumrungrad.

Dental experiences vary greatly. These clinics offer modern equipment and a full range of 'pain reduction techniques'.

- Asavanant Clinic.
- Bangkok Dental Hospital.
- Siam Family Dental.
- The Dental Hospitals on Suk Soi 55, Suk Soi 49 and Suk Soi 39 as well as the Dental clinics at Chula Hospital and Bumagard Hospital are professionally staffed and equipped well.

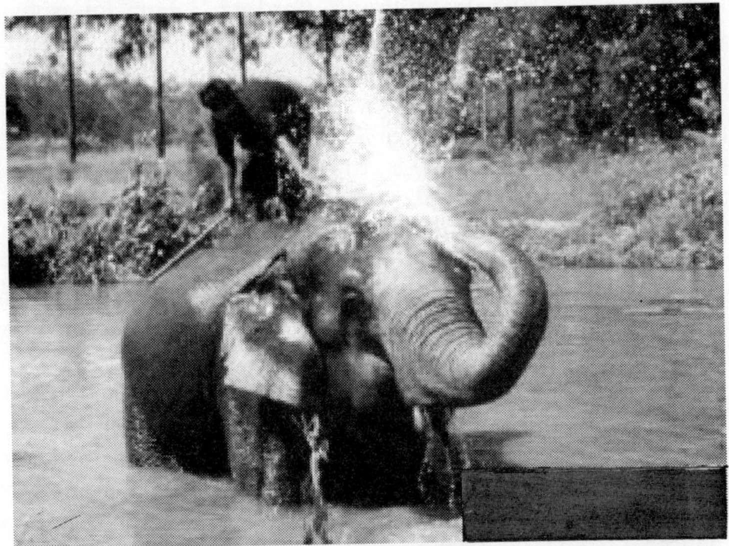

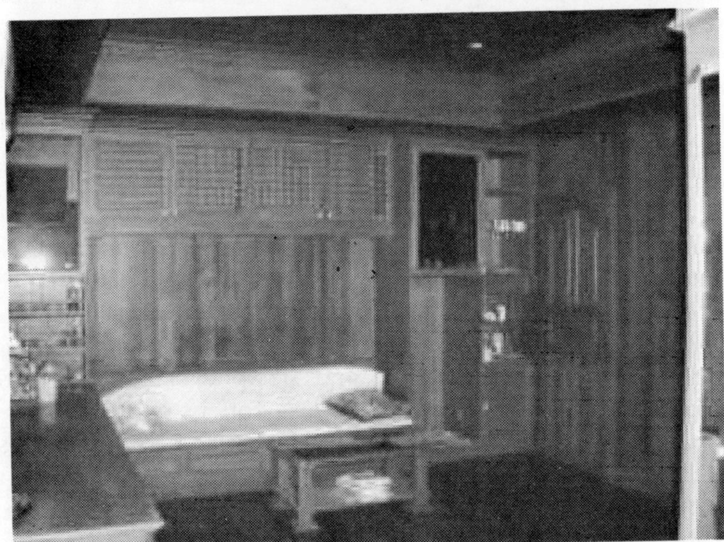

- Bumagard Hospital has serviced apartments adjacent to the hospital.. hospital staffed rehabilitation apartment suites for less than $100 per day.

- Affordable 24/7 out patient nursing. $100. per day can provide luxury hotel accommodations, gourmet meals and 24 hour 'private duty assisting provider' .

More than 150,000 North Americans and Europeans currently seek medical treatment overseas each year, estimates Josef Woodman, author of the forthcoming "Patients without Borders." For invasive surgeries, preferred destinations include India, Thailand, Singapore and Malaysia. Large hospitals, such as Bumrungrad and the Apollo chain in India, actively court American, European and Middle Eastern patients. Bumrungrad arranges limousines to pick up patients at the airport, and sheiks and princes congregate in the Platinum Lounge of Apollo's Delhi hospital. Abacas International, a leading travel facilitator, reports that medical tourism to Asia could generate billions of dollars.

Businesses are taking notice. At least 40 corporations have signed on to the overseas plan that United Group Programs, a health insurer in Boca Raton, Florida, began offering six months ago. Sending an employee abroad can save 80 percent of the costs of a procedure; a $50,000 angioplasty in the United States costs less than $6,000 in Mohali, Chandigarh, India, according to Global Choice Health Care, a firm that arranges foreign medical procedures. Walk-in patients see a specialist in 17 minutes on average. Since 75 percent of hospital revenues are paid by patients directly, health and insurance companies have no say in treatment. Low labor costs allow Thai hospitals to employ more staff.

In Australia, Europe and North America, "complementary and alternative medicine" (CAM) is increasingly being used in parallel to modern medicine, particularly for treating and managing chronic disease. Concern about the adverse effects of chemical medicines, a desire for more personalized health care and greater public access to health information, fuel this increased use. For the past six years, persons from over two hundred countries with difficult and chronic conditions, i.e., diverticulitis, cancer, and incurable autoimmune diseases such as Systemic Lupus Erythematosis (SLE), Multiple Sclerosis (MS), Lou Gherigi's Disease (ALS), have been motivated to explore the options Traditional Chinese Medicine (TCM) offers them at Huai Hua Red Cross Hospital. Since these conditions are chronic and often times incurable, they have led many patients and/ or their family members to seek and decipher complex, baffling, and, obscure medical information and to explore options encountered beyond the diagnostic and treatment scope generally available to them. Despite their diverse cultural backgrounds, many persons reach this intersecting destination at the time-honored tradition of TCM and the Huai Hua Red Cross Hospital for Difficult and Chronic conditions.

Five million tourists for health treatment

According to the Tourism Authority of Thailand (TAT), at least five million tourists come to the country annually for medical treatment. Various plastic surgery clinics could attest that the number of both Thais and foreigners undergoing dental and plastic surgeries, lasik, and other physical enhancement procedures is increasing. Aside from these, Thailand has earned its reputation as an excellent location for spa services. "The growth of spa business is a good sign that tells us that we can respond to customers' needs," Mr. Apichai added pointing to Proud Asia 2008 as an excellent venue where the international community can actually see the advancements that Thailand has taken the field of medical tourism.

"Beauty business will continuously grow as both men and women care about their looks," President of Thai Society of Cosmetic Dermatology and Surgery, Dr. Thada Piamphongsan, said, adding that Thailand has more advantages than other countries in Asia when it comes to offering the best quality medical and beauty services but at cheaper rates.

"Proud Asia 2008 is definitely not just the usual exhibition event on beauty and health care products and services we see here and in other countries. What makes this event extraordinary is the fact that we are going to have a grand showcase of the latest innovations of products and services in the field of medical tourism, spa and wellness. Everybody will be here the expert in medical tourism, the best spa and wellness providers, and the most highly interested buyers. "The event promises to be a big one for both suppliers and buyers and the most important thing is that it will be held right here in Bangkok. This means that the Kingdom will again have the chance to prove to the international community that Thailand has sufficient MICE infrastructure to be the best venue for this kind of trade exhibition and conference. Proud Asia 2007 is a huge event that will help the country achieve its goal of becoming a regional hub for exhibitions and conventions business and Mice market," said Mr. Vithaya.

Health tourism boom takes Singapore by storm

Singapore on the other hand makes world headlines for performing complex neurosurgical procedures and delivering cutting-edge medical treatment by the region's leading health specialists. The Republic's reputation for high quality medical facilities and well-trained doctors pulled in more than 370,000 visitors in 2004. The cost of treatments in Singapore, such as a hip replacement, can be less than a third of the price in the United States. In some cases, the cost is less than a tenth of what people would pay in America or Europe.

Raffles Hospital, has gained fame in recent years for highly publicized operations to separate conjoined twins, exemplifying the highly skilled expertise available.

The tiny island of Singapore, having a populace of 4.4 million, is fast positioning itself as a medical tourism hub. The authorities are ambitious of serving one million foreign patients annually by 2012 and generate USD 3 billion in revenue.

Parkway hospitals group is Singapore's largest private health care group in Asia, owning three tertiary care private hospitals: East Shore,

Gleneagles and Mount Elizabeth. The magnificent façade of these hospitals are complemented by equally competent doctors and excellent services with world class equipment. Incidentally, quite a few patients come from India for liver transplant. Nitin Saxena, who brought his father all the way from Delhi to Gleneagles for a liver transplant, opines unlike Indian hospitals, the services and facilities value for money.

Stem cell transplant is yet another field developing rapidly on the health map of Singapore. The haematology and stem cell transplant centre of Mount Elizabeth Hospital has pioneered stem cell treatment for patients with advanced cancer tumours. Headed by director Dr. Patrick Tan, a world renowned specialist in the field of oncology, cost of treatment here ranges from USD 72,000 to USD 90,000 per person, compared to USD 235,000 for similar treatment in the US. Recently, a 12-year-old girl from Delhi underwent cord blood transplant at the centre. As a mark of hospitality, hospital staff goes to receive patients and their relatives from the airport, make arrangements for their stay and even provide with language whenever required.

The medical tourism boom is just not restricted to Singapore alone. Current trend of economic developments in the Asian region, higher life expectancies, an ageing population and an ever-increasing awareness of the benefits of the quality health care have given a shot in the arm to the Asian health care industry, taking it to witness an unprecedented growth. Presently, there are only 140,000 hospitals serving an Asian population of 3.5 billion. With Asian population expected to grow to 5.6 billion by 2050, the consumer expenditure on health care services and goods will increase from US $90 billion in 1999 to US $188 billion in 2013. Malaysia is targeting the Middle East and China to generate whopping revenue of 2.2 billion by 2010. These emerging markets prove that there's immense potential in the Asian health care business, remarked Ms Tan-Hoong Chu Eng, MD, Parkway Promotions Pte Ltd., a subsidiary company of Parkway-Holdings Ltd. the largest private health care group in Asia.

Demand for health care is rising in the Middle East with millions of dollars spent in establishing specialised hospitals and clinics, expanding existing facilities and adopting world class technology in Bahrain, Kuwait, Yemen, Oman and Qatar. In the UAE, for instance, the government plans to double the bed capacity of public hospitals to achieve a target of one for every 300 people by the end of the decade.

The Philippines Faith healers

The Philippines probably beat other countries to this idea of medical tourism bit many years ago. I recall how in the 1970s, faith healers like Tony Agpaoa were already offering tour packages for people coming in from Europe and Japan who wanted the faith healers' services. Agpaoa even had his own little hotel in Baguio City so patients didn't have to look for their own accommodations. The faith healing packages eventually went into decline, and last I heard, it was our faith healers who were going to Eastern European countries to do their road-show healing.

Earlier this year, then-secretary of tourism Roberto Pagdanganan announced that the Department of Tourism was teaming up with the Department of Health, specifically the Philippine Institute of Traditional and Alternative Health Care, to promote medical tourism. At that time, he said only the St. Luke's hospital had been accredited for their program but Asian Hospital, Capitol Medical Center, and Medical City had also applied. Our medical and nursing curricula are certainly tougher than many of our neighbours' in Southeast Asia. Who knows, maybe medical tourism can convince a few more Filipino health professionals to stay rather than migrate.

Malaysia

Malaysia raked in RM 203.6 million in hospital receipts last year from nearly 300,000 foreign medical patients. Health Ministry parliamentary secretary Datuk Lee Kah Choon said Penang's portion of the takings amounted to RM129.9 million or 63.83 per cent of the total. The other cities involved were Kuala Lumpur, Malacca and Johor Baru. "We are expecting double-digit growth for hospital receipt figures this year," he said after witnessing the signing of a clinical research collaboration between YSP Industries Sdn Bhd and Penang-based Infor Kinetics Sdn Bhd here. Among the types of treatment sought are for heart ailments, cosmetic surgery, and wellness treatment at spas. "Patients include those from Indonesia and Singapore. The government is studying ways to make medical tourism more attractive to invest in." Health Care tourism in Malaysia took off in an aggressive manner in 2002 when Tourism Malaysia began promoting it overseas. "This includes tax-relief on the purchase of medical equipment or capital allowance on costs for new buildings," he said, adding that the proposed breaks were to reduce the "burden" on these institutions to enable them to continuously invest in upgrading their services. The Health Ministry is pursuing international accreditation for two Kuala Lumpur hospitals to boost medical tourism.

Several other countries in Asia and other continents are also working for medical tourism.

COMMON SURGICAL INTERVENTIONS SOUGHT BY FOREIGN MEDICAL TOURISTS

Globalisation has promoted a consumerist culture, thereby promoting goods and services that can feed the aspirations arising from this culture. This has had its effect in the health sector too, with the emergence of a private sector that thrives by servicing a small percentage of the population that has the ability to "buy" medical care at the rates at which the "high end" of the private medical sector provides such care. However, for patients and profits to increase, India must remedy negative first impressions and persuade doubters that millions of the country's poor and ailing won't be left behind.

The following services are visibly noticed:

Bone Marrow Transplant

Major hospitals in India have oncology units comprising surgical oncology, medical and radiation therapy as well as the crucial Bone Marrow Transplantation (BMT). The BMT unit with high-pressure Hipa filters has helped achieve a very high success rate in the various types of transplantation. Cord Blood Transplant and Mismatched Allogeneic Stem Cell Transplant have been performed successfully, a feat that is remarkable and significant, considering the fact that the treatment costs one-tenth of what it does in the west. Special surgeons are available for individual organs. Plastic surgeons of repute provide treatment for head and neck cancer, breast cancer and other malignancies. Facilities offered include tele-therapy, which includes simulation work stations to ensure high precision and safety during treatment at the 18 MV linear accelerator or telecobalt machines, brachy therapy and 3-D planning systems. In orthopedics, the Ilizarov technique is practiced for the treatment of limb deformities, limb shortening and disfiguration.

Cardiac Care

Cardiac care has become a specialty in India with institutions like the Escorts Heart Institute and Research Centre, All India Institute of Medical Sciences and Apollo Hospital becoming names to reckon with. These centres have the distinction of providing comprehensive cardiac care spanning from basic facilities in preventive cardiology to the most sophisticated curative technology. The technology is contemporary and world class and the volumes handled match global benchmarks. They also specialise in offering surgery to high-risk patients with the introduction of innovative techniques like minimally invasive and robotic surgery.

Having accomplished what he set out to do with Escorts, Trehan is planning a multispecialty hospital in Gurgaon, on the outskirts of New Delhi, that's patterned on the Cleveland Clinic in Ohio and the Mayo Clinic in Rochester, Minnesota.

Interventional Cardiology

Interventional Cardiology is a specialty which uses imaging techniques and strategies for the diagnosis of the diseases of the heart and blood vessel. These novel, minimally invasive, non-surgical procedures make use of mechanical treatments for the diseases of the heart and blood vessels. These procedures are mostly performed under local anesthesia, have a considerably short hospitalization and recovery period with minimal post-operative pain and discomfort. Interventional Cardiology includes a number of procedures that can be performed to the heart by means of inserting a 'catheter' either in your heart or in one of your blood vessels of the groin, neck or forearm. Established in 2000, the Krishna Heart Institute and Specialty Clinic is known for its innovative diagnostics and treatment procedures, and its extensive work in areas such as cardiology and joint replacement. Located in Ahmedabad, Gujarat, this institute is one of Gujarat's leading medical facilities. Initially specializing in cardiac care, the institute has grown into specialized areas such as hip and knee replacement surgeries, plastic and reconstructive surgeries, Onco-surgery, and other invasive and minimally invasive procedures. The institute has an excellent record for providing quality medical care for its international visitors at affordable prices. An air conditioned lounge is on each floor and there is a cafeteria with an expert chef serving a selection of cuisines. The institute provides continuous central monitoring and International standard water filtration and distribution systems for pure water, hot and cold. This institute is only one of the several cenres of excellence in the field of interventional cardiology.

Peripheral Angioplasty or Percutaneous Transluminal Angioplasty (PTA)

Peripheral Angioplasty is a minimally invasive procedure which is used to open narrowed arteries of the legs (most commonly iliac arteries causing cramps when walking, known as claudication), those to the brain known as the carotid arteries (causing stroke) and the arteries to the kidneys (causing high blood pressure). These conditions belong to the group of Peripheral Vascular Disease. Another condition may be ballooning of the artery called aneurysm. Aneurysms commonly occur in abdominal aorta where it manifests itself with abdominal pain or tenderness and a throbbing mass in the abdomen. Peripheral Vascular Disease is diagnosed by a procedure called angiogram which is similar to Coronary Angiogram. Peripheral Angioplasty is very similar to Coronary Angioplasty where arteries of the heart are narrowed due to atherosclerosis (Coronary Artery Disease). The blockage in the arteries is caused by deposition of fat in the form of plaques which accumulate along the arterial wall. Cost of procedure performed in the US: $18,171.

What does the procedure for Peripheral Angioplasty involve?

The procedure for Peripheral Angioplasty usually comprises of three steps: Step one of Peripheral Angioplasty, also known as artherectomy involves removal of blockage (plaque) from your peripheral artery either by laser or with specialized instruments to cut the plaque away and clear the arterial channel. The second step of Peripheral Angioplasty makes use of a balloon. An un-inflated balloon is inserted with the help of a guide wire to the site of blockage. The balloon is then inflated, which as a result enlarges the blood channel and increases blood flow through the artery. It is interesting to note that Peripheral Angioplasty can reduce a 70-90% blockage to about 20-30%. Step three of Peripheral Angioplasty consists of implanting a mesh stent which is tightly mounted on the Peripheral Angioplasty balloon into the walls of blocked artery.

If you have been diagnosed with intermittent claudication, i.e. aches, pain, cramps, or tightness in the calves, thighs, hips or buttocks when walking, which is relieved with a few moments rest, if you have leg ulcers or gangrene, if you have an aneurysm (abdominal aorta or cerebral artery), if you are a smoker who experiences numbness, tingling or coldness of legs and feet, if you suffer from high blood pressure, diabetes, high cholesterol, a family history of heart or vascular disease, and are overweight with symptoms of peripheral vascular disease, then you are an ideal candidate for Peripheral Angioplasty.

Peripheral Angioplasty has a success rate of almost 95% with the chances of re-stenosis occurring in 5% of the patients. This procedure is less painful and allows you to go back to your daily activities quickly. This means that you will not have the symptoms of Peripheral Vascular Disease any more. Insertion of Drug Eluting Stents have potentially improved the clinical outcome of the procedure of Peripheral Angioplasty. Peripheral Angioplasty has revolutionized the treatment of Peripheral Vascular Disease. Implantation of stents during angioplasty procedure reduces the chances of re-stenosis of the artery tremendously. The procedure of Peripheral Angioplasty is certainly not a treatment for Peripheral Vascular Disease however, accompanying lifestyle changes can definitely reduce your chances of further problems and complications. Cost of procedure performed in the US $18,171.

What is Coronary Angiography?

Coronary Angiography is a procedure in which a non-ionic contrast dye is injected into the coronary arteries. This allows your cardiologist to visualize the coronary arteries on an x-ray and view the flow of blood through them. Cost of procedure performed in the US $3,000 to $6,000. During the procedure of Coronary Angiography, you might experience some flushing and/or palpitation which will sub-side quickly. If you have chest pain which may or may not be increasing in intensity and duration, if you have unexplained pain in your jaw, neck or arm, if you have congenital heart disease or congestive heart failure, if you are planning to have heart valve surgery, if you have problems with your blood vessels like aortic aneurysm, if you have suffered a traumatic injury to your chest, then you are an ideal candidate for Coronary Angiography. Coronary Angiography is a relatively harmless procedure that can unfold tremendous amount of information and detail about the structure and function of your coronary arteries. Coronary Angiography is a diagnostic procedure that is used to confirm the diagnosis of the diseases affecting your heart and blood vessels. This procedure is also used to determine the extent and severity of your disease, and to help plan your treatment.

Risks of Coronary Angiography:

- Allergic reaction to the contrast dye
- Irregular heart beat (arrhythmias)
- Heart attack and death during the Coronary Angiography procedure

- Stroke
- Injury to the internal wall of the artery where the catheter was threaded in
- Perforation of coronary artery
- Kidney damage
- Excessive bleeding (hemorrhage)
- Infection
- Blood clots

Alternatives to Coronary Angiography

- *Magnetic Resonance Angiography (MRA)*—In this procedure detailed images of your heart are captured using radio waves in a strong magnetic field without the use of catheters or x-rays
- *CT Angiography*—This method does not require catheterization within the heart reducing some. of the risks associated with Coronary Angiography.
- *Digital Subtraction Angiography (DSA)*—This method combines the X-ray techniques of Coronary Angiography with a high-speed computer to improve the resolution of images obtained.
- *Cardiac Catheterization*—This procedure is very similar to Coronary Angiography and consists of passage of a catheter in the coronary artery

What is Coronary Angioplasty?

Coronary Angioplasty or Balloon Angioplasty is a minimally invasive procedure in which the blocked or narrowed coronary arteries are opened (widened) to facilitate perfusion of the heart muscle. Coronary Angioplasty reduces the need for medication and to some extent eliminates chest pain due to Ischemic Heart Disease. Cost of procedure performed in the US $35,000. The procedure for Coronary Angioplasty usually comprises of three steps: Step one of Coronary Angioplasty, also known as artherectomy involves removal of blockage (plaque) from your coronary artery either by laser or with specialized instruments to cut the plaque away and clear the arterial channel. The second step of Coronary Angioplasty makes use of a balloon (thus the alternative term Balloon Angioplasty). In this step, an un-inflated balloon is inserted with the help of a guide wire to the site of blockage. The balloon is then inflated, which enlarges the blood channel and increases blood flow through the artery. It is interesting to note that Coronary Angioplasty can reduce a 70-90% blockage to about 20-30%. Step three of Coronary Angioplasty consists of implanting a mesh stent which is tightly mounted on the Coronary Angioplasty balloon into the walls of blocked artery. The balloon is then deflated and removed leaving the stent in place permanently to hold the artery open. In this procedure of Coronary Angioplasty, the coronary arteries are accessed through a puncture made in the groin (femoral artery) or arm (brachial artery). Usually the femoral artery is used. Depending upon the extent of coronary artery narrowing, all three steps may or may not be carried out. The procedure of Coronary Angioplasty can take 30 minutes to several hours depending on the number of blockages being treated.

Benefits of Coronary Angioplasty

- Quicker and less painful recovery
- Short hospital stay, does not require general anesthesia
- Small incision
- Coronary Angioplasty can be done under local anesthesia
- The chest cage does not need to be opened
- Chances of major post-operative complications like stroke are minimized as heart-lung machine is not used during the procedure of Coronary Angioplasty

Risks of Coronary Angioplasty

- Allergic reaction to the dye
- Ruptured coronary artery
- Bleeding and infection at the site of insertion
- Arrhythmia
- Stroke
- Heart attack
- Kidney failure
- Rupture or dissection of the coronary artery
- Re-stenosis of the coronary artery requiring Heart Bypass Surgery

Why is Coronary Stenting performed?

Coronary Stenting is performed to hold your coronary artery open to facilitate flow of blood to the heart muscle and reduce your chest pain due to angina. The coronary stents physically hold your artery open and create a channel for your blood to flow through it easily. Coronary Stenting is usually performed as part of the Coronary Angioplasty procedure. So if you are an ideal candidate for Coronary Angioplasty, i.e. if one or more of your coronary arteries are blocked, if your chest pain due to angina is not well controlled with medications or if it is severe enough to disrupt your daily activities and also occurs at rest, then you are an ideal candidate for Coronary Stenting. Coronary Stenting has a success rate of almost 95% with the chances of re-stenosis occurring in 5% of the patients. This procedure is less painful and allows you to go back to your daily activities quickly. This means that you will not have chest pain any more and that your tolerance to exercise will increase. Drug Eluting Coronary Stents have potentially improved the clinical outcome of Coronary Stenting.

Benefits of Coronary Stenting

- Quicker and less painful recovery
- Short hospital stay, does not require general anesthesia
- Small incision
- Coronary Stenting can be done under local anesthesia
- The chest cage does not need to be opened
- Chances of major post-operative complications like stroke are minimized as heart-lung machine is not used during Coronary Stenting procedure
- Implantation of drug eluting coronary stents dramatically decreases the chances of re-stenosis and the need for a repeat procedure.

In the procedure for Drug Eluting Coronary Stenting, the implanted stent is coated with a medication that prevents re-stenosis. This type of stent consistently releases a chemical substance that prevents clot formation and narrowing of coronary artery. Drug Eluting Coronary Stenting has been 20-30% more successful than bare metal stenting. Cost of procedure performed in the US $37,000.

Benefits of Drug Eluting Coronary Stenting

- Quicker and less painful recovery
- Short hospital stay, does not require general anesthesia
- Small incision (Minimally Invasive procedure)
- Drug Eluting Coronary Stenting can be done under local anesthesia
- The chest cage does not need to be opened
- Chances of major post-operative complications like stroke are minimized as heart-lung machine is not used during the procedure of Drug Eluting Coronary Stenting.
- Implantation of Drug Eluting Coronary Stenting has dramatically decreased the chances of re-stenosis and the need for a repeat procedure.

Dialysis and Kidney Transplant

Common diseases like diabetes, hypertension and chronic glomerulonephritis can lead to permanent loss of renal functions—with dialysis and renal transplantation being the frequent outcome. The emergence of new therapeutic interventions has created opportunities in India to manage the progression of renal diseases. Major hospitals in India like Holy Family Hospital, Jaslok Hospital, Apollo Hospital, Sir Ganga Ram Hospital, Batra Hospital, Bombay Hospital and Hinduja Hospital have departments of Nephrology and Organ Transplant equipped with the latest computerised dialysis machines, reverse osmosis water plant to provide pure and trace element-free water supply, as well as state-of-the-art facilities in the operating rooms and Transplant Intensive Care Units.

For those who need renal replacement therapy, the following services are also available.

Patients can also avail of the bicarbonate dialysis facility at these centres. Round the clock service is available at these hospitals for the critically ill patients in the intensive care units who may need fluid, electrolyte management and renal supportive therapy.

The cost of getting a dialysis is around Rs. 1700 to Rs. 1800 per dialysis whereas the same costs about $300 in the U.S.A. Similarly a kidney transplant package in India is available for around Rs. 3 Lakhs, which is comparatively much cheaper than what it would cost abroad. Hemodialysis Chronic Ambulatory Peritoneal Dialysis (CAPD) Transplantation. In addition to the basic haemodialysis facilities, the patients' requirements for other modalities of treatment such as—Continuous Arterio-Venous Haemofilteration (CAVH) Continuous Veno-Venous Haemofilteration (CVVH) Continuous Cycler-Assisted Peritioneal Dialysis (CCPD)

Gynecology and Obstetrics

Leading Indian hospitals with gynecology departments and women's hospitals have facilities for the prevention and early detection of gynecological disorders. Many hospitals have women check-up programmes designed to detect the earliest signs of disorders of the breast and the organs of reproduction as well as catering to the contraceptive needs of women. A mammogram, an ultrasound of the pelvis and a pap smear of the cervix are an integral part of any good medical check-up for women. Specialist medical as well as surgical care is available for all types of gynecological problems like menstrual abnormalities, prolapse, fibroids and other tumors of the uterus and ovaries, tubal re-canalization by microsurgery and care of the infertile couple. State-of-the-art gynecological surgery is available with world-class equipment and expertise using minimally invasive techniques.

Ectopic pregnancies, ovarian cysts and tumors, fibroids endometriosis, tubal blocks and even hysterectomies can be performed laparoscopically. Hospitals like Apollo have state-of-the-art IVF labs backed by highly experienced doctors who have been involved in the field of infertility and assisted Reproductive Technologies (ART).

Joint Replacement Surgery

Shoulder/hip replacement and bilateral knee replacement surgery using the most advanced keyhole or endoscopic surgery and arthroscopy is done at several hospitals in India including the Apollo Hospital, Sir Ganga Ram Hospital and Holy Family Hospital in Delhi, Bombay Hospital, Leelavati and Hinduja Hospital in Mumbai and the Madras Institute of Orthopaedics and Trauma Sciences. Some hospitals like Apollo in Delhi have Operation Theatres with Laminar Air Flow System, which compares with the best in the USA and the UK. A knee joint replacement costs only a quarter of what it costs in the UK. In the last 5 years arthroplasty has got established and has changed the face of osteoarthritis patients. More than 10 million people are supposed to suffer from this ailment in India alone. Dr. Dholakia was the first to introduce the technique in 1986. Ranawat performed surgery on the knees of the then prime minister of India in 2000. Now further advancement has occurred and new techniques have come in giving better results.

Neurosurgery and Trauma Surgery

Other routine procedures performed with excellent results are replacement arthroplasty, diagnostic and operative arthroscopy, spinal surgeries including. Harrington Rod Instrumentation for scoliosis, corrective and reconstructive procedure for poliomyelitis and cerebral palsy, micro cascular surgical procedures and automated percutaneous lumbar distectomy. In addition, the advanced Luque technique is employed for the correction of complex scoliosis, and decompression and stabilisation of fractures of dorsal and lumbar spine with paraplegia, by neurosurgeons with excellent training and background. Many super-speciality hospitals in India like AIIMS, Ram Manohar Lohia Hospital, Vidya Sagar Institute of Mental Health and Neuro Sciences, Bombay Hospital, Jaslok Hospital, Nizam Institute of Mental Health and Neuro Sciences and Apollo Hospitals have advanced facilities devoted to the treatment of the entire range of brain and spinal disorders with highly experienced neurosurgeons, neurologists, Neuro-anaesthetists and Neuro-radiologists. Treatment of intra-and juxta-cranial, spinal tumours and vascular malformations, aneurysms and thrombolysis for brain attacks are done at these centres. Hospitals like Apollo employ state-of-the-art LINAC-based stereotactic radio surgery system outside the USA. The Clinic 6000SR Linear Accelerator with XKNIFE system is a highly sophisticated computer-driven technology used for removal of appropriately selected brain tumours, arteriovenous malformations and other abnormalities.

Osteoporosis

Several drug therapies now easily available in the market have been shown to be clinically effective in slowing down or reversing the bone-loss process. Leading hospitals in India are well equipped to detect and treat bone loss in its earliest states, so as to prevent the disease or lessen its impact. Doctors in leading hospitals have the expertise for the diagnosis and treatment of osteoporosis that involves an objective, quantifiable measurement of the patient's bone mass or bone density. Advanced technology called the DXA for bone densitometry is available. During a comprehensive bone valuation with DXA, the patient lies comfortably still on a padded table while the DXA unit scans one or more areas, usually the fractured spine or the hip. The entire process takes only minutes to scan depending on the number of sites scanned. It involved no injections or invasive procedures and the patient remains fully clothed.

Refractive Surgery

Refractive surgery is gaining popularity in India both among the public as well as among ophthalmologists. Till a few years ago only a few centres performed high volume radial keratotomy. Today, the highest international quality of eye care for cornea, cataract, squint and glaucoma is available in over 40 centres all over India. When it comes to reliability, India has the best ophthalmic surgeons with clinico-academic expertise honed to perfection in the best possible institutions. Apollo Hospital, Gurunanak Eye Centre, Dr. Rajindra Prasad Centre For Ophthalmic Sciences and Mohan Eye Centre in Delhi, Shankar Naytralaya in Chennai, L.V. Prasad hospital in Hyderabad are just some of the more popular eye care hospitals. The No Stitch Cataract Surgery with the most modern way of removing cataract through the use of Phacoemulsification procedure can be performed in India for as little as Rs. 20,000, for both the eyes, whereas the same surgery costs $ 45,000 in the USA. Facilities for PRK, myopia and astigmatism are now available in almost all parts of the country. Hyperopic and LASIK are available and even supra hard cataracts are treated using just 1 mm incision instead of the 3 mm incision size. Photo-refractive keratectomy or PRK treats the surface of the cornea with the Excimer laser while LASIK treats the inner tissue of the cornea. For this reason, with LASIK there is less area to heal, less risk of scarring, less risk of corneal haze, less post-operative pain and vision often returns very rapidly.

Urology

Several super specialty hospitals in India offer comprehensive Urologic services to diagnose and treat stone disease, Urologic cancer, incontinence, infertility, impotency and other urinary difficulties. Advanced methods such as lithotripsy for treating kidney and ureteric stones without surgery are available with complementary methods of treating stones endoscopically. Advanced machines like the Lithostar obvert the need for anaesthesia in the treatment of kidney and ureteric stones. High tech facilities for the treatment of prostate, bladder cancers, urethral strictures are also available. Investigation and treatment facilities for impotence and male/female infertility exist with specialized facilities for pharmacotherapy, cavernosometry and cavernosography, in addition to doppler studies for the assessment of blood flow.

Other surgeries

Removal of the gall bladder, the spleen, the bowel and other organs like the adrenals, an operation for prolapse rectum and hiatus hernia repair have become fairly commonplace in almost all the major speciality hospitals in India. Experts are easily available and accessible and the workload at most of these hospitals ensures that the doctors have enormous experience. High intensive care treatment at much cheaper rates than in the west is available at most of these centers.

Preventive Health Care

Preventive health care has been introduced for the first time in the country by Apollo Hospitals with hospitals in the metros of Hyderabad, Chennai and Delhi, within easy international air access. The professional chain also pioneered the concept of lifestyle clinics, established the first organ registry in the country and introduced non-invasive technique for treatment of lesions and tumours of the brain—Stereotactic Radio Surgery and Radiotherapy in the country. It recently installed a state of the art Cobalt Unit. Apollo Heart Hospital provides a complete network for cardiac patients. It has a total bed capacity of 500 beds distributed between Apollo —Chennai, Hyderabad and Delhi. Apollo is linked to the Mayo Clinic and the Minneapolis Heart Institute, a premier heart institute led by the team of doctors who pioneered the Jarvik artificial heart.

Imaging with MRI, a hypertension research centre and facilities for hemodialysis and kidney transplantation are available at Akila Hospitals at Trichy. The hospital boasts a transplant team with 8 specialists, bone marrow transplant team along with five specialists on call to Sri Lanka, Sharjah, Kuwait and major Indian cities.

In Chennai, the Vijaya Heart Foundation's 79 beds have a state of the art cardiology and cardio-thoracic surgical unit manned by competent and experienced staff. The Vijaya Health Centre with 270 beds offers diagnostic facilities in laboratory, X-ray, ultrasound, treadmill, Endoscopy, C.T. Scan, M.R.I. and nuclear medicine.

Fasting

Naturopath doctors at such centres mean a minimalist diet of 300 calories per day—veggie broths and juices-for two weeks to several months, accompanied by blood tests, purges and other treatments. They say many hard-to-treat conditions, from arthritis to allergies and various skin disorders, benefit from the metabolic switch that takes place when the body starts living off its own reserves. Of the thousands guests who come to fast each year (half from southern Europe, America and the Middle East), about one third arrive with serious ailments—the rest come to lose weight or cut stress. Fasting has lately gotten a boost from medical research. Clinical studies in Scandinavia have shown that fasting is an effective treatment for rheumatism—especially if followed by a vegetarian diet. In one study, pain and swelling came down by a third in a week and stayed that way for a year. Other studies have shown success in lowering blood pressure and treating chronic pain like migraine or arthritis. They have shown that when patients fast, stress hormones levels go down and serotonin levels rise (which may explain the "fasting high" many patients report). "The more we look into it, fasting seems to work like a reset button for the body's own self-regulating mechanisms," say Naturopaths.

$800 vs. $18

In the U.S., organisations such as the Joint Commission International

(JCI) on Accreditation of Health Care Organisations, based in Oakbrook Terrace, Illinois, assess infection rates, the width of hospital corridors and the capacity of elevators. Dr. Trehan, Escorts' founder, says the hospital had a mortality rate of 0.8 percent and an infection rate of 0.3 percent in 2003. That compares with an observed mortality rate, or the rate of actual deaths, of 4.77 percent for heart valve surgery or coronary artery bypass surgery that included heart valves at New York—Presbyterian Hospital. Charging foreigners more than Indians is one way hospitals can make money to treat the poor, says Gautam Kumra, a McKinsey and Co. partner in New Delhi. An echocardiogram machine, used to picture the heart, costs about $200,000 anywhere in the world. Doctors can charge $800 per scan in the U.S.; in India, they charge 800 rupees, or $18, Trehan says. Fortis Health Care plans is setting up two hospitals on the outskirts of New Delhi. One will cater to overseas patients and charge them higher prices, says Harpal Singh, who adds the hospitals haven't set fees yet. Fortis is owned by brothers Malvinder and Shivinder Singh, who control India's largest drug company, Ranbaxy Laboratories Ltd. Harpal Singh is Malvinder Singh's father-in-law. One imbalance that works in India's favour is its lower salaries. A top cardiac surgeon in India makes about $330,000 a year compared with $5 million in the U.S., says Anupam Sibal, director at Apollo Hospital New Delhi.

Cosmetic and Plastic Surgery

This is a surgical specialty that corrects disfigurement caused by burns, tumor, congenital defects, developmental abnormalities, trauma, infection, disease or injuries, improves appearance and self esteem and restores function. Cosmetic and Plastic Surgery is mainly concerned with correcting problems and enhancing appearance of exposed areas of the body and the face. Reconstructive Plastic Surgery is another term that is used in this context mainly referring to surgical procedures that correct severe functional impairments, fix physical abnormalities, and compensate for tissue lost to trauma or surgery.

Some disfigurations corrected include hair restoration (hair implants, hair flaps, and scalp reductions), rhinoplasty (reshaping or re-contouring of the nose), stalling of the aging process (face lift, cosmetic eyelid surgery, brow lift, sub-metal lipectomy for double chin), dermabrasions (sanding of the face,) otoplasty for protruding ears, chin and cheek enlargement, lip reductions, various types of breast surgery and reconstruction and liposuction.

The problem of loose upper arm skin usually occurs after weight loss. This problem is more common in people who have lost a lot of weight. If you were over weight, the skin of your arm has to stretch to accommodate the increased volume of your upper arm. After weight loss, the skin usually fails to tighten and sags. Brachioplasty is performed to correct this problem of loose hanging skin of your arms. Brachioplasty is performed as an outpatient procedure in the plastic surgeon's office under local anesthesia with sedation. The entire procedure of Brachioplasty takes about an hour per arm. The surgeon makes zigzag, elliptical or triangular incisions along the inner surface of upper arm. The space contained between the incisions is exactly the area of skin that would be removed. Removal of loose skin tightens the surface of the arm however, it does not remove the fat. That is why it is usually recommended that Brachioplasty be accompanied with liposuction as well to remove extra fat from your arms. Make sure that you make arrangements for some one to accompany you as you will be allowed to go home after a couple of hours following Brachioplasty procedure.

Benefits of Brachioplasty

- Brachioplasty will help you get rid of the extra fat and skin after losing weight. Although this requires you to undergo a Brachioplasty procedure, the results are well worth it. To be able to get the lean and shapely arms that you have always longed for, Brachioplasty is the best option available.
- Brachioplasty is performed under local anesthesia, does not require hospitalization and you can return to work and resume your daily activities within 2 weeks.

What is Body Lift?

Body Lift or Total Body Lift is a Cosmetic and Plastic Surgery procedure performed to reshape your body to it's natural curves and contours. Body Lift is a surgical procedure where the loose and hanging skin of the entire body is tightened and implants are inserted, all in one procedure. Body Lift basically reshapes the breasts, chest, arms, thighs, hips, back, waist, abdomen and knees after losing weight (for example those people who lose lot of weight after undergoing weight loss surgeries like Gastric Bypass, Laparoscopic Gastric Bypass, Gastric Banding), aging and multiple pregnancies. Body Lift can be:

- *Central Body Lift*—This procedure is also called Belt Lipectomy. In Central Body Lift, excess skin and fatty tissue is removed circumferentially from the belly, hips, back, buttocks, and outer thighs.
- *Lower Body Lift*—Lower Body Lift is performed to shape buttocks and thighs by removing excess skin and fat from these areas.

Body Lift can be combined with other Cosmetic and Plastic Surgery procedures like Liposuction, Power Assisted Liposculpture (PAL), Tummy Tuck, Thigh Lift, Arm Lift, Breast Reduction, Breast Augmentation, and Breast Lift. Skin Grafting may also be performed in places of the body where needed. These procedures not only remove excess skin and fat, they also improve the unsightly stretch marks and create an uplifted, shapely, youthful and fuller appearance.

If you have lost large amounts of weight (50-300 lbs.) and have loose, hanging skin on your face, breasts, back, belly and thighs, or if you want to lose weight (especially if you suffer from central obesity) that is resistant to diet and exercise, if you have folds of loose, hanging skin due to aging or multiple pregnancies that might pose a danger of cellulitis or abscess, then you are an ideal candidate for Body Lift. This procedure can either be performed in isolation or in combination with other body contouring and weight loss procedures like Liposuction, Tummy Tuck, etc. If you are severely obese, are a smoker or an alcoholic or do not have a stable mental state to undergo a major surgical procedure and follow post-operative instructions to obtain optimum benefit or if you are allergic to the medication used for general anesthesia, then you are not an ideal candidate for Body Lift.

Body Lift is performed in a hospital setting under general anesthesia and can take about 5-7 or may be 10 hours depending on what other cosmetic surgery procedures are performed along with it. The Body Lift surgery is usually performed to remove excess skin from the belly first, i.e. from the area between the belly button and pubic hair and tightening of abdominal muscles is also performed. Excessive skin is removed, belly button is repositioned, remainder of the skin is approximated and the incision is sutured. The surgeon will then turn you on your side, make incisions in your buttock and back area, remove fat and excess skin to try and normalize the curves and contours of your sides and back. Body Lift also involves Liposuction of the buttocks, thighs and abdomen areas. Lastly your surgeon will work on the flabby arms (commonly called bat wings) and make them shapely. As mentioned above, Liposuction, Power Assisted Liposculpture (PAL), Tummy Tuck, Thigh Lift, Arm Lift, Breast Reduction, Breast Augmentation, Breast Lift and Skin Grafting can all be performed at the same time, whatever your need may be.

Body Lift is a comprehensive procedure that can take care of flabby, bulges in different parts of your body. The best results are obtained when Body Lift is performed by skillful and experienced cosmetic surgeons. This procedure is as safe as multiple shorter cosmetic surgeries. The contours of your body will be better defined and if you commit yourself to exercising regularly and eating sensibly, chances are that the results of Body Lift will be good for the rest of your life. Body Lift is a revolutionary surgical procedure that quickly, safely and effectively re-shapes the normal contours of your body. Most people who undergo Body Lift are quite satisfied with the results. The procedure of Body Lift is unified approach to treat and skin laxity as a result of aging, pregnancy and dramatic weight loss. Body Lift is a remarkable procedure which can help you get started on the way to a new, more fulfilling life of normalcy and a level of self-esteem that you may have never imagined.

Alternatives to Body Lift

- Liposuction is commonly used in both men and women to remove localized excess fat deposits that are resistant to dieting and exercise.
- Power Assisted Liposculpture (PAL)—Power Assisted Liposculpture uses a powerized cannula which moves back and forth through the fat tissue in a rapid motion.
- Tummy tuck, also known as Abdominoplasty or Panniculectomy is a procedure where large amount of skin and fat are removed from the middle and lower part of the abdomen.
- Thigh Lift is a procedure which is performed to remove loose and excessive (hanging) skin around your thighs and buttocks, thus to tighten them and improve it's appearance and texture.
- Arm Lift—Brachioplasty or Arm Lift is a procedure where loose and excess skin are removed from your arm.
- Breast Reduction is a surgical procedure designed to remove excessive fat, glandular tissue, and skin from large and pendulous breasts, making them smaller, lighter, and firmer.
- Breast Augmentation or Breast Implant Surgery is a surgical procedure in which the size and shape of a woman's breast is enhanced by inserting an artificial breast implant behind each breast.
- Breast Lift or Mastopexy is a surgical procedure which is commonly performed in men and in women to reshape sagging or drooping breasts and to give them a firm, youthful contour.
- Skin grafting is a surgical procedure by which skin or a skin substitute is used to replace the damaged skin or provide a temporary wound covering.

Body Lift is fondly called the Face Lift of your body. The resulting body contour shows a remarkable and significant improvement in the areas of the belly, pubic region, hips, back, and buttocks and will bring you to the range of normal body contour.

What is a Breast Implant?

A breast implant is a soft shell or a rubber sac that is filled with silicone gel or saline (salt-water). The feel of the implant is very natural and close to the feel of the normal breast tissue. They are available in several different sizes to accommodate different patient's needs and surgeon's preference. The surface texture of the implant can be smooth or contoured. There are different approaches used for Breast Augmentation surgery: (1) Infra-mammary Breast Augmentation—This is the most commonly used approach for Breast Augmentation operation. In this approach an incision is made in the crease just below the breast where the breast tissue meets the chest wall. (2) Peri-areolar Breast Augmentation—In this approach a semi-circular incision is made around the lower part of the areola (areola is the dark area of skin surrounding the nipple). (3) Trans-axillary or Axillary Breast Augmentation—In this approach an incision is made in the armpit to insert the breast implant. (4) Trans-umblical or Umblical Breast Augmentation—In this approach, a breast implant is inserted through the umbilicus or belly button with the help of an endoscope.

Breast Augmentation surgery takes about 2-3 hours. Most commonly you can go home the same day or the following day. The sutures are covered with a gauze dressing to promote speedy healing. The outcome of Breast Augmentation is very satisfactory and successful. Your breasts will be enlarged for life. Clothes fit better and it certainly boosts your self confidence and self esteem. Some cases of leakage or breaking of the breast implant have been reported. In this case, a second Breast Augmentation surgery may be needed. The breast tissue is actually pushed to the surface as the breast implant is inserted behind the breast tissue. Following Breast Augmentation surgery it might become easier to perform breast self examination to gain familiarity with your breast tissue. Of course the obvious benefit Breast Augmentation is improved look of your breasts and your overall body image remains undisputed without any doubt. Breast Lift is designed to regain you youthful look and vigor. This procedure of Cosmetic and Plastic Surgery is used world wide by women as well as men to improve the appearance of drooping, sagging breasts. Breast Lift is performed in conjunction with Breast Augmentation to increase their size and give firmness. Breast Lift is a very popular surgery and the number of men and women undergoing Breast Lift has increased tremendously (214%) in the past five years. The beauty of Breast Lift is that it enhances your body image and maintains the normal shape of your breast as closely as possible. The operation for Breast Lift is an excellent option that reverses the changes that occur in your breast due to weight loss, pregnancy, breast feeding and aging. The goal of your plastic surgeon will be to restore the normal contour and firmness of your breasts as closely as possible. You will be extremely pleased with the results of Breast Lift surgery if you completely understand the procedure and make an informed decision but at the same time have realistic expectations.

What is Breast Reduction?

Breast Reduction is a surgical procedure designed to remove excessive fat, glandular tissue, and skin from large and pendulous breasts, making them smaller, lighter, and firmer. During Breast Reduction, the size of the areola is also reduced in proportion to the breast size. Breast Reduction is also performed in men for the correction of Gynecomastia. Breast Reduction surgery is performed to alleviate both your physical and psychological problems due to large breasts. Physical problems include upper back and neck pain and discomfort, deep and sore indentations on the shoulder from bra straps, rashes on the under surface of the breast due to sweat and moisture and difficulty finding clothes or bra that fit you well.

Psychological problems include feeling self-conscious due to large breasts. All the above reasons are definite indications for Breast Reduction surgery. Breast Reduction is also performed in men who have large breasts. Although certain health conditions and medications are known to cause male breast enlargements (Gynecomastia), there is no other known cause for this problem in men. If you are a woman who has large, pendulous breasts and are not planning on having any more children, if you have chronic headache, upper back or neck pain, then you are an ideal candidate for Breast Reduction surgery.

Benefits of Breast Reduction

- Breast Reduction surgery not only alleviates your anxiety of being self conscious about large, sagging breasts but it also relieves physical discomfort like chronic neck and back pain and skin rashes. Of course to say the least, Breast Reduction adds tremendously to your self-confidence and self-esteem as it enhances your body image and allows you to enjoy wearing clothes that you might have avoided to wear in the past. Breast Reduction also allows you freedom to enjoy sports and physical activities that might have been painful or uncomfortable due to bouncing of large and heavy breasts.
- You can feel the breast tissue better during Breast Self-Examination as the surrounding excessive fat surrounding the glands and ducts has been diminished

HOW MUCH CAN YOU SAVE BY YOUR WORLD-CLASS TREATMENT IN INDIA?

The best part about treatment in India is that you enjoy world-class medical advantages at a fraction of the cost in comparison with destinations like US, Europe, Africa and the Middle East. The greatest cost savings is typically found in orthopedic/cardiac procedures (75-90% lower fees outside of the United States). If you have received quotes in the US for $10,000, you can expect the same procedure to cost between $2,500 and $5,000 or less. If one is uninsured or under insured for medical treatment in U.S.A., the better option is to come to India. The significant cost reduction enables you purchase a round trip air ticket, recuperative holidays post-treatment in a exotic beach location in India and return home saving money. India aims to replicate the Thai model, which is still the first Asian destination for International Patients. Here are some examples of your medical price savings.

Nature of Treatment	Approximate Cost in India ($)	Cost in other Major Healthcare Destination ($)	Approximate Waiting Periods in USA / UK (in months)
Open heart Surgery	4,500	> 18,000	9 - 11
Cranio-facial Surgery and skull base	4,300	> 13,000	6 - 8
Neuro-surgery with Hypothermia	6,500	> 21,000	12 - 14
Complex spine surgery with implants	4,300	> 13,000	9 - 11
Simple Spine surgery	2,100	> 6,500	9 - 11
Simple Brain Tumor - Biopsy - Surgery	 1,000 4,300	 > 4,300 > 10,000	6 - 8
Parkinsons - Lesion - DBS	 2,100 17,000	 > 6,500 > 26,000	9 - 11
Hip Replacement	4,300	> 13,000	9 - 11

Bargain Prices

Treatment	*India*	*US*
Coronary Artery Bypass Grafting	$6,600	$60,000
Knee Replacement (single knee)	$6,500	$22,000
Rhinoplasty (nose job)	$2,000	$10,000
Bone Marrow Transplant	$26,000	$2,50,000
Root Canal Treatment	$100	$1000

Procedure	*Cost (US$)*	
	United States	*India*
Liver Transplant	3,00,000	69,000
Cataract Surgery	2,000	1,250

Where do the cost savings come from?

The answer lies in the economics of health care in the United States and the amount of fraud and waste that is present in the U.S. health care system. 80% of all health care dollars that go through their office cover nothing but paperwork. As a medical tourist in another country, you eliminate these paperwork shufflers. And right there, you can save as much as 80% right off the bat. In the United States, your money is going to the insurance company and then the insurance company money is being used to pay paper shufflers.

Dental procedure	*Cost in US (US$)*		*Cost in India (US$)*
	By General Dentist	By Top End Dentist	By Top End Dentist
Smile designing	-	8,000	1,000
Metal Free Bridge	-	5,500	500
Dental Implants	-	3,500	800
Porcelain Metal Bridge	1,800	3,000	300
Porcelain Metal Crown	600	1,000	80
Tooth impactions	500	2,000	100
Root canal Treatment	600	1,000	100
Tooth whitening	350	800	110
Tooth colored composite fillings	200	500	25
Tooth cleaning	100	300	75

Some cost saving figures in dental treatment at a glance!

Case Study: An 87 year old US citizen who needed a mitral valve replacement turned to Madras Medical mission hospital Chennai, India as no hospital would touch him being a high risk patient. He underwent a triple by-pass surgery years ago that cost him $40,000 in contrast the mitral valve surgery, a more complex and expensive surgery cost only $8,000 here in India. (The patient's damaged mitral valve was replaced with a bio-prosthetic valve whose life is said to be 15 years.) (The India Post Newspaper Publication, USA; Feb. '05)

Uninsured, Uninsurable or Underinsured: Americans increasingly traveling overseas

In the United States, health care is exorbitantly expensive, and each year millions of Americans find themselves unable to pay for the health care they want or need because they are either uninsured, uninsurable or underinsured. Over 47 million Americans have no health insurance at all, and millions more are forced to forgo 'elective procedures' that do not qualify for coverage by insurers. An estimated 120 million Americans live without any form of dental insurance. A recent study describes fifty-percent of bankruptcies in 2001 as being related to medical crises and each year millions of Americans are forced to choose between incurring crushing debt or foregoing medical procedures.

Medical Tourism has emerged as a viable health care alternative for many Westerners for a variety of reasons. Furthermore, an increasing number of Western-trained physicians from the developing world have returned to their country of origin to practice. The result is that a "perfect storm" of positive factors have come together to offer real, high quality medical alternatives to Westerners faced with significant costs or waiting times at home. What may accelerate the trend is that some pioneering U.S. corporations, swamped by rising health care costs, are taking a serious look at medical outsourcing. Blue Ridge Paper Products of Canton, N.C., a manufacturing company, may soon offer employees outsourcing as a health care option. The carrot? The patient would get to pocket some of the firm's substantial savings.

Americans looking to save money on medical procedures are increasingly traveling overseas for surgeries not covered by their insurance to avoid costly hospital stays in the United States. The trend is being driven by rising health care costs and frustrated ranks of uninsured American workers, said John Knox, a spokesman for MedSolution, a Vancouver, B.C.-based company that brokers transactions between American patients and foreign hospitals. Surgeries are cheaper in Third World countries where salaries and litigation expenses are lower, Lindland said.

Service providers

There are several service providers; some of them are mentioned elsewhere. One website, www.mediescapes.com that aims to be an extensive resource for International patients needing affordable medical care in India at the same level one could expect from a "first-world" country service but with an third world prices tag!. The three main steps to complete successfully a treatment abroad are:

(a) Your medical insurance (private or governmental) or if any other, and be sure of having sufficient funds.
(b) Your medical travel itinerary.
(c) Your treatment procedure well explained itself.

Many major employers in the U.S. are self-insured, which means they pick up the tab for much of their employees' medical care. That's why three major corporations that collectively cover 240,000 lives asked Dr. Arnold Milstein, national health care "thought leader" at the consultancy Mercer

Health and Benefits, to assess the best places to outsource elective surgeries. Procedures in Thailand and Malaysia, he found, cost only 20% to 25% as much as comparable ones in the U.S.; top-notch Indian hospitals sell such services at an even steeper discount. The bottom line: If more private payers sent patients abroad for uncomplicated elective surgeries, the savings could be enormous. "This has the potential of doing to the U.S. health care system what the Japanese auto industry did to American carmakers," says Princeton University health care economist Uwe Reinhardt.

Employees who opt for India would get to take along a family member, says Darrell Douglas, vice president of human resources, and the whole experience, including a recuperative stay at a hotel, would be covered. IndUShealth, a medical tourism start-up in Raleigh, N.C., will make all arrangements and coordinate care between U.S. and Indian providers. The sweetener: the company will share with these intrepid employees up to 25% of savings garnered from the outsourcing.

Would people actually travel 10,000 miles for medical care just to make a few bucks? Polls commissioned by Milstein suggest that few consumers would opt for surgery abroad for incentives below $1,000. But raise the ante above $1,000, and the equation changes. Among people who have sick family members, about 45% of the underinsured or uninsured declare they would get on the plane; even 19% of those who have insurance say they're game. Above $5,000, the percentage of takers climbs to 61% and 40%, respectively.

Is the quality of care in foreign hospitals high enough? To cater to an international clientele, many private hospitals abroad are applying for accreditation (many of them successfully) from the Joint Commission International, the global arm of the institution that accredits most U.S. hospitals.

A corresponding boom is taking place among Western agencies that funnel patients to Asia. Eight have popped up in Canada, where national health care can mean a yearlong wait for elective surgery. In the U.S. several firms are aiming at the roughly 61 million people who are uninsured or underinsured. Planet Hospital's founder, "Rudy" Rupak Acharya, says his agency, which in the past seven months has sent some 200 patients abroad, got 11,000 inquiries in March alone. He has just retained Mercer to help him develop an insurance plan for the uninsured that will combine primary and emergency care in the U.S. with surgery abroad.

Patrick Marsek, managing director of the agency MedRetreat, says his company sent 200 people abroad last year and is already processing 320 this year. He is demanding a deposit of $195 from customers because people posing as patients have been looking for information to start up their own agencies.

Why would someone travel to India and not to Thailand?

The cost difference between treatment in India and Thailand is favourable to India. Also India offers what you call a language advantage—

a patient would surely prefer a country where English is widely spoken. Also, it is believed that the facilities in India are more suited for International patients.

How can you trust Indian Doctors?

Well, many highly qualified doctors have had some form of training from abroad, especially USA and UK. Indian surgeons and doctors are known for their skill and research throughout the world.

Why is India most suitable?

Indian corporate hospitals excel in cardiology and cardiothoracic surgery, joint replacement, orthopedic surgery, gastroenterology, ophthalmology, transplants and urology to name a few. The various specialties covered are Neurology, Neurosurgery, Oncology, Ophthalmology, Rheumatology, Endocrinology, ENT, Pediatrics, Pediatric Surgery, Pediatric Neurology, Urology, Nephrology, Dermatology, Dentistry, Plastic Surgery, Gynecology, Pulmonology, Psychiatry, General Medicine and General Surgery

The various facilities in India include full body pathology, comprehensive physical and gynecological examinations, dental checkup, eye checkup, diet consultation, audiometry, spirometry, stress and lifestyle management, pap smear, digital Chest X-ray, 12 lead ECG, 2D echo colour doppler, gold standard DXA bone densitometry, body fat analysis, coronary risk markers, cancer risk markers, carotid colour doppler, spiral CT scan and high strength MRI. Each test is carried out by professional M.D. physicians, and is comprehensive yet pain-free.

There is also a gamut of services ranging from General Radiography, Ultra Sonography, Mammography to high end services like Magnetic Resonance Imaging, Digital Subtraction Angiography along with intervention procedures, Nuclear Imaging. The diagnostic facilities offered in India are comprehensive to include Laboratory services, Imaging, Cardiology, Neurology and Pulmonology. The Laboratory services include biochemistry, hematology, microbiology, serology, histopathology, transfusion medicine and RIA.

All medical investigations are conducted on the latest, technologically advanced diagnostic equipment. Stringent quality assurance exercises ensure reliable and high quality test results.

CUTTING-EDGE VACATIONS

In the U.S. insurers negotiate discounts, but the uninsured pay retail rates for medical procedures. Here's how the prices of one surgical tourism agency compare. Its packages include airfare and hospital and hotel rooms, but costs can climb if there are complications.

Procedure	*U.S. Insurer's cost*	*U.S. Retail price*	*India/Thailand/Singapore*
Angioplasty	$25,704 to $37,128	$57,262 to $82,711	11000 13000 13000
Gastric bypass	$27,717 to $40,035	$47,988 to $69,316	11000 15000 15000
Heart bypass	$54,741 to $79,071	$122,424 to $176,835	10000 12000 20000
Heart-valve replacement (single)	$71,401 to $103,136	$159,326 to $230,138	9500 10500 13000
Hip replacement	$18,281 to $26,407	$43,780 to $63,238	9000 12000 12000
Hysterectomy	$9,591 to $13,854	$20,416 to $29,489	2900 4500
Knee replacement	$17,627 to $25,462	$40,640 to $58,702	8500 10000 13000
Mastectomy	$9,774 to $14,118	$23,709 to $34,246	7500 9000 12400
Spinal fusion	$25,302 to $36,547	$62,778 to $90,679	5500 7000 9000

SOME OTHER SERVICES

Tummy tuck

Tummy tuck or abdominoplasty surgery is a major surgical procedure that involves the abdominal area. The abdominal skin is trimmed and excess fat is removed. The stomach muscle is also tightened by stitching them together. The end result is a slimmer waistline. Being a major surgical operation, the recovery period can take anywhere from 6 to 12 months before you can enjoy the full benefits of a tummy tuck. A major surgery like a tummy tuck normally entails spending a few nights at the clinic or hospital so be prepared to fork out a bit more cash for a room. Once you have been discharged from the room or clinic, be prepared to budget for follow up visits to the tummy tuck specialist. The first few visits will be to remove the dressing and to check on the healing of the scar while monitoring your overall recovery progress. The doctor will also be prescribing you some medication to help you through the rest of your recovery.

Gynecology services and women's hospitals

Many hospitals have women check-up programs designed to detect the earliest signs of disorders of the breast and the organs of reproduction as well as catering to the contraceptive needs of women. A mammogram, an ultrasound of the pelvis and a pap-smear of the cervix are an integral part of any good medical check-up for women. Specialist medical as well as surgical care is available for all types of gynecological problems like menstrual abnormalities, prolapsed, fibroids and other tumors of the uterus and ovaries, tubal recanalization by microsurgery and care of the infertile couple. State-of-the-art gynecological surgery is available with world class equipment and expertise using minimally invasive techniques.

Abnormal Uterine Bleeding

Heavy or irregular bleeding can disrupt your life. Having to be constantly on guard with pads can distract you at work, an evening out with friends and worse still you may feel worn out. You may wonder if this is normal and if so what is causing this. Normal menstrual cycle ranges from 24-35 days length, with an average bleeding for 2-8 days. The menstrual cycle is governed by a hormone "Estrogen" in the first half of the cycle which helps the lining of the uterus to grow. Mid-cycle hormonal surge causes the ovary to usually release an egg, which triggers the 2nd hormone called Progesterone to act on and nature the endometrium. At the end of the cycle, the hormone levels drop when there is no pregnancy and the lining is shed with blood, which is called Menstruation.

Executive Health Check-up

It's designed for busy professionals on the go (okay, so I'm faking it a bit) and involves several hours of all sorts of tests, and a follow-up session a few days later. It starts at 8:30 a.m., after 12 hours of fasting. The reception area looks like hotel lobby, in fact the entire place is spic n' span, with lots of natural light, potted plants, marble floors and views of the gardens.

I quickly check-in and am introduced to Mr. Singh, the hospital traffic co-ordinator. He leads me from appointment to appointment; readjusting my schedule depending on line-ups to make sure wait time is minimal.

The near-painless blood-taking is followed by a glass of glucose and the handing over of a cute and discrete little bag containing my sample containers. Then, it's off for a chest X-ray. The room looks like every other X-ray room on the planet, sterile and steely. The gowns aren't exactly award-show great, but they cover all the essential bits with more flair than usual. The radiologist cheerfully chats about Toronto doctors he's worked with as he takes snaps of my inner being.

From there, Mr. Singh takes me to my electrocardiogram test in the garden-view diagnostic centre. As she wires me up, the nurse tells me it's International Women's Day and that I should do something special with my friends. She is going to the movies later with her pals. She also administers my pulmonary function test, and cheerleads as I huff and puff, encouraging me to greater windy heights than I thought possible.

Next door is my ultrasound. Another nice gown and clean, professional room. Again the doctor has colleagues in Canada, and we commiserate about the weather as she pokes and prods.

Mr. Singh takes my lunch order and then, in quick succession, I have my bone density tested, a post-glucose blood test, a treadmill test and a meeting with a G.P. The G.P. answers all my questions with patience—so much so that I start making up problems just to see if he'll kick me out, like my G.P. back home does. He doesn't, he just answers in a relaxed and friendly way, which is why I now know that toenails grow slower than fingernails (seems that circulation is poorer in the feet.) Time well spent, I think.

The same level of professional care holds through my next batch of appointments with the gynecologist, cardiologist, ophthalmologist and physiotherapist. Finally, a break for lunch, a nice light sandwich and juice that I eat in the garden.

Then, more appointments. The ear, nose and throat man discovers my deep (because it is several centimetres inside my head), dark (because, contrary to popular belief, there are no light bulbs in there) secret. Apparently I have slighted retracted eardrums. All the flying, probably. He prescribes some medicine, which I get for a few dollars at the hospital pharmacy. Then more tests. I barely spend any time in the waiting room, but what little I do, I end up next to a couple from Arizona who are on the same check-up circuit. They are more experienced, though.

Having been to India before, they also knew to stock up on cheap medicine, prescription glasses (she got two pairs, including prescription sunglasses, for $40 U.S.) and to see a dentist (he is contemplating nine teeth implants for $2,000 U.S.)

End result: Seven hours of tests, half a dozen doctor appointments, a personalized diet plan, all my charts and scans to take back home, a nice lunch and a couple of slightly retracted eardrums. Total cost: $100 (U.S.) Sitaram Bhartia, an excellent non-profit research institute, is a favourite of Indian politicians and bureaucrats, but is less well known to tourists.

Talks and views

Niraj Sharan: In Australia, medical tourism is a new concept. We are tying up with our hospital chains in India.

Stan Correy: And the Indians have done their research on what may attract Australians to medical tourism.

Niraj Sharan: Yes, especially the dental surgery—no doubt there's a lot of opportunities, especially as it's not covered under the insurance policy overseas, and in comparison to costs overseas it's very cheap in India.

Stan Correy: There's been a plethora of Australian media stories in recent weeks about long waiting lists in our public hospitals, higher fees in private hospitals and not enough dentists. So will the Indian corporate hospitals find a lucrative market? "In certain cases, it would make economic sense if you wanted to have a holiday and combine it, say, with having your teeth done." And with the money you save, you can pay for a little holiday afterwards. Dentistry is now a major cost for families, and most of the private insurance programs restrict you to a number of visits or a number of procedures per year.

Stan Correy: Poland and Hungary offer special cheap dental tours to other Europeans. India, Thailand, South Africa and the Caribbean also offer the joys of being an 'orthodontal tourist'.

Ian Crombie: So I got out there, met at the airport, VIP treatment, taken to a private hospital in Chennai, which is the modern name for Madras. I had a suite, which was a room with an en suite bath, choice of menu, daily newspapers, and it was like staying in a resort hotel. I got to meet Dr. Reddy; he is the founder of the Apollo Hospital Group, and he wanted to know how I'd been treated, whether I was satisfied and all that, and he took a great sort of interest. And there were other expats there at the same time, having hip replacements. There was a Kuwaiti having something done to his spine, etc. the anaesthetist was British trained, the cardiologist was British trained, and of course Dr. Vijay himself was British trained. So based on that, I thought, Why the hell not? I mean there is nothing the Apollo Group doesn't do. "The anaesthetist was British trained, the cardiologist was British trained, and of course Dr. Vijay himself was British trained. So based on that, I thought, Why the hell not?" In other words, I want competent people. It turned out.

Stan Correy: Ian Crombie didn't feel lonely as he waited for surgery. There were several other non-Indian medical tourists.

Pauline Gately: Trade in services itself is not an area that's well understood, and part of the reason it's not well defined or understood, it's not like trade in other commodities. Part of the reason also that health services and health expenditure has risen is because of course of rising incomes, demographic changes, ageing populations. And the development and diffusion and uptake of new drugs and new technologies.

Stan Correy: Countries like Australia have been slower than other parts of the world to build themselves up for the potential business opportunities. As well, there's a general suspicion of Australians going to other countries for medical treatment.

Aadiyta Mattoo: if you were able to buy these services from other countries, it's not difficult to see that the ability to buy a service more cheaply outside your country than in your own country, can make you better off.

Stan Correy: In the Gulf State of Dubai they've built a luxurious

Health Care city. Western health care corporations such as the Mayo Clinic, and Harvard Medical International are falling over themselves to get into this medical city.

Stan Correy: That health conference in Dubai took place last week. Dean of Surgery at the University of Sydney is Professor Andrew Coats. He's recently returned from the Middle East where he visited Dubai Health Care City.

Andrew Coats: I think what we're seeing is very much part of the development of the Middle East; Dubai is a prime example, where we're seeing an area staking a place in the marketplace say for high quality area within the Middle East where people can get First World quality, hotels, resources, infrastructure, and health is a very major aspect of that. They have traditionally gone to the UK or the US, and the people in Dubai believe that if you set-up First World quality health care in Dubai, people will travel from the adjacent Middle East, and I think that's probably a fairly safe bet.

Stan Correy: So in a sense, it's not only what's happening in India or Asia, that kind of centre, or medical city, is also driving the competition in this medical area.

Andrew Coats: Yes. For some countries it will be good quality health care at low cost, in other countries it will be the highest quality health care at a higher cost, and others will offer a geographical advantage, and that's where Dubai might fit in where they can say, We can offer you a US, UK, Australian quality health care, but you don't have to fly eight to twelve hours to get there.

Derek Morgan: This is probably what we're now seeing as the development of a second wave in terms of medical tourism.

Stan Correy: The second global wave of medical tourism is creating new players, new companies, that are not health specialists, but facilitators, brokers between the international patient and the hospital networks.

Derek Morgan: There are two forces I think, that are external to the health care market, which are really contributing to this. The first I mentioned earlier on, is the relative decline of the cost of air travel across the world. And the second is the rise of the internet. "The internet enables increasingly knowledge-rich patients to seek out service providers, to make comparisons for themselves, or for specialist firms to grow up in order to broker patients and specialist services."

Stan Correy: Medical insurance and medical broking are not the same thing. A medical broker is someone who operates as a middleman who, for a fee, will act as a go-between to find the best deal for your personal needs. Medical insurance is self explanatory, but there are very few medical insurers who will let you take your insurance cover to another country.

Leslie Smith: We then found individuals calling us, asking us for help, saying that they were on an NHS, National Health Service waiting list, couldn't get surgery and were suffering considerable pain levels.

Stan Correy: India is becoming a popular destination for Americans, and there are 47-million poor Americans who have no medical insurance at all, and who might simply die because they can't pay for treatment.

Bob Couch: And you know, you've got to remember we're retired. I mean I'm 81 you know. We're not broke, but these are big sums of money to take out of the bank, because we haven't got the income, we're just living on our savings all the time.

Stan Correy: Before his operation he had to fill in a questionnaire regarding his medical history and the normal documents that patients sign before surgery.

Leslie Smith: I'm particularly concerned always with hundreds and hundreds of patients, you're going to get things go wrong because they're under the surgical knife and anesthesia. So things will go wrong, and I just want to make sure the patients are fairly treated, they can sue properly in the appropriate country, they can be reimbursed, they can be brought home.

Stan Correy: How do you come under as a financial company?

Leslie Smith: No, we're still under the insurance regulator here for our insurance advice. But so far, the industry of facilitating patients to other hospitals around the world, without giving medical advice, there's no regulator for that as far as I'm aware in Europe at this time. I think there will be in the future.

Stan Correy: Acting as a broker for international patients is in its early days, and Leslie Smith admits that there are large regulatory issues involved. Many countries don't have the protective legal systems westerners are used to.

Derek Morgan: You've identified a difficult issue within this whole sort of boutique market that's now developing. What is the legal status? we don't really know. We're not entirely sure. Complications do arise in any potential operation that is undertaken. You can't guarantee that health care and the sequelae to operations are always going to run smoothly, there will always be issues about problems that arise. And how one deals with those on a patient who, let's say, has made a contract with a company or a broker in London to travel to Johannesburg for surgery, to travel on to another country for recuperative holiday and such like, and something goes wrong in the operation itself, trying to resolve these legal issues really is going to become a quite fundamental issue over the next 10 or 15 years. And of course it's going to differ from jurisdiction to jurisdiction. It may even differ from where the patient comes from.

Stan Correy: You can have a hip replacement in India, or heart surgery in Dubai, or dental work in Malaysia, but you may find it hard to get insurance, or a legal comeback if you're badly treated.

Leslie Smith: The interesting thing about Singapore and in Thailand, is the involvement of state government, where they're investing millions of dollars in state-of-the-art hospitals, recognizing that the kind of health tourism from Australasia or Japan is hard currency, which is dollars. "They have all the skills there, they have huge numbers of nurses and they can do this just as good as the westerners, if not better."

Stan Correy: So let's hitch a ride on one of those big white aeroplanes, full of medical tourists from UK, Canada and the US, refugees from overstretched and expensive health care systems. Waiting with open arms and beds are a whole chain of new Indian health care corporations. The Escorts Group, Fortis Health Care, Max Health Care, Wockhardt, and the largest, the Apollo Group, which is the most aggressive in promoting its business abroad. They're also lobbying the Indian government to make India more attractive for medical tourism.

Sangita Reddy: I think in any other sector some things can wait, it's not as critical. But health care is life. And also we come from a culture of people expecting the government to provide health care, as we transition from a country where the private sector is playing such an important role. It's important for the private sector and the public to work together and try and give more efficient solutions, reach people quicker, extend our reach, and there are many examples of win-win solutions when we work together.

Stan Correy: Indian corporate hospitals say business is good and they offer world class treatment. But there are critics who see medical tourism as a sick concept. In India, NGOs say the reason we're hearing so much about medical tourism is that too much money is being spent on building expensive hospitals, and that the vast majority of ordinary Indians can't afford them.

Ravi Duggall: Without regulated health care market insurance will find it very difficult to operate because the younger people are not insuring themselves. So you have a very small, about 2%, of the population which seeks this kind of voluntary insurance, and the private sector has stayed away, the study that they did, the private insurance companies said they've gone into life insurance or other general insurance, but they have stayed away from health because they realise that the people who are insuring themselves are high risk people. So that would have been a good base for many of these elite hospitals to fill up their vacant occupancies. But that has somehow not worked. So the other option is now looking to developed countries to cater to their over-supply of patients which they can't handle.

Stan Correy: Apollo and other Indian hospital corporations have recently asked the Indian government to relax foreign investment guidelines to allow international health insurance companies to set-up in India. But insurance companies demand better government regulation of health care. In India, the only accreditation these relatively new groups have isn't by any health authority. Apollo, for example, is accredited by Crisil, an Indian financial and credit rating company which isn't really the same thing.

Ashok Ananthram: if you look at the Apollo Group, we are touching 60,000 cardiac surgeries to date. At a success rate of well past 95%, 98%. Now JCI et cetera is a tangible proof of the fact that the systems, your processes, your entire hygiene, perhaps the quality of blood, et cetera is at international levels. I think we need to get international accreditation to be counted amongst the world's best.

Stan Correy: And after you had the operation, what was the experience like then?

Ian Crombie: I spent a couple of weeks in Chennai. In the Taj Hotel, where I came across Warnie and Gilchrist and all the other lot about to play the second Test Match down there, and we had a great time. And during that time that I was in the hotel, every day they sent over a nurse to make sure the dressing, the stitches were OK. They also sent a physio across every day to make sure I was doing my exercises. I mean, you couldn't have asked for better care.

Stan Correy: In the Bloomberg's article, it says you paid a total of 5,000 pounds for the trip.

Ian Crombie: By the time I would have paid for my air fare, plus my hotel stay, yes, it would have come out at about 5,000 pounds.

Stan Correy: Outsourcing of IT has already given the Indian economy a huge boost, and it's no secret that India has turned around from being one of the poor countries of the world to an emerging economic power. There's talk of Indian medical care being worth billions of dollars.

Guy Ellena: I don't believe that they've established management of hospitals in such a strong way, that they can guarantee consistent quality of health care, a consistent quality of services around health care. They have fantastic doctors, no doubt, I mean OK a lot of them being trained either in India, but also trained in the US, in the UK, in Australia, and different countries, if something was to happen, or people started to be dissatisfied, because, if big numbers were really to flock into India I think the system would be very much stressed.

Stan Correy: He's concerned that the Indian health care corporations may be over-hyping the market for medical tourists.

Guy Ellena: the private sector is not going to address the needs of the entire population, because they have private hospitals, they need to generate profits, if not OK they would close the doors. Clearly they need to sell their services to a population that can pay.

Stan Correy: Ellena's more critical perspective on the profits to be made from medical tourism comes from first-hand experience.

Guy Ellena: I'm traveling all around the world. We are financing hospitals in Latin America, in Central Europe, in Russia, in East Asia, Africa, all over the world. They all believe that they have a comparative advantage. There have been, up to 9/11, it's true, a trend where wealthy patients from the Middle East felt reluctant, or a difficulty, to be treated in the US because of getting a visa, or they didn't feel comfortable to go, and they have moved back to other places where is easier. Europe, and/or to some extent the subcontinent or Thailand. But still these are very, very small numbers.

Stan Correy: Once a trend and hype bubble gets rolling in the global economy, it's hard to stop. Everyone wants to be a health care hub. The surgery itself, it seems, is first class in the best places. And it's much cheaper than what you pay in the UK, the USA and Australia. But it's not only all about providing better health care. It's about business and commerce and trade.

Debra Lipson: Our members, along with thousands of unrepresented workers, are now being confronted with proposals to literally export themselves to have certain "expensive" medical procedures provided in India. When you're there, you give up your legal rights that you have here. You can't sue if there's malpractice. Who would send their 7-year-old child or their 80-year-old grandmother to a foreign country for surgery and you couldn't do anything if something goes wrong? Exacerbating this crisis by attempting to outsource health care is not only shameless; it does nothing to solve the nation's skyrocketing health care costs.

So America is also aware of its shortcomings and wants to improve its health care. If it does it may have impact the medical tourism plans of countries across the globe.

APPENDIX

BUMRUNGRAD HOSPITAL (BANGKOK, THAILAND)

Since its inception, this hospital has achieved a high status based upon its quality operations.

Milestones

• Opened 200-bed facility	September 17, 1980
• Listed on the Stock Exchange of Thailand:	1989
• Expanded facility commissioned:	January 1, 1997
• Joint Commission International Accreditation: Reaccredited	February 2002; April 2005
• Joint Commission International:	October 2006
• Disease or Condition-Specific Care Certifications	October 2006

Mission

The hospital has a loudable objective of serving patients. The hospital has its mission to provide world class health care with care and compassion.

Ownership

Burmrungrad Hospital (BH) is a Government Hospital run as a public company traded on the Stock Exchange of Thailand. The majority shareholders are Bangkok Insurance Public Company Limited and the Sophonpanich family, one of Thailand's most respected business families. The company form of organisation provides flexibility and autonomy to the hospital and the day-to-day interference of the Government is avoided. The hospital is running efficiently in a company form. There is a new set-up that our Indian hospitals at territory level should be run in company or corporation form to avoid day to day political interference and promote efficiency.

Patients are considered the VIPs and they are the main focus of hospital authorities. The mission is put in practice and is not merely a decorative piece.

The hospital is progressing fast. It expands its area of operation frequently. For example in 1997, it promoted the following additional facilities.

Facility (Opened 1997)

- Largest private hospital in South East Asia
- One million square feet

- 12 stories plus basement parking
- Fully licensed medical heliport
- US Hospital (NFPA) building/fire standards
- Hospital 2000 information system
- Hospital wide wi-fi network coverage

Patient Volumes and Revenues

- The result of efficient running of hospital can be seen in the increase of patients and revenue.
- Over 1.2 million patients treated per year (outpatient and inpatient).
- Over 430,000 are international patients from over 190 different countries.
- US$ 220 million turnover in 2006.

The success and failure of any organisation depends upon the quality of personnel especially at its top level. The hospital is very careful in the selection of medical experts to meet the needs of the patients. It has been rightly said that human rather than capital is the key to development. The hospital is staffed with the following human resources:

- American-led international management team.
- Over 3,000 employees.
- Over 900 physicians and dentists, most with international training/certification.

The hospital has inpatient capacities and outpatient facilities of high quality.

- 554 Inpatient Beds
  - 500 Medical/Surgical/OB/Pediatrics
  - 26 Adult Intensive Care
  - 14 Cardiac Care (CCU)
  - 9 Pediatric Intensive Care
  - 5 Level III Neonatal Intensive Care
- 57 Deluxe rooms, 21 VIP Suites and 2 Royal Suites.

Outpatient Facilities

- 135 examination suites
- Capacity 3,500 OPD patients per day
- Ambulance and mobile critical care fleet
- Outpatient Surgery Center
- 24-hour emergency care including emergency cardiac catheterization.

Outpatient Centers

- Allergy Center
- Eye and ENT Center
- Plastic Surgery Center
- Aviation Medicine Center
- Eye Laser Refraction Center
- Pulmonary Physiology Center
- Behavioural Health Center
- Fertility Center
- Radiology Center
- Breast Screening Center
- Health Screening Center
- Rehabilitation Center
- Children Center
- Heart Center
- Skin Center
- Dental Center
- Horizon Regional Cancer Center
- Skin Laser Center
- Diabetes Center
- Medical Center
- Sleep Disorder Center
- Dialysis Center
- Neurology Center
- Stroke Center
- Digestive Disease Center
- Orthopedic Center
- Surgical Center
- Early Intervention Center
- Pathology Center
- Urology Center
- Emergency Center
- Physiotherapy Center
- Women's Center
- Endoscopic Center

Special Facilities

- 2 Cardiac Catheterization Laboratories
- 2 Cardiac Operating Theaters
- 19 Operating Theaters
- Interventional Radiology
- MRI, CT and Lithotripsy
- Neonatal Critical Care Transport
- Nuclear Medicine

- Radiation Therapy (Linear Accelerator)
- PACS Radiology
- Vital Life Wellness Center
- 64-slice CT Scanner
- Surgical Navigation System

International Representative Offices

Australia, Bangladesh, Cambodia, Canada, Ethiopia, Hong Kong, Indonesia, Macau, Mongolia, Myanmar, Nepal, Netherlands, Nigeria, Oman, Seychelles, Sri Lanka, Sweden, Taiwan, Vietnam, Uganda, Ukraine.

Special Interracial Services

- International Patient Center: interpreters, international/airport concierge service, embassy assistance, VIP airport transfers, e-mail correspondence, international insurance coordination and international medical coordinators, vise extension counter, Diet helm Travel Thailand counter, airline ticket counter, prayer room.
- Bumrungrad Hospitality Residence: 74 fully serviced apartments connected to the hospital
- Bumrungrad Hospitality Suites: 51 fully serviced apartments with pool and fitness facilities.

Quality and Certification

- The first private hospital awarded Thailand Hospital Accreditation.
- Asia's first hospital accredited by the US-based Joint Commission International (JCI); the first hospital in Asia to be reaccredited.
- First hospital outside the US to receive two JCI Disease or Condition-Specific Care Certifications (Primary stroke Programe and Acute Myocardial Infection with ST Segment Elevation (STEMI) Program.
- Awarded the Best Small Cap Company by Asia Money's 2003 Survey.
- Internationally Certified Laboratory

Social Responsibility

Established in 1990, Bumrungrad Hospital Foundation is dedicated to helping the underprivileged in Thailand access free health care services. The Foundation has provided over 100,000 Thais with free medical services ranging from check-up programs to heart surgery for children.

HEALTH SCREENING CENTRE

Keeping your health in check

The hospital has developed an innovative centre which can prevent major risks. It is rarely available in any hospital. We, in India, should follow this and set-up health screening centre.

Prevention is the best medicine and annual health screenings are key to your well-being. Often the early stages of diseases present no symptoms, or the symptoms may be so mild that they go unnoticed. The earlier a problem is detected, the more effectively it can be treated.

Preparing for your Visit

General Instructions

- Do not eat or drink anything except plain water for at least 9 hours prior to check up in case of Upper GI X-ray, please keep fasting.
- Please bring along your ID card or passport and arrive 10 minutes before the scheduled appointment time.
- Stool and urine samples will be collected on the day of examination.
- If you have a pre-existing medical condition, please bring along any test results or reports you have for the doctor to review.

If you schedule a stress test

- Please bring your jogging shoes.
- If you need to eat before the stress test, then eat a light snack only and avoid fatty foods, caffeine, and alcohol.
- If you are under treatment or taking medication for any medical or physical condition, please notify the nurse in advance.
- If you are suffering any chest pain or breathing difficulty, please notify the nurse in advance.

Instruction for abdominal ultrasound

Drink plenty of water before the ultrasound exam. The test requires a full bladder for best results. Do not void prior to the ultrasound examination.

Payment

Pre-payment is required for all check up programs.

Location

The Health Screening Center is located on the 11th floor of Bumrungrad International Clinic.

Hours of operation

07:00-15:00 hrs everyday.

Appointments

Please make your appointment at least 3 days in advance.
To make or change an appointment:
Tel: 66(0)2667 1555 Fax:+66 (0) 2667 295
Online appointment:www.bumrungrad.com

BONES AND JOINT CENTRE

Some of life's greatest pleasures are simple things—a walk along the beach, a round of golf with friends or a good night's sleep. But the simple pleasures we often take for granted remain out of reach for people living with painful, debilitating bone and torturous joint problems.

Longer life expectancies have made joint pain—especially in the knees and hips—a growing problem in Thailand and around the world. Serious bone-related conditions, whether caused by aging, injury, or diseased like arthritis and osteoarthritis, can quickly wreak havoc on one's ability to do normal daily activities and enjoy a decent quality of life.

In the past, treating serious bone and joint conditions often required traumatic and complex major surgery, with up to a full year of recovery time, and frequently left significant scarring.

What a difference a few years has made! Advances in medical technology and techniques have revolutionized technology and techniques have revolutionized the treatment of bone and joint problems. Joint replacement is a prime example of these exciting changes. To learn more, Better Health spoke to Dr. Sitthiporn Orpain, an orthopedic surgeon specializing in joint replacement.

The sources of joint pain

Joints are where two bones are joined by connective tissue called cartilage. Cartilage acts as a protective cushion to allow the joint to support body weight and move comfortably. But when the cartilage is damaged by disease, infection, wear-and-tear or injury, the result is often painful inflammation, stiffness and reduced mobility.

"While there are many causes of joint pain," explained Dr. Sitthiporn, "Osteoarthritis and other degenerative joint diseases are among the most common. These conditions cause a break-down in the cartilage that affects the normal workings of the joint. As the cartilage wears away, the two bones rub against each other, causing great pain.

Aging is a key risk factor for developing osteoarthritis, especially after the age of 50. Obesity, a family history of osteoarthritis and being in overall poor health also increase one's risk.

"The first symptoms people usually notice are pain, stiffness, and reduced flexibility of a joint," Dr. Sitthiporn noted. "The area around the joint may become swollen as an unusual fluid builds up, and that can

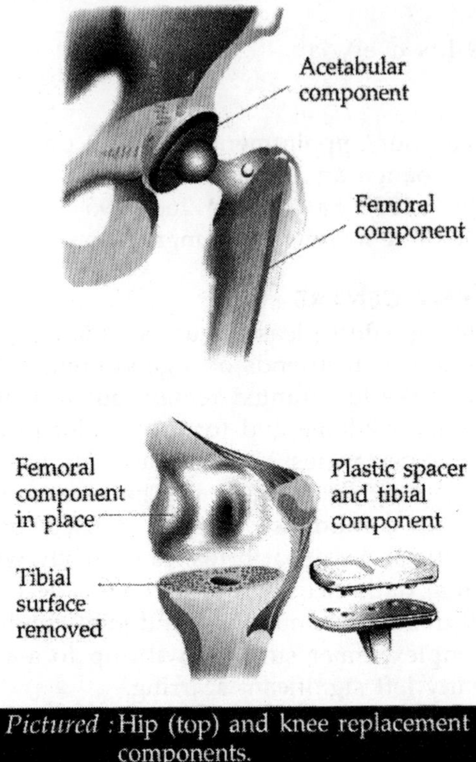

Pictured : Hip (top) and knee replacement components.

worsen the pain, each time weight is exerted on the joint," Osteorathritis is a progressive disease whose symptoms and severity worsen over time, so early detection is very important to successful treatment.

Rheumatioid arthritis also leads to serious joint damage. This condition causes chronic inflammation of the joint that results in pain, stiffness, and swelling. "The repeated inflammation causes damage to the bone and cartilage," Dr. Sitthiporn added. "While joint pain and stiffness caused by osteoarthritis usually affect one knee or one hip, the pain and stiffness from rheumatoid arthritis tends to affect both hips or both knees at the same time."

Diagnosis and Treatment

To diagnose the cause of joint pain, your doctor will usually begin with a through physical examination and ask about your medical and family histories. Specialized tests, such as a biopsy, X-rays, MRI scans, and arthroscopy help confirm the diagnosis and determine the severity of the condition. Blood tests are sometimes used to check for the presence of rheumatoid arthritis of infection.

Patients diagnosed with mild to moderate osteoarthritis can usually be treated without surgery. Doctors may recommend a combination of options including.

- Weight reduction for overweight or obese patients
- Rest or activity modification
- Medication to relieve pain and inflammation
- Physiotherapy
- Using a brace or walking aid.

The Joint Replacement Revolution

More serious cases may require the complete replacement of the damaged joint. As Dr. Sitthiporn explained, "For many people, joint problems become so severe to the point where the patient suffers a serious decline in quality of life. In many of these cases, a good option is to replace the damaged knee or hip with an artificial joint."

Ten years ago, the idea of replacing a real hip or knee joint with an artificial one may have seemed quite radical. Today, joint replacement is among the most successful treatments for serious joint conditions; it has already brought great relief to thousands of long-suffering patients. Here's detailed look at the knee and hip replacement procedures.

Knee Replacement

The knee joint is formed where the lower part of the thighbone (femur) connects with the upper part of the shinbone (tibia) and the kneecap (patella). Shock-absorbing cartilage covers the surfaces of these bones.

During a typical knee replacement surgery, the damaged areas of the thighbone, shinbone and kneecap are first removed. The surgeon then smoothes and reshapes the ends of the remaining bones to ensure an optimal fit of the artificial knee components.

Major knee surgery used to require long hospital stays and up to a year of recovery time. That's no longer the case, as Dr. Sitthiporn explained: "knee replacement usually requires 4-7 days in the hospital. The recovery period depends on a patient's general health, age, and other factors, but many patients resume their normal activities within three months."

Once the knee has sufficiently healed, patients are often advised to incorporate a comprehensive exercise programme into their daily routine. Low-impact activities like swimming and walking are highly recommended, as they can help improve blood circulation, endurance, flexibility and muscle strength, without putting too much pressure on the knees.

Hip Replacement

The hip is a large "ball-and-socket" joint that bears much of the body's weight and movements. The ball of the joint at the top of the thighbone (femoral head) moves within the hollow socket (acetabulum) of the pelvis. A layer of cartilage allows the ball to glide smoothly inside the socket.

During the total hip replacement procedure, the surgeon removes the ball part of the joint and replaces it with a prosthetic ball. The ball is attached to a stem that fits into the hollowed-out space in the thighbone. Damaged cartilage and bone are removed from the socket, and a cup-like component is inserted in its place.

Hip replacement surgery has rapidly become a leading choice for treating severe hip problems, with shorter hospital stays and faster recovery times compared to traditional hip surgery.

Younger patients with less-serious hip problems are also benefiting from major advances in technology and techniques through a procedure called hip resurfacing. According to Dr. Sitthiporn, "Hip resurfacing is a less-invasive, bone-conserving surgical technique that has already allowed thousands of people in their 40s and 50s to resume active lives and delay or eliminate the need for total hip replacement.

Unlike the prosthesis used in total hip replacement, the resurfacing prosthesis allows the head to be preserved and reshaped. The resurfaced bone is then capped with a metal prosthesis. As with total hip replacement, the socket is fitted with a prosthesis.

Is joint replacement right for me?

As people pursue active lifestyles well into their 60s, 70s and 80s, joints need to stay strong and healthy. But the added years means more wear-and-tear on knees and hips, and increased risk of serious disease and injury.

Joint replacement surgery has established an impressive record for safety and successful post-treatment results, eliminating pain and restoring mobility in patients who don't respond to other treatments. All medical procedures, including joint replacement and resurfacing, involve some level of risk and may not be suitable for every patient. Your doctor will explain the treatment options and recommend the best course of treatment for your individual situation.

"It's important for patients to have realistic expectations about joint replacement surgery," said Dr. Sitthiporn. "While most patients are able to resume most normal activities without pain, it won't enable them to run a marathon! Not all patients are good candidates; for example, people who are obese may have to be excluded."

Exercise and Healthy Joints

The right exercise is essential for keeping bones and joints healthy. Even for people being treated for joint problems, regular exercise can still help reduce joint pain and stiffness. Be sure to consult your doctor before starting any exercise program.

It's best to choose non-weight bearing, low-impact exercises like walking or swimming as they are safer for joints compared to more vigorous high-impact exercises such as jogging.

Stretch: Warm up by gently stretching the muscles in the front of the thigh (quardriceps), the side of the thigh, and the back of the thigh (hamstrings); stretching reduces pressure on the knees and hips that occurs during exercise.

Strengthen: Strengthening exercise increase muscles strength, a key to supporting bones and joints.

Swimming is an ideal exercise for those with arthritis as it can increase mobility and build muscle strength. An unlike exercise on dry land, the water helps reduce the amount of stress on the body's hips, knees and spine.

You don't have to be a fitness fanatic or "gym rat" to reap the benefits of regular exercise. Look for opportunities in your daily routine to add some exercise and increase your level of activity. Take the stairs instead of the elevator, or try a nightly after-dinner walk with your family. Your bones and joints will be glad you made the effort.

Minimally-invasive: Less trauma, faster recovery

Dramatic advancements have been made in recent years in the effectiveness and durability of prosthetic replacement joints thanks to better design, materials and production methods. At the same time, similar advances have come in the way of new and improved surgical techniques that require smaller incisions and causes less trauma to surrounding areas.

"The minimal-incision surgery technique minimizes trauma to muscles, tissue and tendons and results in less bleeding during surgery," explained Dr. Sitthiporn, "Patients typically experience less pain after surgery, so they can be up and walking around sooner, and their hospital stay is usually shorter as well.

IMAGE GUIDED NAVIGATION SYSTEM—POINTS THE WAY TO HIGH-TECH SURGERY SUCCESS

Joint replacement surgery has quickly become one of the most popular and successful treatment options for patients with serious joint and bone conditions. A successful joint replacement operation depends on several factors, most notably the precise and accurate alignment of the joint component. Accurate alignment during surgery is critical to a patient's future mobility, and its helps maximize the longevity of the prosthetic components. A new generation of image-guided navigation systems like the one in use at Bumrungrad is giving surgeon a powerful tool to perform many successful procedures including joint replacement.

Real time 3-D positioning

Image-guide navigation systems for surgery operate in a similar way to the latest navigation systems for cars and ships that help pinpoint the driver or captain's precise location and guide them on their journey. The system provides surgeons with clear and detailed images and positioning calculations, in 'real-time' on a computer screen, giving the surgeon a clear view of the area where the operation is being performed.

Computer navigation gives the surgeon visual information on the precise positioning during a surgical procedure, including joint replacement surgery which is performed using smaller incisions. As a result, the minimally invasive procedure can be highly reliable and accurate.

During a joint replacement procedure, the surgeon first places temporary markers on and around the joint bones at the positions that have been located using the system's infrared camera. Next, the system tracks the position of each marker while the surgeon guides the joint through a variety of motions. The computer processes the data and generates a highly detailed 3-dimensional image of the joint.

A complement of the minimally-invasive surgery

This new technology is a perfect complement to minimally-invasive surgical procedures, that give patients an easier and faster recovery. Traditional surgery usually involves large incision that cut through muscles tissue and cause a lot of bleeding during surgery. On the other hand, minimally-invasive surgery uses small punctures in the skin to perform the surgery. Lesser trauma to the surrounding tissue means less post-operative pain, quicker restoration of mobility, and shorter hospital stays. Patients can now look forward to a much faster return to their normal lifestyle.

FIRST IN ASIA: SWISSLOG PHARMACY ROBOT—NOW SERVING BUMRUNGRAD PATIENTS

The pharmacy of the future has arrived in Asia. Bumrungrad International recently introduced the region's first 'Pharmacy Robot'—a fully-automated drug management system being used by many leading medical centers around the world.

The accuracy of the system is one of its unique strengths. The traditional system of preparing and dispensing medications in hospitals is inherently complex; there can be more than 100 steps from the time a prescription is written to the time a patient receives the medication. Technology reduces errors by reducing complexity, avoiding over-reliance on memory, simplifying critical processes, and increasing efficiency. The system will allow highly-trained pharmacists and technicians to spend less time on routine tasks, and more time on patient care.

Automated packaging and dispensing systems for filling patient orders are becoming common in US hospitals as a result of increased public knowledge about medication crrors. Bar coding helps reduce medication errors during dispensing and administration. A unit-dose drug is created when a single drug is taken from its bulk container and put into a labeled package. Bar coding of unit doses allows nurses to easily verify that the right dose of the right drug is being given to the right patient at the right time.

The automated robot system will help Bumrungrad care for the more than 1 million patients from 190 different countries who come to the hospital each year. "The automated drug management system is part of the hospital's continuing commitment to patient safety," explained Dr. Karoon Mekanontchai, Bumrungrad's Medical Director. "The system should increase patients' confidence in the hospital's quality."

HEPATITIS PREVENTION

The hepatitis B virus has been around for generations, but it receives relatively little attention from the media or from the public at large. Most people are unaware that they're infected, and the serious, sometimes deadly consequences can take decades to appear. But make no mistake, hepatitis B has quietly become a major health threat to millions of people in Thailand, and millions more throughout Asia and around the world.

The ABCs of Hepatitis

The word hepatitis means inflammation of the liver, which is usually caused by a viral infection. There are many types of hepatitis (A, B, C, D, and D). While hepatitis A is the most prevalent, it goes away on its own and does not lead to long term liver damage. Hepatitis B has far more serious consequences, including liver scarring, cirrhosis of the liver, and liver cancer. It can also be fatal.

It's estimated that more than 350 million people around the world have been infected with the hepatitis B virus, and nearly 75% of them are Asian. Thailand has one of the highest rates of infection; nine million Thais have the HBV virus.

To gain a better understanding of this serious threat, Better Health spoke with Dr. Virasak Wongpaitoon, M.D., a gastroenterologist and hepatologist with many years' experience treating patients infected with hepatitis.

How does infection occur?

The hepatitis B virus is transmitted through three main routes; unprotected sexual contact, exposure to blood or bodily fluids such as semen or vaginal secretions of a person who carries the virus, and 'vertical' transmission from mother-to-child during childbirth. Most patients diagnosed with chronic hepatitis B as adults became infected during infancy or childhood. In addition to the risk of mother-to-child infection during childbirth, Dr. Virasak noted that children are at higher risk due to normal activities and surrounding. "There is a high incidence of hepatitis B infection in places with lots of children," he explained. "At school or on the playground, children play together, and it's common that they scrape or cut themselves and expose an open wound. Because children's immune systems are still developing, they're more vulnerable to infection. "Many children's immune systems are strong enough to completely kill the virus. In others, most of the virus is killed off, but they still carry the virus and can infect others. In serious cases, the HBV virus proves too strong for the immune system, and symptoms of chronic hepatitis B will eventually become apparent during adulthood (usually between the ages of 20 and 40).

Dr. Virasak stressed one of the most dangerous aspects of the HBV virus; Most people don't realize they've been infected. "Infection typically produces no symptoms at all, or only mild symptoms such as a fever or aches and pains that go away within a few days", he explained. "There is a high prevalence of hepatitis B in Thai people because there are few symptoms at the time of infection. As a result, patients don't seek medical treatment, the disease continues to progress, and they can spread the virus to others."

The dangers of Hepatitis B

- More than 9 million Thais—and nearly 300 million people across Asia—carry the hepatitis B virus (HBV).
- Most people don't know they're infected, and they can spread the virus to many others.
- Infants and children are at the greatest risk of infection.
- Chronic hepatitis B can lead to serious, potentially fatal liver problems including cirrhosis, liver cancer and liver failure.

Infant and Childhood Dangers

In the majority of infections that occur during adulthood (termed 'acute'), the body's strong immune system is able to produce antibodies that completely kill off the HBV virus within a few months after infections. These antibodies provide lifetime protection against becoming re-infected. Patients who are unable to kill off the virus within six months face the future health threats of 'chronic' hepatitis such as cirrhosis and liver cancer. And as HBV carriers they can pass the infection on to others.

When infection occurs during infancy or childhood, the hepatitis B virus is much more threatening. With few or no symptoms at the time of infection, it's often years before an infected child has a blood test for hepatitis B. That's more than enough time during the critical years before the immune system has fully developed for the HBV virus to multiply and progress to the point of inflicting serious liver damage—usually without any noticeable signs or symptoms of the disease.

Vaccination and Prevention

Despite its serious nature, hepatitis B can be easily prevented through vaccination, regular medical check-ups, and avoiding the risk factors for transmitting the virus.

The vaccine against hepatitis B has proven highly effective in offering a lifetime of protection against the virus. These days, most newborns receive the vaccine soon after birth.

Avoiding the major risk factors for transmission of the virus is critical to reducing the rate of HBV infection. In addition to practicing safer sex, "if you haven't been tested for the virus." Dr. Virasak advised, "or if you haven't been vaccinated, talk to your doctor. And don't share personal items such as razor blades and toothbrushes."

If You Think You Are Infected...

For patients who worry that they may be infected with the HBV virus, a simple blood test is used to check for the presence of the virus in the bloodstream. If the virus is detected, additional test may be recommended to check for the presence of antibodies, and your doctor may also prescribe a liver function test and ultrasound examination to determine the extent of any damage to the liver.

Recently-infected patients (i.e. those with acute hepatitis B) require a lot of rest until any symptoms go away. Among patients diagnose with chronic hepatitis B, those who show no symptoms and have normal liver function usually don't require medication. Some patients with chronic hepatitis B may need medication that can effectively reduce or completely eliminate the HBV virus. Your doctor will set-up a schedule for regular check-ups and monitoring of the disease's progression to ensure earlier detection of potential problems including cirrhosis, scarring and cancer.

To lessen the risk of future health problems, Dr. Virasak recommends that all patients with HBV "should consult their doctor before taking any medication, abstain from drinking alcohol, get regular medical check-ups, and lead a healthy lifestyle. That means reducing stress, practicing good nutrition and exercise habits, and avoiding the risk factor that can spread the virus to others."

STEM CELL TREATMENT

Stem cell transplantation has received worldwide media attention and has shown great potential for treating many serious illnesses. To provide more insight and understanding on this very complex topic, Bumrungrad's website (www.bumrungrad.com) now includes a section that provides information and Bumrugrad's position on stem cell treatment issues.

Clinical studies have already shown stem cell treatments to be effective for treating certain blood-related disorders, and experienced Bumrungrad physicians offer treatments in those proven areas.

To learn more about developments in stem cell treatment, simply visit www.bumrungrad.com/stemcell. You'll find a special briefing on Stem Cell Treatment that answers the most frequently-asked questions on this important and fast-developing topic.

HYPERBORIC OXYGEN THERAPY UNIT

Bumrungrad International's new Hyperbaric Oxygen Therapy (HBOT) Unit is now open, offering therapeutic benefits to inpatients and outpatients who suffer from certain illness and conditions. The HBOT (high pressure) treatment is a non-invasive and painless course of treatment originally developed to treat scuba and deep-sea divers with the dangerous condition called decompression sickness. However, it is now being used to treat several other conditions. For example, HBOT can reduce the effects of toxic substances, alleviate gas-bubble obstructions, promote wound healing, increase oxygen delivery to injured tissue, and improve infection control.

"Breathing 100 percent pure oxygen, under higher-than-normal atmospheric pressure, increases the amount of oxygen in the blood," noted

Dr. Karoon Mekanonthchai, Bumrungrad International's Medical Director. "This can help and fight off infection, reduce swelling and aid the growth of new blood vessels-benefits that cannot be achieved by breathing oxygen in a regular room."

MEN'S HEALTH

If you are a man over 40 and you answered "yes" to more than two questions, it's time to take action. Our men's health experts can help you with problems that threaten your life, or just diminish your lifestyle:

- Andropause
- Back and knees
- Diabetes
- Erectile dysfunction
- Infertility
- Fitness and weight
- Hair loss
- Heart disease
- Prostate problems
- Stroke

Andropause is the result of a decline in male hormone (testoterone) levels which can occur with aging.

The decline in hormones, coupled with unhealthy diet, stress, and lack of exercise, can cause health problems. You don't have to accept these problems as investiable and unmanageable. You can do something to remain in control of your health and lifestyle.

Men Center at Bumrungrad International is a team of doctors who study, understand, and treat the health issues faced by men as they age. You start with an initial evaluation with a Men Center doctor. He will give you advice and may recommend appropriate treatment by a specialist on the Men Center team. The team includes experts in cardiology, urology, orthopaedics, hormones, psychiatry, nutrition, anti-aging medicine—whatever you need to get back to looking, feeling, and living better.

Our experts enjoy access to the hospital's stat-of-the-art technology. For example, laser treatment of the prostate to relieve painful urination; 3-D imaging of bones and joints; and sophisticated blood testing that profiles hormone and micronutrient levels.

ANDROPAUSE AND ERECTILE DYSFUNCTION (ED)

For men over 40, getting older doesn't have to mean living with declining health. Thanks to extensive research and new treatment advances, male andropause can be diagnosed and treated successfully.

There's a ring of truth to the old saying that "Life begins at 40," Entering the middle part of life is supposed to be a positive experience, and a time to feel more settled, established and comfortable.

But for a great number of men, life beyond the age of 40 can feel more like the end of good health, with unexplained fatigue, insomnia, depressed feelings and a general lack of enthusiasm for living—not unlike the difficulties many women encounter during menopause. For some middle-aged men, the physical and mental toll of everyday living means a profound decline in quality of life.

Given the similarities to the symptoms of female menopause, this condition has been referred to as "male menopause", or "mid-life crisis." Some used to believe it was just a normal part of the male aging process. Others questioned whether it was all just a state of mind.

So what exactly is it that these men are experiencing? And what is the best way to deal with it? For answers, Better Health turned to Dr. Pansak Sugkraruek, an endocrinologist and fertility expert with vast experience treating men for what is now called andropause.

What is Andropause?

Years ago many doctors believed that male 'menopause' symptoms were merely an unavoidable part of the aging process; consequently, relatively little research effort was made to understand what exactly was causing the condition. Thanks to intensive research in recent years, science now has a clear understanding that andropause results from declining levels of several male hormones.

"People used to equate these symptoms in men with those that occur during female menopause, and so the term 'male menopause' was coined," says Dr. Pansak. "Extensive research in recent years has shown that the term doesn't properly describe the male condition. While the symptoms are similar in both men and women, the causes are very different.

For women, menopause begins when the ovaries stop functioning and no longer produce hormones. "In men, hormone production continues," Dr. Pansak explains, "but certain bodily conditions impair a man's hormone production to such an extent that this hormone deficiency begins to have a noticeable effect on some important body function."

"The correct term to describe this process is testosterone deficiency syndrome or androgen deficiency of the aging male," says, Dr. Pansak. "In simple terms, this is andropause."

Andropause and Hormone Deficiency

The impact of hormone deficiency in men is usually gradual and often goes unnoticed at least initially. "As the condition progress it can lead to a significant impact in both physical and psychological terms on a man's quality of life," Dr. Pansak explains. "Andropause affects a man's self-esteem and how he relates to others. Men with hormone deficiency often feel frustrated, irritable, subdued and pessimistic. Their muscles contract while body fat increases. They often experience insomnia, emotional turbulence, less sharp thinking, a decreased sex drive and erectile dysfunction. Serious cases can eventually lead to clinical depression."

Andropause affects more than just testosterone. "All hormones experience a decline," Dr. Pansak continues. "One of the first to decline is melatonin, the so-called 'hormone of the night.' Melatonin is normally secreted after sundown and helps a person feel sleepy as bedtime approaches, allowing him to fall into deep healthy sleep around midnight. In a healthy man, the pituitary gland produces a variety of hormones during deep sleep. The first of these is the growth hormone which preserves one's youthfulness and counters the aging process."

"The thyroid gland then produces a hormone that converts food into energy," explains Dr. Pansak. "A healthy thyroid hormone function gives a man energy to enthusiastically engage in activities. The adrenal gland produces the antioxidant hormone DHEA that slows the aging process."

The male sexual hormone testosterone is the last hormone produced. "This hormone helps one think decisively, reasonably and positively as a healthy man should," says Dr. Pansak. "It also supports bone and muscle strength and regulates body fat and body contour. That's why men with normal hormone levels usually don't have 'beer belly.' Their bodies are strong and their mood is good."

The Dangers of Male Hormone Deficiency

If left untreated, male hormone deficiency poses a number of potentially serious health risks, including fragile bones, weak muscles, erectile dysfunction, hypertension, heart disease and stroke.

"With decreased hormone levels, body at increase and accumulated around the waistline," notes Dr. Pansak. "The beer belly is one sign of male hormone deficiency. The criterion is a waistline in excess of 94 centimeters for westerners and 90 centimeters for easterners."

Beer Belly Dangers

While most of us are aware of the health risks that come with being overweight, the specific dangers for men with excessive fat accumulation around the waist are less well understood, but no less serious

"Think about it: When a man has a 'spare tire' around his waist, he's unlikely to have the energy or the desire to stay active," Dr. Pansak explains. "This lack of activity means he's not using enough energy to burn his daily calorie intake, and that leads to even more fat buildup. This increased fat clogs blood vessels and leads to hypertensions. It can also cause dyslipidemia, the condition of having too much 'bad' cholesterol and not enough 'good' cholesterol. This can significantly raise a man's risk for stroke, a potentially deadly condition."

This unhealthy state can also affect a man's sexual health. "Clogged blood vessels affect the supply of blood to the genitals," says Dr. Pansak. "This can cause erectile dysfunction. Excess fat accumulates in the genital muscles, further worsening the symptoms. This is a prime example of how the body's many systems are interconnected."

Dr. Pansak stresses the importance of consulting a doctor at the first sign of difficulty in achieving a normal erection. "Your doctor may recommend a hormone level test to check for possible deficiencies," he explains. "Your doctor can recommend a treatment strategy for sexual impotency as well as other steps to address one's overall health situation."

Treating Hormone Deficiency

Hormone Supplement Therapy

The old saying "Getting old is natural, feeling old is optional" certainly applies to male hormone deficiency. Today's modern lifestyles are far different from earlier generations. People tend to spend more time working and less time sleeping, and most of us endure greater stress from everyday living. Our fast-paced world leads to eating on-the-run and sleeping just a few hours a night, while leaving less time for exercise and relaxation. These factors all contribute to premature hormone deficiency.

Dr. Pansak shares his experience: "I see more and more men in their 30s who come to me because of loss of sexual desire and erectile dysfunction, hair loss or obesity. Dealing with their problems requires a holistic approach, to diagnose and treat the full range of health issues to produce a successful treatment outcome."

"Sexual impotency is an important indicator of male health problems, so we have to check blood sugar and body fat levels, hormone levels, the health of the prostate gland, and understand a patient's lifestyle and family history to see what changes may be needed," says Dr. Pansak. "Hormone supplement therapy is often recommended as part of the treatment plan. After a period of taking hormone supplements, patients usually experience noticeable improvements to their health and wellness, which are often accompanied by weight loss and improved sexual function. A patient's mood and overall happiness usually also improves."

Hormone supplement therapy has an impressive record of safety for effectively treating men suffering from andropause. All medical treatments and procedures involve some level of risk and may not be suitable for everyone. Your doctor will explain the risks involved and recommend the course of treatment that's right for your individual situation.

Lifestyle Modification

Dr. Pansak emphasizes the hormone-related differences between men and women. "The female body stops producing female hormones during menopause", he explains. "Replacement therapy is usually recommended to mitigate the negative effects. On the contrary, the male body never stops producing male hormones. The levels of hormones decline, but they can be restored. Doctors will advise their patients on specific lifestyle changes that can help increase hormone production. For some patients—usually older men with greater hormone deficiency—doctors will also prescribe male hormone supplements to be taken on a regular basis".

Do you have hormone deficiency? Find out by taking this quiz.

Are you experiencing these symptoms?

Sexual health:	Yes	No
1. Decreased sex drive	☐	☐
2. Difficulty achieving and/or maintaining an erection	☐	☐
General health:		
3. Decreased strength and stamina	☐	☐
4. Fatigue or lack of energy	☐	☐
5. Depression	☐	☐
6. 'Shrinking' or having a hunched back	☐	☐
7. Difficulty concentrating at work	☐	☐
8. Feeling unhappy or pessimistic about life	☐	☐
9. Decreased athletic capabilities	☐	☐
10. Falling asleep or nodding off during the day	☐	☐

If you answered YES to questions 1 or 2, or if you answered YES to at least 3 of the general health questions, you may be experiencing male hormone deficiency. Consult your doctor for a physical examination and a hormone level test.

Source: www.andropause.com

There are simple guidelines that all men can follow to improve their overall health and limit the effects of hormone deficiency. Dr. Pansak recommends:

- Going to bed early enough to ensure that you fall into deep sleep by midnight;
- Exercising most days for 45 minutes per workout (or 300 total minutes each week) as opposed to the 30 minutes per workout guideline for the general population;
- Eating a healthier diet; and
- Adopting a positive attitude in order to avoid depression and insomnia.

According to Dr. Pansak, unhealthy living is often the biggest single factor in causing male hormone deficiency. So making healthy lifestyle changes under the supervision of a medical specialist can prove highly effective in returning to better health. Middle age really can be the beginning of a happier, healthier life. As the famous comedian George Burns said, "You can't help getting older, but you don't have to get old".

Erectile dysfunction (ED)

Q: What are the most common myths and misconceptions about ED?

A: One common misconception is that emotional and psychological problems are the main causes. In truth, it's just opposite; research has shown that physical causes account for over 80% of ED cases.

Another popular myth is that ED is an unavoidable part of the aging process. Yes, a man's hormone levels diminish with age, and he may need more stimulation to achieve a healthy erection. But age alone does not cause ED.

Q: What are the most common causes of ED? What are the key risk factors?

A: Difficulty achieving an erection can be caused by any number of factors, either physical, psychological, or a combination of the two. A number of medical conditions are known to cause ED, including some arterosclerosis, heart and vascular diseases, diabetes, prostate conditions including enlargement and cancer, disease affecting the nerves and brain (e.g. multiple sclerosis, Parkinson's disease, Alzeimer's disease), and vascular conditions that affect blood vessels and circulation.

Unhealthy living-excessive stress, obesity and poor nutrition lack of exercise tobacco use, excessive alcohol consumption and drug use, among other's can lead to ED. It's also a potential side effect resulting from a number of prescription medications, medical procedures and surgeries.

Age also plays a role; studies show ED affects about one out of 20 men aged 40, but about one out of four men aged 65.

ED can also be a symptom of a potential undiagnosed medical

condition; which is one of many reasons why it is important for men to talk to their doctor about ED.

Q: What treatment options are most effective?

A: There has been tremendous progress in the number and effectiveness of treatments of ED. The best treatments include medications (taken orally), penile implants, and penile pumps. Doctors often recommend lifestyle modifications such as exercise, smoking cessation, and stress reduction, all of which help improve erectile function and overall health.

Q: What advice should be given to men who may be suffering from ED but are reluctant to seek help?

A: Men should know that it's normal feel anxious about talking to your doctor about ED. Men have always been less likely than women to make regular doctor visits, and there's a stigma in almost every society that men should be able to handle their problems by themselves, and that feeling vulnerable or seeking help is a sign of weakness.

Doctors have been successfully treating men with ED for many years. With even more effective treatment option available now, whatever anxiety men may feel about seeking help always pales in comparison to the anxiety and potentially serious medical problems that can result from not seeking help.

PET/CT

Every year, cancer claims the lives of millions of people. It continues to be a leading cause of death among Thais. But it doesn't have to be that way. Many types of cancer are treatable and curable if detected early.

Recent advances in technology are helping detect cancerous cells earlier and with greater precision and accuracy, making it possible to save potentially millions of lives. One of the most exciting innovations in cancer detection is PET/CT (Position Emission Tomograph/Computed Tomograph) technology. In the few short years since its introduction, PET/CT has become one of the most highly effective tools for early detection of cancerous cells.

PET/CT provides an anatomical map of the body with 64 slices per revolution in only 0.33 seconds. It produces high resolution 2-dimensional and 3-dimensional images capable of revealing even tiny traces of cancerous tissue—as small as 3 millimeters in size. Its effectiveness helps doctors to plan medical treatments and scheduled suitable to each patient individually.

Dr. Narongsak Kiatikajornthada, Hematology and Oncology specialist at Bumrungrad International Hospital, explains how PET/CT technology is used to pinpoint the exact location and size of tumors and to quickly determine the exact stage of cancer. "The procedure begins with an injection of FDG, an analog of glucose that is tagged to the radionuclide F 18," Dr. Naraongsak says. "Tumors trap more FDG than other organs, so PET/CT can identify gamma rays in the rapidly growing tumors. This helps doctors to detect and diagnose cancer faster and easier."

The scanner pinpoints the exact location of tumors that may have gone unnoticed by other CT or MRI diagnostic tools. Besides cancer, PET/CT can also detect some brain diseases such as Alzheimer's disease and epilepsy.

With early detection being among the most important factors for successful cancer treatment, Bumrungrad patients are already reaping significant benefits through more successful and less traumatic treatment regimens.

NEW INTERNATIONAL CLINIC

Following its July 31 grand opening, the brand new 53,000-square meter Bumrungrad International Clinic is now delivering an unrivaled patient experience in a warm, comfortable and friendly environment.

The 22-storey building was designed to be the ideal place for patients and doctors to meet for consultation and medical services. The clinic is equipped with world-class medical technology and equipment and offers a full range of facilities, including spacious lobby and seating areas, an international food center, retail shops, and a lounge for Bumrungrad patients and Healthy Living Club Members.

The Bumrungrad International Clinic delivers on its promise of a one-stop, one-location service with ease and convenience from start to finish. New technology delivers more streamlined patient registration and online medical records availability. More convenience is offered with diagnostic imaging services available right inside patient consultation rooms, and expanded laboratory automation to provide faster and more accurate test results. Patients can even pay their bills and pick-up prescribed medicine on the same floor.

With the opening of the new outpatient building. Bumrungrad International is Thailand's largest private hospital, with 250 outpatient consultation rooms and the capacity to welcome upto 6,000 patients each day.

The Bumrungrad International Clinic incorporates many medical services and specialist centers, including:

- Medical Coordination Center
- Health Screening Center
- Respiratory Efficiency Testing
- Rehabilitation Center
- Surgical Clinic
- Men Center
- Endocrinology Services
- Nutrition therapy
- Diagnostic radiology
- Heart Center

- Dialysis.
- Specialists in infectious disease, lung disease, internal medicine, allergies, orthopedics and rheumatism, hematology, urology, neurology, neurosurgery and breast surgery.

Bumrungrad International now serves more than 12 million Thai and International patients each year from 190 countries all over the world and is acknowledged as a pioneer in Medical Tourism. More recently, *The Wall Street Journal Asia* named Bumrungrad one of the best companies in Thailand.

WELLNESS PROGRAMMES; VITAL LIFE

Anti-Aging Programs

A thoughtful anti-aging program will lead to optimal health

It is a way to manage health risks so you can be sure that you are as healthy as can be.

The Vital Life approach is an integrated and personalized plan that combines nutritional, hormonal, and physical therapies to slow the aging process and improve your functionality.

Make it your way to a longer and healthier life.

I. EXECUTIVE ANTI-AGING

Consultations

- Physician: Anti-Aging Medicine
- Physician: Functional Medicine
- Physician: Sports Medicine
- Registered: Dietician

Laboratory Evaluations

Antioxidants

Vitamin C (Ascorbate), Vitamin A (Retinol), Vitamin E (Alpha-Tocopherol), Gamma-Tocopherol, Beta-Carotene, Alpha-Carotene, Coenzyme Q 10 (Ubiquinone), Lycopene

Vitamins and Minerals

Folate (Vitamin B9), Vitamin B12, Chromium Copper, Ferritin, Magnesium, Selenium, Zinc.

Hormones

LH, FSH, Estradiol, Testosterone*, Progesterone**, TSH, Free T3, Free T4, DHEA-S

General

Complete Blood Count (CBC)

Inflammatory Markers

ESR, CRP

Cardiac Profile

Cholesterol, Triglycerides, HDL, LDL (calc)

Insulin Resistance

Fasting Plasma Glucose (FPG), Insulin

Liver and Kidney Function

AST, ALT, Alkaline phosphatase, Creatinine

Gout

Uric Acid

Tumor Markers

CEA, AFP, PSA

Other Laboratory Evaluations

Urine Analysis (UA), Stool Analysis

Investigations

- Bio-Physical Assessment
- Chest X-Ray
- EKG
- Bone Scan (hip and spine)
- Ultrasound of the Whole Abdomen
- Ultrasound of the Prostate (trans-rectal)*
- Mammogram with ultrasound breast**
- Pap Smear**

THB 35,000 (Female)
THB 34,000 (Male)

* Male only
** Female only

2. COMPREHENSIVE ANTI-AGING

Consultations

- Physician: Anti-Aging Medicine
- Physician: Functional Medicine
- Physician: Sports Medicine
- Registered: Dietician

Laboratory Evaluations

Antioxidants

Vitamin C (Ascorbate), Vitamin A (Retinol), Vitamin E (Alpha-Tocopherol), Gamma-Tocopherol, Beta-Carotene, Alpha-Carotene, Coenzyme Q 10 (Ubiquinone), Lycopene

Vitamins and Minerals

Folate (Vitamin B9), Vitamin B12, Chromium Copper, Ferritin, Magnesium, Selenium, Zinc

Hormones

LH, FSH, Estradiol, Testosterone*, Progesterone*, TSH, Free T3, Free T4, DHEA-S, IGF-1

General

Complete Blood Count (CBC)

Inflammatory Markers

ESR, CRP

Cardiac Profile

Cholesterol, Triglycerides, HDL, LDL (calc)

Insulin Resistance

Fasting Plasma Glucose (FPG), Insulin

Liver and Kidney Function

AST, ALT, Total Bilirubin, Alkaline Phosphatase, Albumin, BUN, Creatinine

Gout

Uric Acid

Iron Study

Serum Iron, Ferritin

Tumor Markers

CEA, AFP, PSA*

Special laboratory Evaluations

Oxidative Damage Markers

MDA (Malonyldiadehyde)
Carbonyl Proteins
Allantoins
80 HdG (8-Hydroxy deoxyguanosine)
Gluathione

Essential and Metabolic Fatty Acids

Omega 3, Omega 6, Omega 9,
Saturated Fatty Acids
Even Carbon Atom Fatty Acids

Urinary Organic Acids

Functional Deficit of Vitamins
Metabolite Indicators of Energy Production
Gut Dysbiosis Markers
Sulfate Detoxification
Neurotransmitters

Other Laboratory Evaluations
Urine Analysis (UA) Stool Analysis.

Investigations

- Bio-Physical Assessment
- Chest X-Ray
- EKG
- DEXA Scan (whole body)
  Body Fat Analysis
  Bone Mineral Density
- Ultrasound of the Whole Abdomen
- Ultrasound of the Prostate (Trans-rectal)*
- Mammogram with ultrasound breast**
- Pap Smear**

THB 69,000 (Female)
THB 68,000 (Male)

* Male only
** Female only

A healthy body is one in biochemical balance with nature.

A personalized VitalLife supplement program will replenish your body's reserves, strengthen your immune system, and make up for deficiencies that come from poor diet or a hectic daily schedule.

We custom design and compound nutritional supplements to ensure your body has the right balance of vitamins, minerals, and antioxidants to achieve peak physical and mental performance.

I. ANTIOXIDANTS

Consultations
Physician: Functional Medicine

Laboratory Evaluations

Antioxidants

Vitamin C (Ascorbate), Vitamin A (Retinol), Vitamin E (Alpha-Tocopherol), Gamma-Tocopherol, Beta-Carotene, Alpha-Carotene, Coenzyme Q 10 (Ubiquinone), Lycopene

THB 5,800

2. MICRONUTRIENTS

Consultations

Physician: Functional Medicine

Laboratory Evaluations

Antioxidants

Vitamin C (Ascorbate), Vitamin A (Retinol), Vitamin E (Alpha-Tocopherol), Gamma-Tocopherol, Beta-Carotene, Alpha-Carotene, Coenzyme Q 10 (Ubiquinone), Lycopene

Vitamins and Minerals

Folate (Vitamin B9), Vitamin B12, Chromium Copper, Ferritin, Magnesium, Selenium, Zinc

THB 9,200

3. ANTIOXIDANTS-LIFESTYLE

Consultations

- Physician: Functional Medicine
- Physician: Sports Medicine
- Registered Dietician

Laboratory Evaluations

Antioxidants

Vitamin C (Ascorbate), Vitamin A (Retinol), Vitamin E (Alpha-Tocopherol), Gamma-Tocopherol, Beta-Carotene, Alpha-Carotene, Coenzyme Q10 (Ubiquinone), Lycopene.

Investigation

Bio-Physical Age Assessment

THB 10,300

4. MICRONUTRIENTS-LIFESTYLE

Consultations

- Physician: Functional Medicine
- Physician: Sports Medicine
- Registered Dietician

Laboratory Evaluations

Antioxidants

Vitamin C (Ascorbate), Vitamin A (Retinol), Vitamin E (Alpha-Tocopherol), Gamma-Tocopherol, Beta-Carotene, Alpha-Carotene, Coenzyme Q 10 (Ubiquinone), Lycopene.

Vitamins and Minerals

Folate (Vitamin B9), Vitamin B12, Chromium, Copper, Ferritin, Magnesium, Selenium, Zinc

Investigation

Bio-Physical Age Assessment

THB 13,700

5. EXECUTIVE WELLNESS

Consultations

- Physician: Functional Medicine
- Physician: Sports Medicine
- Registered Dietician

Laboratory Evaluations

Antioxidants

Vitamin C (Ascorbate), Vitamin A (Retinol), Vitamin E (Alpha-Tocopherol), Gamma-Tocopherol, Beta-Carotene, Alpha-Carotene, Coenzyme Q 10 (Ubiquinone), Lycopene.

Vitamins and Minerals

Folate (Vitamin B9), Vitamin B12, Chromium, Copper, Ferritin, Magnesium, Selenium, Zinc

General

Complete Body Count (CBC), Fasting Plasma Glucose (FPG).

Inflammatory Markers

ESR, CRP

Cardiac Profile

Cholesterol, Triglycerides, HDL, LDL (calc)

Liver and Kidney Function

AST, ALT, Alkaline Phosphatase, Creatinine

Gout

Uric Acid

Tumor Markers

CEA, AFP

Other Laboratory Evaluations

Urine Analysis (UA), Stool Analysis.

Investigation

- Bio-Physical Age Assessment
- Chest X-Ray, EKG, Ultrasound of the Whole Abdomen

THB 19,500

6. COMPREHENSIVE WELLNESS

Consultations

- Physician: Functional Medicine
- Physician: Sports Medicine
- Registered Dietician

Laboratory Evaluations

Antioxidants

Vitamin C (Ascorbate), Vitamin A (Retinol), Vitamin E (Alpha-Tocopherol), Gamma-Tocopherol, Beta-Carotene, Alpha-Carotene, Coenzyme Q 10 (Ubiquinone), Lycopene.

Vitamins and Minerals

Folate (Vitamin B9), Vitamin B12, Chromium, Copper, Ferritin, Magnesium, Selenium, Zinc

General

Complete Body Count (CBC).

Inflammatory Markers

ESR, CRP

Cardiac Profile

Cholesterol, Triglycerides, HDL, LDL (calc)

Insulin Resistance

Fasting Plasma Glucose (FPG), Insulin

Liver and Kidney Function

AST, ALT, Total Bilirubin, Alkaline Phosphatase, Albumin, BUN, Creatinine

Gout

Uric Acid

Iron Study

Serum iron, Ferritin

Tumor Markers

CEA, AFP

Special Laboratory Evaluations

Oxidative Damage Markers

MDA, Carbonyl Proteins, Allantoins, 80 HdG, Glutathione

Essential and Metabolic Fatty Acids

Omega 3, Omega 6, Omega 9, Saturated Fatty Acids, Even Carbon Atom Fatty Acids

Urinary Organic Acids

Functional Deficit of Vitamins, Indicators of Energy Production, Gut Dysbiosis Markers, Sulfate Detoxification, Neurotransmitters

Other Laboratory Evaluations

Urine Analysis (UA), Stool Analysis

Investigation

- Bio-Physical Age Assessment
- Chest X-Ray, EKG, DEXA Scan (whole body), Ultrasound of the Whole Abdomen.

THB 54,000

Weight-Loss Programs

The VitalLife weight loss program is designed to help you lose pounds but not feel hungry... to keep your energy levels up without stimulants!

Our system begins with a thorough diagnosis of your weight status and the reasons for it. Then we will prescribe nutritional supplements just right for you. Enjoy the VitalLife food supplements, and after you have reached your goals, we will give you a maintenance plan to keep you looking and feeling your best.

1. WEIGHT LOSS INITIAL SCREENING

Consultations

Physician

Laboratory Evaluations

- Complete Blood Count (CBC)
- Serum Iron
- Thyroid Function
  TSH, Free T4, Free T3
- Insulin Resistance
  FPG, Insulin
- Cardiac Profile
  Cholesterol, Triglycerides, HDL, LDL (Calc)
- Liver Function
  AST, ALT, Alkaline Phosphatase
- Kidney Function
  BUN, Creatinine
- Electrolytes
  Sodium, Potassium, Chloride, Bicarbonate
- Uric Acid, Calcium
- Urinary Microalbumin/Creatinine Ratio

Investigations

- EKG
- Dexa Scan
  Body fat analysis
  Bone mineral density

THB 10,000

2. HIPRO RAPID WEIGHT LOSS

HiPro—4 Month Program

1 month	Hi-Pro Rapid Weight Loss
3 months	Maintenance
Consultations	
• Physician	5 sessions
• Exercise Physician	6 sessions
• Registered Dietician	7 sessions

Investigations

• Blood Tests	2
• Urine Tests	2
• DEXA Scan	1

Supplements

• Nutraceuticals	4 months supply
• Vitallife Functional Food (Protein Shakes)	1 months supply

THB 58,000

HiPro—5 Month Program

2 months	Hi-Pro Rapid Weight Loss
3 months	Maintenance

Consultations

• Physician	7 sessions
• Exercise Physician	6 sessions
• Registered Dietician	7 sessions

Investigations

• Blood Tests	4
• Urine Tests	4
• DEXA Scan	2
• EKG	1

Supplements

• Nutraceuticals	5 months supply
• Vitallife Functional Food (Protein Shakes)	2 months supply

THB 88,000

HiPro—6 Month Program

3 months	Hi-Pro Rapid Weight Loss
3 months	Maintenance

Consultations

• Physician	9 sessions
• Exercise Physician	6 sessions
• Registered Dietician	7 sessions

Investigations

• Blood Tests	7
• Urine Tests	6
• DEXA Scan	2
• EKG	2

Supplements

• Nutraceuticals	6 months supply
• Vitallife Functional Food (Protein Shakes)	3 months supply

THB 118,000

3. FOUR-MONTHS WEIGHT LOSS PROGRAM

Consultations

• Physician	1 session
• Exercise Physician	5 sessions
• Registered Dietician	5 sessions

Investigations

• Blood Tests	1
• DEXA Scan	1

Supplements

• Nutraceuticals	4 months supply

THB 42,000

4. TAILORED WEIGHT LOSS PROGRAMS FOR SPECIAL NEEDS

For individuals who are not residents of Bangkok and need to return home after the screening test.

Consultation with

Physician via e-mail or telephone

Supplements

As prescribed

Price based on actual

Vitality Programs

Hormone replacement therapy results in a more active and vital life

It counters the effects of andropause in men and menopause in women. A hormone replacement program increases sexual desire and fulfillment, generates a higher level of motivation, and helps you be more focused and affirmative in your daily decision-making.

We start with a comprehensive screening to know your levels of wellness, prescribe an appropriate program designed specifically for you.... then monitor your state of wellness on a regular basis so that you maintain maximum vitality.

Signs and Symptoms of Hormone Deficiency

Male

- Fatigue, loss of energy
- Loss of memory or concentration
- Loss of sex drive or libido
- Loss of morning erections or sexual performance
- Backache, joint pains or stiffness
- Loss of fitness
- Depression, lacking motivation
- Irritability, anger or bad temper
- Anxiety or nervousness
- Feeling over-stressed

Female

- Hot flashes and sweats
- Lethargy, loss of energy
- Depression, moodiness
- Tension, irritability, anxiety
- Loss of memory or concentration
- Headaches
- Droopy breasts
- Loss of sex drive or libido
- Vaginal dryness, urinary symptoms
- Hair and skin changes

I. VITALITY

Consultations

Physician: Anti-Ageing Medicine

Laboratory Evaluations

Hormones

LH, FSH, Estradiol, Testosterone*, Progesterone**, DHEA-S

General

Complete Blood Count (CBC)

Liver Function

AST, ALT

Tumor Marker

PSA*

Other Laboratory Evaluation

Urine Analysis (UA)

Investigations

- EKG
- Bone scan (hip and spine)
- Ultrasound of the Prostate (trans-rectal)*
- Mammogram with ultrasound breast**
- Pap Smear**

THB 13,000 (Female)
THB 12,000 (Male)

2. VITALITY-LIFESTYLE

Consultations

- Physician: Anti-Ageing Medicine
- Physician: Sports Medicine
- Registered Dietician

Laboratory Evaluations

Hormones

LH, FSH, Estradiol, Testosterone*, Progesterone**, DHEA-S

General

Complete Blood Count (CBC)

Liver Function

AST, ALT

Tumor Marker

PSA*

Other Laboratory Evaluation

Urine Analysis (UA)

Investigations

- EKG
- Bio-Physical Age Assessment
- Bone scan (hip and spine)
- Ultrasound of the Prostate (trans-rectal)*
- Mammogram with ultrasound breast**
- Pap Smear**

THB 17,000 (Female)
THB 16,000 (Male)

3. EXECUTIVE VITALITY

Consultations

- Physician: Anti-Ageing Medicine
- Physician: Sports Medicine
- Registered Dietician

Laboratory Evaluations

Hormones

LH, FSH, Estradiol, Testosterone*, Progesterone**, TSH, Free T3, Free T4, DHEA-S, IGF-1

General

Complete Blood Count (CBC), Fasting Plasma Glucose (FPG)

Cardiac Profile

Cholesterol, Triglycerides, HDL, LDL (calc)

Liver and Kidney Function

AST, ALT, Alkaline Phosphatase, Creatinine

Gout

Uric Acid

Tumor Marker

CEA, AFP, PSA*

Other Laboratory Evaluations

Urine Analysis (UA), Stool Analysis

Investigations

- Bio-Physical Age Assessment
- Chest X-Ray
- EKG
- Bone scan (hip and spine)
- Ultrasound of the Whole Abdomen
- Ultrasound of the Prostate (trans-rectal)*
- Mammogram with ultrasound breast**
- Pap Smear**

THB 24,000 (Female)
THB 23,000 (Male)

4. HORMONE SCREENING PANEL

Consultations

Physician: Anti-Ageing Medicine

Laboratory Evaluations

Hormones

LH, FSH, Estradiol, Testosterone*, Progesterone**, TSH, Free T3, Free T4, DHEA-S, IGF-1

THB 9,000

*Male only
**Female only

HEALTHY LIVING CLUB

Bumrungrad International hospital offers the Healthy Living Club program to provide affordable international-standard health care—with additional privileges.

Care benefits

Register for a Main Membership Card and pay only 6,300 baht for 3 years and receive a privilege coupon for the Executive Health Check-Up program valued at 6,300 baht. You are then eligible for a Supplementary Card for any member of your family for only 3,000 baht for 3 years—and receive an additional privilege coupon worth 3,000 baht towards an Executive or Comprehensive Check-Up.

Value benefits

For inpatients : 30% discount for an inpatient room*
For outpatients : 15% discount for medicine and medical supplies**, Laboratory Test***, X-ray

Remarks: Discounts exclude doctors' consultation fees and special medical equipment.

* Except meals, nursing services and other services
** Except special medicine such as Chemotherapy
*** Except special lab

Members are eligible for outpatient discounts upon registration. Inpatient discounts may be received starting 7 days after registration.

Convenience benefits

- Free access to Wi-Fi internet
- Access to the Napa Lounge in the Bumrungrad Clinic building
- Receive Better Health magazine, delivered to your home free
- Pre-booking privileges for our public health seminars
- Other additional privilege programs are offered to members only.

Other benefits*

Get special discount privileges from retailers at Bumrungrad, such as Booskorn Flower Shop, New City, Baby and Children, Get The Books, Ayame Japanese restaurant and Portofino Italian Restaurant. Also get special giveaway privileges when purchasing food and beverages at Au Bon Pain and McDonald's.

CONCLUSION

The hospital is providing preventive, promotive and curative services efficiently and promptly. The reasons for this are:

(a) Patient centered approach
(b) Excellent staff
(c) A combination of preventive and curative approach
(d) Subsidized services to weaker sections
(e) High Tech specialized centers
(f) Special arrangements to foreigners.

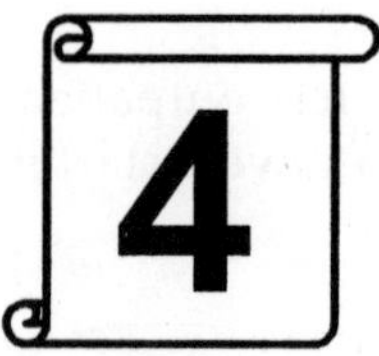

Indian Hospitals: Destination of International Patients

India's tertiary care hospitals are on the road to global fame. It is an ironic outcome of economic reforms that in spite of failures in public health, India is increasingly seen as an attractive international health care destination. That potential is based, in part, on the low cost of care in international price terms, competent medical personnel and absence of long waiting times for procedures, says a CII report. Stories of foreign nationals undergoing complicated surgery in the country are frequently featured in the media. Those who come now are not just from other developing countries, but also from the United Kingdom, Europe and North America. Tanzania and Iraq have a Memorandum of Understanding with the Madras Medical Mission.

DE-STRESSING AND HEALTH-BUILDING

The CII-McKinsey report says that the modern system can offer treatment in specialties such as cardiac, liver, renal and orthopedic procedures, while Indian systems of medicine could attract patients from even the developed world to treat "lifestyle diseases" such as stress and rheumatism. Many visitors who come for such de-stressing and health-building treatment may also choose to visit tourist spots. Such tourism potential holds the key to Kerala's plans. The Ayurveda State had declared 2006 the year of medical tourism and is actively supporting its well-known traditional medicine and tourism sectors, as they reach out to more potential visitors. Nepal plans to step up health tourism investment along the lines of Kerala, a hot tourist destination for ayurvedic treatments and health packages. "Being a source of rare Himalayan herbs and oils, we are looking keenly at wellness tourism," Nandini Lahe-Thapa, the Nepal Tourism Board's director of marketing and promotion said.

"Inspired by the success of Kerala (in southern India), Thailand and Malaysia, we will be looking at more investment in the wellness sector," she said. "As an offshoot of our rich herbal heritage, we are planning to promote the wellness theme. We already have the Kunfen organisation with branches all over Nepal and even overseas where healing is done through mantras, chants and medicines prepared with a blend of herbs and metals, including precious metals and stones," she said. Indian health products major Dabur is one of the major enterprises that is engaged in cultivation of rare herbs and manufacture of herbal products in Nepal targeting the growing interest in ayurvedic products.

Karnataka, which gets about 8,000 patients a year and forecasts an annual growth rate of 25 per cent, will promote a massive health park/ medi city near a new international airport in Bangalore; non-resident Indians have formed a medical tourism company in Vadodara and international property developers are venturing into the health care sector to participate in the construction boom. In Maharashtra, the State Government is part of the Medical Tourism Council that has members from Association of Hospitals and FICCI. In New Delhi, Naresh Trehan, executive director of the Escorts Heart Institute and Research Centre has proposed a Medicity on the outskirts of the capital to develop a 1,500-bed health care centre of international standards with 20 super specialties. It will incorporate traditional medicine too and have such facilities as hotels, serviced apartments, clinical and biotechnology laboratories. The corporate health care sector views such support as critical, considering that it is competing with Thailand, Singapore, Malaysia and South Korea for a bigger share of Asia's medical tourism market. "Medical tourism can be a much bigger business, if we have infrastructure and networking among hospitals, hotels and tourism agencies.

Joint Commission International, a benchmarking body lists Indraprastha Apollo, New Delhi, and Wockhardt, Mumbai, as accredited hospitals. Accreditation apparently brings immediate benefits. "There has been a steady increase in the number of patients, particularly from the U.K. and U.S. The numbers have been increasing after accreditation, particularly from the U.S.," says Vishal Bali, chief executive officer of Wockhardt.

See Appendix 5 for more on JCI accreditation and other aspects of medical tourism promotion.

It is also important to have systems that meet the criteria of insurance companies. Says cardiac surgeon V.V. Bashi of MIOT Hospital, Chennai: "Our medical standards are world class, but if we have to get more patients from the U.S. and other developed countries, we must match their hospital documentation standards. This is really important because the insurance companies must cover all the risks in the event of an adverse treatment outcome."

Says Anil Maini, president, corporate development, Indraprastha Apollo, "We have 64 slice CT scans, PET CT and 3 TELSA MRI machines which most hospitals abroad cannot boast of." Some observers fear an exodus of highly skilled doctors from the atrophied public health system to high paying private hospitals. "Many States are not even ready to fill vacancies in government medical service, compounding the problem," says a surgeon in Chennai's Government General Hospital. The Karnataka Tourism Department says it has been receiving about 8,000 patients annually, mostly for cardiac and orthopedic procedures. Manipal gets 3,000 foreign patients a year, some of them for dental care. With increased activity to build hospitals in the corporate sector, foreign patient arrivals are expected to rise significantly.

The top hospitals like Apollo and Sir Ganga Ram are providing travel facilities akin to the best offered by the hotel industry. Patients and their families are not just assured of a pleasant and comfortable experience throughout their stay, the hospitals arrange for everything they need from the time they arrive in India till they board their flight home. From airport pickups and drops to making available language translators, hospitals even arrange accommodation for patients' families. Some hospitals also take care of the visa and forex requirements of foreign tourists. 'We have been helping our foreign patients by providing them money exchange facility,' said S.K Sama, chairman of the Sir Ganga Ram Hospital. Multi-cuisine facilities are available in almost all big hospitals. 'Some hospitals are even running their own air ambulance services,' said Sohail Kadri, an agent with Akbar Travels in Gujarat that caters to tourists coming to super-specialty hospitals located in Ahmedabad.

A Synergy between Government and private care

The perceived potential of medical tourism is apparent in the fact that even the Ministry of Tourism (MoT) has included health care in its campaigns. CII on its part has provided a list of hospitals to the ministry, which has come out with a special medical tourism brochure under its Incredible India campaign. It, together with CII, plans to develop a strategy to market these services overseas as well. While these efforts validate the health tourism phenomenon, there is still a very fragmented approach by the stakeholders viz. tour operators, health institutes and tourism boards—barring Kerala. Kerala tourism board has once again proved to be a pioneer by taking its international patients, health facilities and its oldest stronghold—tourism, seriously. It has formed a forum with about eight major health institutions and has applied to NABH for accreditation and is considering looking at an international accreditation as well. E.K. Bharat Bhushan, Kerala tourism's principal secretary, says that the Kerala government and the state tourism board are preparing a project report in consultation with CII to evaluate the potential of medical tourism. However, there seems to be a lack of synergy between health care professionals and travel agents with the former preferring to restrict their roles to getting patients to their hospitals, instead of exploring the tourism potential as well. Even Dr. Trehan insists that health care is serious business and "we do not want to make it cheap". Similarly, Chennai-based Apollo Hospitals restricted itself to a marketing tie-up with the Tamil Nadu Tourism Development Corporation, where tourists were given coupons for master health check-ups. But visiting international patients or relatives were not being offered travel packages by the tourism board or the hospital.

In Malaysia, a strong contender for medical tourism, the holiday packages offered vary depending upon the choice of treatment desired and are planned keeping in mind the patient's state of health and amount of post-operative recuperation. In order to create the perfect health care package, the hospital sends strict guidelines regarding recuperation and permissible post-operative activities for each procedure. Based on this, the tour operator creates holiday packages for each individual procedure with suitable itineraries and sends it back to the hospital for approval. After careful scrutiny, the hospital selects a final holiday package which is the safest and most advantageous for the particular treatment. Hospitals could probably make a start with providing a link on their websites to tourism boards, travel agents and tour operators, who in turn need to customize their packages according to the patient's needs.

Health tourism can be India's next big story

As the concept of medical tourism continues to gain momentum in India, the Ministry of Health and Family Welfare, following a meeting with the Ministry of Tourism, has stated that a NAHB has to be set-up for maintaining international standards in our medical facilities. The intricacies discussed include price banding, hospital accreditation, quality control, categorization and selection of hospitals, etc. Minister of Health and Family Welfare Dr. Anbumani Ramadoss said that the government has cleared medical visa and there is tremendous potential for tourism as well as for the health sector, with India specially being cheapest destination for medical care of highest standards. He also emphasized on modern diagnostics with Indian systems of medicinal care, which has been accepted as an effective system of health care worldwide.

Dr. Ramadoss said that some measures like fast track clearance for medical patients at the airport are in the offing in coordination with other Ministries that would be of great help to foreign tourists coming to India for medical treatment. In this regard, the Minister also mentioned development of appropriate health packages for traditional therapies like yoga, meditation, ayurveda and other traditional systems of medicine, which would not only attract high-end tourists from European and Middle East countries but also give a boost within the country.

Some people might ask, "What if something goes wrong during the surgery?" Well, here you have the reputation of the hospital and the surgeon at stake. They know that they must offer you outstanding, high-quality service. Otherwise, word will spread via the internet and elsewhere, and tourists won't come visit their hospital. Things can go wrong, but they can go wrong anywhere. Something like one percent of all people undergoing gastric bypass surgery die on the operating table. That's going to happen in any country, anywhere you are. And whether or not there's medical insurance and malpractice insurance in effect at the time of your surgery doesn't affect your outcome. All it does is it gives people a chance to sue when they don't get the outcome they want.

Deterioration of the U.S. health care: Opportunities for India

The U.S., for its part, tends to be rather protectionist about all of this. Similarly, the FDA wants to regulate and even outlaw most nutritional supplements and medicinal herbs. That's once again a protectionist strategy to protect the profits of the pharmaceutical industry. I wouldn't be surprised if sooner or later someone in organized medicine argues that outsourcing our offshore surgical procedures is hurting the U.S. economy, and they might try to pass a law that makes it illegal to go overseas to get surgery. There have already been many attempts to arrest people traveling to anti-cancer clinics in Mexico, or to seize their medicinal herbs as they come back across the border.

The specialty hospitals excelling in the medical tourism are:

- Escorts/fortis Heart Institute and Research Centre Limited, Delhi
- All India Institute of Medical Sciences, Delhi and PGI Chandigarh
- Manipal Heart Foundation, Bangalore
- B.M. Birla Heart Research Centre, Kolkata
- Breach Candy Hospital, Mumbai
- Wockhardt Hospitals, five in number
- Christian Medical College, Vellore
- Asian Heart Institute, Mumbai
- PD Hinduja National Hospital and Medical Research Centre, Mumbai
- Jaslok Hospital, Mumbai
- Apollo Hospital, Delhi
- Apollo Cancer Hospital, Chennai

Apollo has been a forerunner in medical tourism in India and attracts patients from Southeast Asia, Africa, and the Middle East. The group has tied up with hospitals in Mauritius, Tanzania, Bangladesh and Yemen besides running a hospital in Sri Lanka, and managing a hospital in Dubai. Another corporate group running a chain of hospitals, Escorts, claims it has doubled its number of overseas patients—from 675 in 2000 to nearly 1,200 in 2005. Recently, the Ruby Hospital in Kolkata signed a contract with the British insurance company, BUPA.

The next big wave

The cost differential across the board is huge: only a tenth and sometimes even a sixteenth of the cost in the West. Open-heart surgery could cost up to $70,000 in Britain and up to $150,000 in the US; in India's best hospitals it could cost between $3,000 and $10,000. Knee surgery (on both knees) costs 350,000 rupees ($7,700) in India; in Britain this costs £10,000 ($16,950), more than twice as much. Dental, eye and cosmetic surgeries in Western countries cost three to four times as much as in India.

Several benefits in India include:

(i) *Cost Benefit*: Many of the Indian hospitals, serving international patients, have state-of-the-art infrastructure, highly educated doctors and top-notch services but the figure on that price tag is a fraction of what it would be in developed countries.

(ii) *Timeliness*: Another advantage is the possibility of getting immediate medical attention. There are no waiting lists or delays to contend with, due to insurance issues or unavailability of doctors, etc.

(iii) *Quality Health Care*: Indian doctors and paramedics are well trained and are one of the best in the world. Many professionals, at most of the lead hospitals in the country, have been trained abroad prior to working in India.

(iv) *Personalized Care*: It is relatively easy to find quality personalized care for critically ill or aged patients.

(v) *Technological Sophistication*: State-of-the-art equipment and infrastructure is the order of the day at most of the top corporate hospitals.

(vi) *Facilitation by Government*: The Government of India has recognized the economic potential of medical tourism. It has facilitated travel by introducing a special visa category known as 'medical visa' for patients as well as introduced tax incentives for hospitals.

(vii) *Ease of Travel and Communication*: Travel in India has become easier and much faster due to introduction of private airlines. Access to Internet in India is considered to be one of the cheapest in the world and communication facilities are well established. Travel agencies have a great online presence and can offer you package deals that include travel costs, boarding as well as treatment costs.

(viii) *Easy Availability of Medicine and Drugs*: Certified drugs and medicines are easily available in India, at comparatively lesser prices.

(ix) *Modern and Traditional*: This is India's USP. Modern medical aid as well as traditional therapy, such as ayurveda, yoga, naturopathy etc, is available at different locations across the country including Bangalore.

(x) *Tourism Potential*: People who come for relatively simple, but important procedures, can consider packing in some travel too, with their doctor's permission! This is an added advantage. Every part of the country is rich in history and diverse in geography.

Quest MedTourism

Quest MedTourism facilitates uninsured and underinsured North American patients seeking affordable medical treatments along with an opportunity to explore mystic Asia and near by tourist locations. We help our clients with completion of their travelling documents, departure from their home country, arrangements at the airport, hotel accommodation and assist them choosing the best, cost effective medical procedures at various hospitals across India along with can exhilarating vacation package. Healing begins when the mind and body are relaxed. Let us help you start the healing process. Medical Treatment-India. com (MTI) is an Indian Company, established to help people with Medical needs, schedule Medical Treatment and Travel Arrangements in India. Some of the Medical Treatment Packages offered by MTI are Open Heart Surgery, PTCA (Percutaneous Transluminal Coronary Angioplasty), Total Knee Replacement, Total Hip Replacement, Cervical Spinal Decompression, Bone Marrow Transplant, Spinal Fusion, Spinal Tumor, Craniotomy-Arterio, Micro Vascular Decompression, Excision of Brain Tumor, Breast Reduction, Breast Augmentation, Face Lift, Whipples, Lap Hernia Repair, Nephrectomy, PCNL, Hysterectomy, LSCS with Tubectomy and Kidney Transplant to name a few. Prerana Health Care Services (PHS) is another managed care service organisation providing innovative services towards health care requirements. Delhi-based Beachcomber Tours and Travel that has a tie-up with 'doctors' working in hospitals in and around Delhi. It helps international patients fix appointments with these doctors and facilitate the entire travel, stay and treatment process, besides arranging tours for relatives and patients, including yoga, and ayurvedic treatments. Kerala-based Great Indian Tour Company has however opted for a more professional approach, thanks to its tie-up with one of the most reputed hospitals, Kerala Institute of Medical Sciences. The travel company also helps smoothen the entire process for the patients by acting as a facilitator between the hospital and the patients, besides suggesting holiday destinations.

Some treatment's may not be available in their home country like Hip Resurfacing, less radical than Hip Replacement, but not yet approved by the US Food and Drug Administration, can be availed over here through Medical Treatment India. India also offers a unique variety of Rejuvenation services like Yoga, Meditation, Ayurveda, Allopathy, Homeopathy and other systems of medicines. What makes us a favourable destination is the ease and affordability of international travel, favourable currency exchange rates in the global economy, rapidly improving technology and standards of care.

The various facilities in India include full body pathology, comprehensive physical and gynecological examinations, dental checkup, eye checkup, diet consultation, audiometry, spirometry, stress and lifestyle management, pap smear, digital Chest X-ray, 12 lead ECG, 2D echo colour Doppler, gold standard DXA bone densitometry, body fat analysis, coronary risk markers, cancer risk markers, carotid colour Doppler, spiral CT scan and high strength MRI. Each test is carried out using world-class facilities and infrastructure by professional physicians and trained paramedics, and is comprehensive. There is also a gamut of services ranging from General Radiography, Ultra Sonography, and Mammography to high-end services like Digital Subtraction Angiography along with intervention procedures, Nuclear Imaging. The diagnostic facilities offered in India are comprehensive to include Laboratory services, Imaging, Cardiology, Neurology and Pulmonology. The Laboratory services include biochemistry, hematology, microbiology, serology, histopathology, transfusion medicine, etc.

All medical investigations are conducted on the latest, technologically advanced diagnostic equipment. Stringent quality assurance exercises ensure reliable and high quality test results. Local populace has English-speaking skills; hence communication is not a hurdle. India has kept pace with the latest in technology and its application has been widely felt in the health industry. The strong pharmaceutical sector has gained international recognition. Renowned for ancient alternative therapies like Ayurveda, Yoga, Therapeutic Massage, an exotic tourist destination—India offers beaches, mountains, cosmopolitan cities, quaint villages, and a pilgrimage to suit every palate. These ancient therapies have proved their mettle in the modern age and are most sought after for total wellness.

India seems to have made its mark on the world travel map. Overseas holidayers and travelers have put India in the big league, ranking it as the fourth most attractive and satisfying holiday destination in the world. It stands ahead of several developed and traditional hot spots like US, France, Singapore, Thailand and South Africa. Thanks to CII's proactive role in recognizing the pressing need for standardization in health care. CII has therefore constituted the National Accreditation Board for Hospitals and Health Care Providers (NABH) in January 2006 as a constituent board of Quality Council of India (QCI), set-up with the cooperation of Ministry of Health and Family Welfare, Government of India and Indian Health Industry. According to NABH, there are about 100 standards to be obtained and over 500 measurable objects. The entire procedure of accreditation is a three-cycle process, beginning with the hospitals seeking a pre-assessment procedure. Accreditation of a hospital would be valid for two years, after which it would have to undergo another assessment. They would have to score 70 per cent on the scoring card to get accreditation. The rest of the 30 per cent would have to be covered over the two-year period. Dr. Naresh Trehan, formerly ED of Escorts Heart Institute and now at Apollo hospital, New Delhi and chairman of CII National Committee on health care, reasons that the glaring deficiency in health care standards in the country has resulted in the birth of NABH, which would lend the much required credibility to these hospitals. "We have invited hospitals to get themselves accredited and have received about 50 applications. It is a process and the general standards of delivery will improve in the next couple of years. It is just a matter of time before patients start looking for accredited hospitals," he observes. This in turn will enthuse hospitals, interested in luring international patients, to equip themselves with accreditation. CII has also come out with a price band, in consultation with 16 states, for specialties such as cardiology, minimally invasive surgery, orthopedics and oncology. Veering towards a more sticky issue of insurance, insurance companies are now tying up with Indian hospitals so that international patients can get their expenses covered. What we need is for the medical fraternity as well as the insurance companies to apply for standard accreditation. CII has already started interacting with insurance companies towards this cause and it won't be too long before these companies start recognizing NABH accreditation. Although a standard for accreditation has been set in place by the NABH, there is no mandate that forces hospitals to apply for it if they want to join the health tourism fray.

Health Tourism, the Indian enterprise

Health Tourism India is a professionally managed, diversified enterprise engaged in four core segments of life—Health Care, Biotechnology, Information technology and Education. www.health-tourism-india.com is part of the health care division of Health Tourism India, registered with Government of India as a limited company. Health Tourism India is being managed by a group of medical professionals with an experience of 18 years in the Indian Health Care industry. At Health Tourism India, our commitment is to deliver high quality services always; our belief in values and dedication towards achieving the best is reflected in our work and client satisfaction. At Health Tourism India we commit and dedicate ourselves to our core values of always extending smiling services to the humanity with respect to every individual and the entire existence.

The hospitals are selected on a number of parameters including experience in specific health care segments, panel of doctors, certifications, infrastructural base and past records. Our panel of consultants and surgeons are highly trained and experts in their fields. Most of the doctors have graduated from top US and UK universities and have vast experience in the critical surgeries and procedures they perform. They offer assistance at every stage including pre-travel arrangements and pre-and post-medical treatment support, including passport and visa assistance, itinerary planning, selection of hospital and surgeons, treatment procedure, suitable accommodation, sight seeing of various tourist destinations and finally the much-awaited homecoming.

A large percentage of the overseas public does not have financial access to major medical procedures. These procedures can be a quality of life procedure such as orthopedic, dental cosmetic or a life saving procedure such as cardiac or oncology.

Some of the services offered are:

- Suggesting Hospitals/Clinics as per treatment required/budget.
- World-class Treatment by UK/USA trained Doctors in India.
- Fixation of appointment with Chief Doctors on top priority prior to arrival.
- Arranging consultations with doctors.
- Assisting in planning treatment/check up with appointment fixing and travel scheduling..
- No waiting time for surgical procedures.
- Packages offered only for Medical Treatment till discharge from hospital.
- Coordinating all appointments.
- Nurses/Guide.
- Online assistance to the Patients.

Optional Services

- Stay arrangements, pre-hospitalization and post hospitalization
- Arranging accommodation for family members and attendants.
- Package Tours can be organised at very reasonable cost to various places of interest in places like, Delhi, Chennai, Bangalore, Hyderabad, Mumbai, Agra, etc.
- Can fix-up guides/escorts to accompany if willing.
- All these optional services can be availed, if desired, at nominal service fees.
- Post treatment medical check-up before departure.
- Airport transfers.

A new trend of health care tourism overseas is Corporate or Institutional medical tourism where corporations are coming up with employee health care benefits strategies that would save on corporate medical treatment costs; particularly the corporate are concerned about the rising cost of business health insurance that comes with high premiums to cover surgical interventions and hospitalization expenses for their employees. The corporate surgery treatment abroad and wellness plans provide an easy alternative to save the costs incurred on employee health care and this also keeps the employees happy when they enjoy a family vacation overseas, in privacy, comfort and relaxed setting with the experience of the world-class, advanced health care treatments.

United health group spreads its wings to India

United Health Group began investing in India in 2002 through the acquisition of a health management and administration company, today called United Health Care India. In 2006, United Health Group's commitment to India grew substantially with the start-up of United Health Group Information Services headquartered in Gurgaon. United Health Group employee strength in India will exceed 2100 by the end of 2007 in these two entities. A key strategic location, United Health Group Information Services, Gurgaon is the largest international location outside America for the enterprise. They provide expertise in software development, health care claims adjudication, and biopharmaceutical services.

United Health Care India, headquartered in Mumbai, provides health plan management and administration services. It also provides medical provider management and underwriting solutions to the life insurance industry in India. Its network of health care providers spans 600 cities across India, and includes 1,100 multi-specialty hospitals and over 1,500 diagnostic centers.

The type of work handled by the IT team in Gurgaon includes:

- Health care claims processing systems architecture, development and maintenance targeted at optimally matching claim detail, benefit eligibility and contractual structures.
- Provider systems that enable contract creation and management between hundreds of thousands of doctors, hospitals and United Health Group.
- Eligibility and billing systems that allow customized consumer benefits configuration, billing schemes, and eligibility and benefit matching to patient and provider needs.
- Consumer, employer and other portals providing real-time access to health claim status, care quality information, physician or hospital proximity to consumers and other critical information.
- Data warehouse and health care analytics experience with one of the largest, production data warehouses in the world.
- Commercial software product development for many of our Ingenix solutions.
- Testing Center of Excellence with an emphasis in cross application testing utilizing automated, white box, black box and smoke testing methods.
- Customer Relationship Management (CRM) systems innovation, development and maintenance.

The Health Care business services

The Health Care Business Services team at United Health Group is at the forefront of knowledge and expertise in providing services to the members, health care providers and other key constituents in the health lifecycle. Presently, these are provided through five distinct disciplines:

- *Claim Adjudication*: Manual Claim Adjudication for multiple

health care specialties, places of service, benefit and plan types inclusive of both core medical and ancillary care services.
2. *Network Intelligence*: Reimbursement analysis for competitive markets and efficiency ratings in delivery of health care services.
3. *Member Benefit Analysis*: Analysis of member benefit details and policy changes in support of member usability and access and the efficiency of the claim adjudication cycle.
4. *Member Benefit Creation and Database Management*: Workflow focused on detailed creation of multiple benefit types for the member community and management of changes to same.
5. *Back-end Rule Setting*: Setting proper rule structures to the end of driving higher efficiency and accuracy in the automatic and manual adjudication processes.

Destination Bangalore/Chandigarh

Chandigarh and Bangalore were planned and set-up as new modern cities after independence. Chandigarh has become a hub of medical tourism for the domestic patients of northern India. Now it is in the forefront of planning facilities in the private sector to attract medical tourists from abroad. The concept of a Medical city, with a cluster of hospitals in every discipline is being explored.

Bangalore has professional experts, technological sophistication and health care services that easily match the best in the world. Bangalore has a pleasant weather all through the year. Some of the lead institutes and private hospitals in Bangalore with regular patients from abroad include: Hosmat, Recoup, Soukya, Narayana Hrudalaya, NIMHANS, Wockhardt, Advanced fertility centre, Sagar Apollo, Kidwai Memorial Institute of Oncology, Sri Jayadeva Institute of Cardiology, St. John's Hospital, St. Martha's Victoria Hospital and Sri Sathya Sai Institute of Higher Medical Sciences, Mallya Hospital, Manipal Hospital and The Bangalore Hospital.

Popular specializations for medical consultation, treatments and surgeries in Bangalore include Cardiology, Orthopedics, Nephrology, Neurology, Neurosurgery, Dentistry, Oncology, Infertility, Gynecology, Homeopathy, Ayurveda, Naturopathy, etc.

Wockhardt's hospital in Bangalore, which has a Harvard Medical International tie-up, gets half of its foreign patients (about 900), from the U.K. The media reported the story of one such patient with coronary heart disease, 73-year old George Marshall last year. This violin repairer from Bradford was operated upon at the hospital for a quarter of what he would have paid for private care in the UK, including the airfare. When he arrived in India, he was initially shocked by the traffic chaos and urban squalor, but it appeared to be a better decision than having to suffer a long delay for bypass surgery in a state-supported National Health Service hospital. Another 35 per cent of Wockhardt's patients come to Bangalore from the U.S. and the rest from the European Union and South East Asia. Another heart care institution in Bangalore, Narayana Hrudayalaya, has a record of

15,000 surgeries performed on patients from 25 foreign countries, half of them children.

India's islands of medical and surgical excellence

India has state of the art Hospitals, good infrastructure, the best possible surgical facilities, with the most competitive prices. A patient will come to India where he will undergo surgical treatment and recuperatrate in resorts having world class facilities. The whole thing would save him a lot of money and he will get to discover India at the same time. A number of private hospitals in India offer packages designed to attract foreign patients, with airport-to-hospital bed transfer service, Internet access, and other facilities. Some packages include add-ons, such as a yoga holiday or a trip to the world-famous Taj Mahal. However, the sight of the country's overcrowded public hospitals, open sewers and garbage-littered streets can unsettle visitors' confidence about sanitation standards in India. Private health care providers argue that foreigners can be sheltered from such nastiness. "In a corporate hospital, once the door is closed you could be in a hospital in America." Vishal Bali, President of Wockhardt Hospitals, points out as proof of quality that the US private health insurers Blue Cross and Blue Shield insure patients treated at his group's hospitals. The British health insurer Bupa also insures the costs of treatment at Wockhardt hospitals.

Some Indian Hospitals of repute are:

- *AIIMS*: A public sector hospital; source of trained manpower and research.
- *Apollo Hosptials group*: Most well organized and with JCI accreditation.
- *B.M. Birla Heart Research Centre*: A specialized hospital dedicated exclusively to the diagnosis, treatment and research related to cardiovascular diseases. It has established itself as India's most advanced heart center.
- *Christian Medical College, Vellore*: Occupies a prominent place among medical institutions in India as a 1,700-bed multi-campus complex.
- *Tata Memorial Cancer Hospital*: Located at Dr. Ernest Borges Marg, Parel, in the Central District of Mumbai, a short taxi ride from the local stations, the hospital has private and deluxe rooms.
- *Apollo Cancer Hospital*: The first hospital in the country to be awarded the ISO 9002 certificate.
- *Indraprastha Medical Corporation*: India's first corporate hospital and the third largest corporate hospital outside the USA.
- *Institute Cardiovascular Diseases*: Has gained a reputation for being one of the most advanced centers in the world.

- *Escorts Hospital and Research Centre*: One of the most frequented hospital for heart ailments.
- *Nehru Hospital, PGI*: A centre of excellence for trained manpower and research.
- *Sahaj Dental Clinic*: Experience Mystic India with World Class Dental Treatment.
- *Inspiration Kerala*: Kerala tour operator, offering ayurveda packages.
- *Advent Medical Services*: Medical service provider with vast experience in medical field.
- *Prerana Health Care Services*: A managed care service organisation.
- *Hinduja Hospital*: Indian National Hospital and Medical esearch Centre.
- *MediEscapes India*: Indian Medical Tourism operator which offers world class medical treatments.
- *Care and Cure Medi-Tours*: Facilitate ailing patients in neighbouring countries to Chennai (India).
- *Longfield Management*: World Class Economical Health Care.
- *Dr. Agarwal Vasans Eye Hospital*: One of the leading eye hospitals in Tamilnadu.

India aims to replicate the Thai model, which is still the first Asian destination for International Patients. A case study done by CII has revealed that Thailand with a population of 60 millions has been successful in attracting 1 million health tourists last year because of the development of world-class infrastructure. It was possible due to aggressive international marketing in conjunction with tourism authority. It has also been integrated with traditional medicine. Government should encourage medical tourism by increasing air connectivity linking major cities like Delhi, Chennai, Bangalore, Hyderabad, Chandigarh and Kolkata, and create health support infrastructure. Setting up of a chain of world class hospitals, i.e Medi city model of health care will not only attract medical tourists from all over the world but also solve the problem of health care of the Indian people.

CII says that it is also essential to establish the Indian health care brand synonymous with safety, trust and excellence. There is also a need to streamline immigration process for medical visitors. If India develops its infrastructure to international levels, it will be able to benefit medical services sector and moreover help the world access the Indian medical services. India has to move into a new area of "medical outsourcing" where sub-contractors aim to provide services to the overburdened medical care systems in western countries. Medical tourism industry in India would bring in revenues worth USD 25 billion by 2020. One of the best-managed health care groups in India with about 6,000 beds, has revenue of about USD 125 million. Going with these numbers, the assumption based on crude mathematical projection is that, it would require about 60,000 beds, to reach USD 1.25 billion revenue and 12,00,000 beds to obtain a revenue of USD 25 billion exclusively from health care services.

In 2003, about 2,726,000 tourists visited India and the revenue from the same was USD 3.5 billion. Well, if that many relatives of patients (about 3 million) travel to India, we could manage another USD 3.5 billion from tourism services.

Currently, the bulk of the patients come to India from neighbouring countries such as Bangladesh, Pakistan, other Asian countries, Africa and the Middle East. A segment of patients sponsored by the governments in their respective countries such as Middle East and Africa come to India; relatively a cost-effective option compared to Europe or the US. Unsponsored patients from these countries look at India as value for money option *vis-a-vis* Europe and US. Moreover, post 9/11 there has been a dramatic drop in patients from Middle East to the US. The market segment that the health care industry is targeting is the patient population from Europe and the US. There are several patients of Indian origin residing in UK and US, who are already using the services of hospitals in India, when they are on vacation, etc. Apart from this we have the widely-publicized cases of patients from the US and Australia. We may want to recognize that a strategy which works for attracting patients from Bangladesh may not work for patients from Britain, since the expectations and drivers are different. What is a good reason for an average senior citizen in the US to fly 18-20 hours to get his hip replaced? Can he even travel with hips in such bad shape? Obviously if he is not covered by insurance and cannot afford the same in US he has to look at options. What if this can be done in Mexico or Costa Rica at comparable rate and a shorter flight? Would a patient be willing to trust his heart, kidneys, hips and face if there is an iota of doubt regarding the quality of care? This segment of high yielding procedures is where the Indian medical tourism market is looking forward to for better profits.

The Apollo Hospitals Group

The Apollo Hospitals Group's hospitals are Located at Delhi, Chennai, Hyderabad and Madurai. Its history of accomplishments, with its unique ability of resource management and able deployment of technology and knowledge to the service of its patients, justifies its recognition in India and abroad. India could earn more than $1 billion annually and create 40 million new jobs by sub-contracting work from the British National Health Service, says Apollo Hospitals. This includes surgery for hip and knee replacements and coronary bypass that would slash waiting times dramatically, reducing the queues of British patients waiting to see their doctors, Dr. Reddy said.

Apollo group alone has so far treated 95,000 international patients, many of whom are of Indian origin. Reddy cited two recent cases of UK nationals who opted for private health care at the Apollo network. One of them—Cyril Parry, a 50-year-old man from Birmingham—successfully underwent hip replacement surgery at Apollo, Chennai. The other—Buckingham Palace employee Elaine Ackrill—was also treated at the Chennai Apollo for cancer of the uterine cervix. Apollo was represented at a London meeting that was also attended by a UK government health adviser and private health care providers from South Africa, Australia, India and the UK. The Apollo team offered a medical tourism package that would cut waiting times for surgery in the UK. "They have a one million waiting list for all kinds of things, especially orthopaedic surgery," explained an Apollo spokesman.

In Apollo hospital group, about 100 beds are usually occupied by foreign patients, mostly from the Middle East, Africa and countries of south Asia. Indeed, demand for medical tourism is most likely to come from among the 25 m-strong Indian diaspora, says Deep Kalra, chief executive officer of travel agency makemytrip.com. NRIs would combine regular visits to India and save time and money by undergoing non-emergency procedures such as eye operations, dental work, cosmetic surgery and knee surgery.

For follow-ups of the medical tourists, Apollo has set the telemedicine centres, where through video-conferencing patients get in touch with their patients, informs Anjali. Last year in November, the group opened a telemedicine centre at the Om Hospital in Nepal. Incidentally, Apollo opened its first international Apollo Health and Lifestyle Ltd. (AHLL) clinic at Doha in 2005. Apollo is looking to branch in South-east Asia, West Asia, Africa, UK and USA through this model, informs Mr. Jalan. Talking about challenges; competition from Singapore and Thailand. However, the cost in India is one fifth of Singapore and half of Thailand. The cardiac success rate here is more than 98.6 per cent. "We are planning to work with insurance providers and health care providers abroad in the UK and the US", they add. Patient break-up at Apollo from various countries is as follows: US and other countries—10.5 per cent, Maldives—46 per cent, Nepal—16.6 per cent, Oman—10.1 per cent, Sri Lanka—22 per cent, Bangladesh—27 per cent.

- o Among the few providers of quaternary care for complicated medical conditions.
- o Touched the lives of over 10 million patients till date.
- o Over 4,00,000 Preventive Health checks done.
- o Has the largest and the most sophisticated sleep laboratories in the World.
- o Pioneered procedures like Total Hip and knee replacements, and the Birmingham Hip Resurfacing technique.
- o Has performed over 750,000 major surgeries and over 10,00,000 minor surgical procedures till date.
- o Has performed over 49,000 cardiac surgeries at a 98.5% success rate.
- o Has performed over 2,00,000 angiograms, 16,200 angoplasties (PTCA) and 3,500 mitral balloon valvuoplasties.

- First heart transplant patient is alive, 7 years after the operation.
- Has performed over 9,400 renal transplants.
- 130 Bone Marrow Transplants performed at high success rates.
- Over 30 Liver transplants done (Live and cadaver).
- Has over 4,000 specialists and super specialists, 3,000 medical officers spanning 53 clinical departments in patient care.

International Affiliations

- Apollo Hospitals is recognized as a training centre by the National Board of Examination in India for post-graduate training in 16 medical departments.
- The Department of Radiology at Apollo is recognized by the Royal College of Radiologists, United Kingdom for training for fellowship examinations like FRCR.
- Recognized as a centre for conducting research work leading to Ph.D. of the Anna University, Chennai, in medical physics and digital signal processing.
- Apollo Hospitals is recognized by the Royal College of Physicians and Surgeons in Edinburgh for training postgraduates in radiology, surgery and trauma care.
- Apollo Hospitals is the only International training organisation for the American Heart Association Technical support from Texas Heart institute and Minneapolis Heart Institute for Cardiology and Cardio Thoracic surgery.
- Apollo Hospitals have exchange programs with the Hospitals in the US and Europe.
- Apollo Hospitals have an association with Mayo Clinic and Cleveland Heart Institute, USA.
- Apollo Hospitals is also associated with Johns Hopkins University.

Apollo launches Asia's first health city: Hyderabad, Tuesday, 12 June, 2007

Going beyond the realm of curative care it offers, the health city is an integrated facility offering solutions across the health care space including preventive care, holistic medicine, research, information technology and education. Spread over 33 acres at Apollo Hospital in Jubilee Hills here, the health city encompasses a 300-bedded multi-specialty hospital with over 50 specialties and super specialties along with 10 centres of excellence. Centres of excellence for heart diseases, cancer, orthopaedics and joint diseases, emergency, renal diseases, neurosciences, eye, minimally invasive surgery, trauma and cosmetic surgery are coming up in the integrated facility.

The Apollo Group plans to apply for a special economic zone (SEZ) status to the health city. "It is not a medical city where you treat only the illness. The Apollo Health City takes care of totality of wellness," Prathap C. Reddy, Chairman, Apollo Hospitals Group, told media hours before the formal launch of the city. He said Rs. 1000 crore were already spent in creating the existing infrastructure for the health city while another Rs. 150-Rs. 250 crore would be invested in setting up research institutes over the next six months. "Once Britain dominated the health care space, then US and now India is emerging as the global health care destination and Hyderabad with the Apollo Health City will lead the way for that," he said. He pointed out that research and technology had always been the thrust of Apollo. Apollo Health City has a variety of initiatives including medical BPO services for offshore customers (health street), online education for medical professionals (Medvarsity) and telemedicine services. The health city has already tied up with Tata Consultancy Service (TCS) for hospital information system. The system connects all Apollo Hospitals and 100 telemedicine centres in India and in Dubai, Kuwait, Doha, Nigeria, Dhaka and Sri Lanka. "We plan to connect 52 African countries through telemedicine," he said. Reddy said Apollo Group was focussing on research in key areas like cardiology, oncology, diabetes and neuro sciences. Apollo has joined hands with Johns Hopkins Medicine International, US, to undertake a collaborative study on cardiovascular diseases in India. "We want to find out why Asians are more prone to heart diseases," he said. He said Apollo created many benchmarks since its inception. "We have performed more than 59,000 heart surgeries with a success rate of 99.6 per cent," he said. Apollo Health City is equipped to create a global talent pool of medical professionals. It will have institutes of PG education for doctors, nursing school and college, hospital administration, medical informatics, emergency medicine and paramedics. The focus at the health city will be on holistic health and facility will offer alternative forms of medicine, the benefits of which have been demonstrated across the world.

One of Asia's largest health care groups, Apollo runs 41 hospitals in India and abroad. It has an annual turnover of Rs. 600 crore.

ESCORTS HEART INSTITUTE AND RESEARCH CENTRE, DELHI

Dr. Naresh Trehan worked as a heart surgeon in Manhattan from 1968 until 1988, and then returned to India to start the Escorts Hospital Group in India. He says the success of the operations performed and the care dispensed at his hospital have established the institute's credibility: "Now we do over 4,000 heart operations a year, and the mortality, which is an index of how well things are, is 0.8% which is even better than most places in the world. The other thing that we measure is infection rate. Ours is 0.3% as compared to the world average of 1%." Escorts is steadily consolidating its presence in health care, which is likely to emerge as the largest service sector industry. Currently, Escorts is operating three large hospitals in New Delhi, Faridabad and Amritsar. Together with 11 heart command centres and associate hospitals, Escorts is managing nearly 900 beds. Escorts excellence in providing health care services has received due recognition. Escorts Heart Institute and Research Centre (EHIRC), New Delhi, has been ranked as the best cardiac hospital in India by an Outlook survey and has been given the highest grade by CRISIL—an acknowledgement of the quality of delivered patient care. EHIRC is a leader in the fields of cardiac surgery, interventional cardiology and cardiac diagnostics. The Institute has introduced innovative techniques of minimally invasive and robotic surgery. The Institute's latest addition of state-of-the-art Cardiac Scan Centre providing a combined power of CV-MRI and Smart Score CT Scanner to diagnose coronary artery disease at its very early stage. This facility is the first of its kind outside America. State-of-the-art infrastructure and equipment has made this set-up technically the largest and the best dedicated cardiac hospital in the world. The 332-bed Institute has nine operating rooms and carries out nearly 15,000 procedures every year.

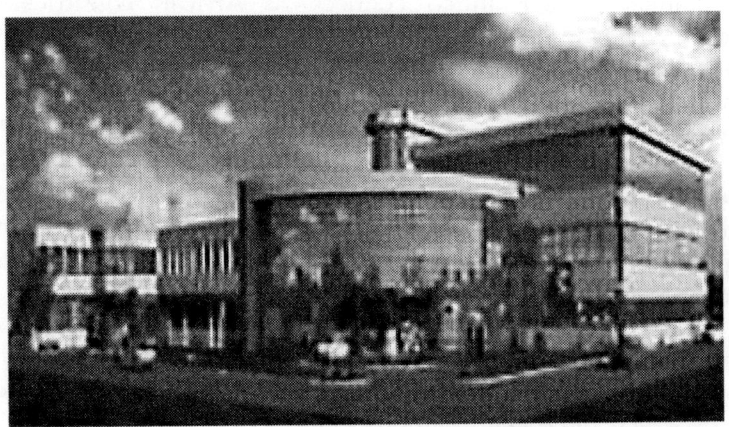

NM EXCELLENCE, MUMBAI

NM Excellence was formed from one man's vision to provide a healthier future for the citizens of Mumbai. Established in 2001 by Dr. Nilesh Shah, this modern and sophisticated preventive health checkup centre aims to revolutionize the way health care is perceived and practiced in India. Backed by over two decades of diagnostic experience under the banner of NM Medical, NM Excellence employs the latest, top-of-the-line imagining modalities, operated by qualified and professional doctors, with a friendly and efficient staff to make a client's experience as memorable as possible. Having viewed the vast range of diseases that can be prevented if detected early enough through its diagnostic experience, NM Excellence philosophizes that a preventive health checkup in today's day and age is an absolute must. NM Excellence is one of Mumbai's foremost preventive health care centers boasting of top-of-the-line diagnostic equipment, highly qualified doctors, a well-trained service staff, and a professional yet warm environment that makes one feel at home immediately.

Health Plan for NRI's and Foreigners

The Plan Price starts from US$ 225+ and includes the following:

Pathology Tests	Complete haemogram, test for diabetes, test for liver disease, test for kidney disease, test for heart disease.
Diagnostic Tests	Digital Chest X-ray, ECG, Sonography, Stress Test, 2D Echo, Spirometry, Dexa Bone Densitometry, Body Fat Analysis, Mammography, Transvaginal Sonography.
Consultations	Physical Examination by Physician, Dental Checkup, Eye Checkup, Diet Consultation, Gynecological Checkup, Pap-Smear.

PD HINDUJA NATIONAL HOSPITAL AND MEDICAL RESERCH CENTRE, MUMBAI

An ultramodern hospital on the busiest artery in Central Mumbai, PD Hinduja National Hospital and Medical Research Centre was established by the Hinduja Foundation in collaboration with Massachusetts General Hospital (MGH), Boston. The fulfillment of Founder Parmanand Deepchand Hinduja's dream, the 351-bed hospital offers comprehensive services covering the gamut from diagnosis and investigation to therapy, surgery and post-operative care. As a tertiary care hospital, the services offered are comprehensive covering investigation and diagnosis to therapy, surgery and post-operative care. According to Dr. Gustad B. Daver, director, professional services, Hinduja Hospital, "A good set-up in a hospital like pre-operative evaluation, an extensive lab set-up and operation theatre facilities, good post operative, intensive care and radiological facilities will be of major help to boost health tourism." Besides this, a proper civic infrastructure needs to be in place like airports and good roads. "There should be proper visa facilities and preferential treatment at immigration," opines Verma. Experts cite that medical insurance, alternate wellness concepts and BPO in diagnostics are other upcoming businesses, which will give a boost to medical tourism in the coming years. Apollo's business began to grow in the 1990s, with the liberalization of the Indian economy.

The inpatient services are complemented with a day centre, out-patient facilities and an exclusive center for health check for executives. Hinduja Hospital was the first multi-disciplinary tertiary care hospital to have been awarded the prestigious ISO 9002 Certification from KEMA of Netherlands for Quality Management System

The Hinduja Foundation's quest for upgradation of health care facilities in India has prompted it to join hands with the 45,000 member American Association of Physicians of Indian origin (AAPI), with the objective of bringing to India well qualified and experienced doctors from USA to upgrade the expertise of HNH doctors, provide quality medical care and continuing medical education; to ensure co-operation in research and pursue joint projects in the fields of: Coronary artery disease, Osteoporosis and Asthma; and to provide consultancy, technology and treatment support to AAPI dispensaries in India on case to case basis. Hinduja Hospital has a fully automated Laboratory Medicine Department. The Laboratory offers over 500 different types of tests some of which are exclusive. It also offers an emergency/Stat menu of tests with a very short turn around time. The department participates in International Quality Control programme conducted by the College of American Pathologists, WHO and National Quality Control Programme where it has achieved and maintained a high ranking consistently for a number of years. Imaging forms a key part of the diagnostic facility at the hospital.

The hospital keeps upgrading its technology by acquiring new state-of-the-art diagnostic and therapeutic equipment. Hinduja Hospital was the first in India to acquire the Gamma Knife-gold standard in Radio surgery, a non-invasive neurosurgical tool. The hospital was also the first to acquire the Holmium Laser in the country thus replacing the surgeon's scalpel. The Oncology Services are wholistic and complete with installation of the Linear Accelerator with Multileaf Collimator (MLC) and Micro MLC. The hospital is the first centre in India to have installed the sophisticated state-of-the-art GE-LCA Digital Subtraction Angiography System. In keeping with the quest for continuous improvement in quality and technological advancement, the hospital has recently commissioned the Bone Mineral Densitometer (DEXA), an addition to the Imaging department.

LV PRASAD EYE INSTITUTE, HYDERABAD

In October 1987, LV Prasad Eye Institute began the work of realizing its mission to achieve excellence, equity and efficiency in eye care. In addition to treating patients dealing with a wide range of vision problems, LVPEI began to conduct research into eye diseases and vision-threatening

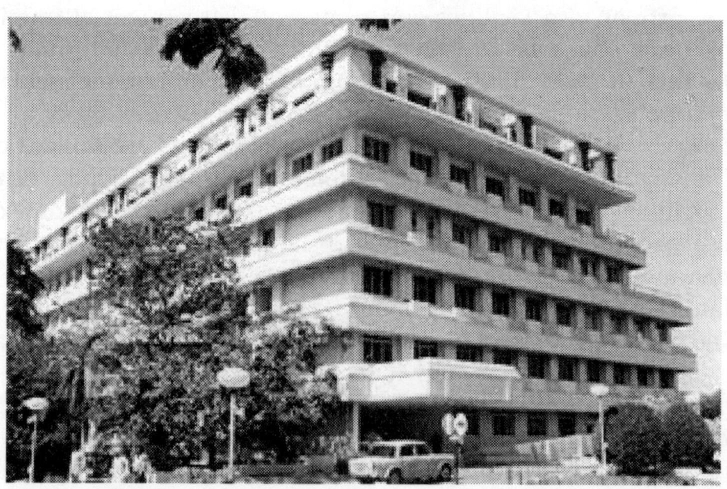

conditions, train eye care workers, product development and rehabilitate those with incurable visual disability. The focus, right from the start, has been on providing eye-care services to underprivileged populations in the developing world

Set up as a not-for-profit trust, LVPEI has now come a long way in its journey towards realizing these goals. However, our changing world continues to throw up new challenges and new threats to health, and LVPEI too continues to search for ways in which these challenges can be overcome, in the field of eye health. In partnership with international health organisations such as the World Health Organisation and the International Agency for the Prevention of Blindness, LVPEI designs and implements innovative eye health programmes that reach people in the most remote rural areas. While the range of our research and training activities is international, our focus is on bringing this quality of care to the poorest segments of India and the developing world. Our successes include the establishment of rural eye health centers that provide high-quality eye care at the lowest possible cost, or at no cost to those to whom such care would otherwise be inaccessible. In fact it is this same model that operates successfully in our nodal center in Hyderabad, Andhra Pradesh. At the LV Prasad Eye Hospital, nearly 50 percent of our patients are treated free of cost. The Eye Hospital forms the nucleus of the Institute's activities. Designed along the lines of the finest eye hospitals in the world. Patients with a wide range of eye disorders are treated which is staffed by a world-class team of dedicated doctors representing all ophthalmic sub-specialties and a highly competent support staff. The Hospital's comprehensive facilities also include the in-house expertise of physicians, microbiologists, pathologists and biochemists trained to apply their knowledge and skills to eye care.

INDIA'S MOST-FAVOURED HEALTH CARE DESTINATION, BANGALORE

Around Rs. 2,000 crore has already been invested in the city's health care and medical infrastructure. It houses four medical colleges (two more are coming up), three super-speciality hospitals, development bases of medical equipment manufacturers like GE Medical, Siemens and Philips, research outfits of Novo Nordisk (diabetic) and AstraZeneca (TB), in addition to a large number of pharma and biotech companies. Increased direct air connectivity brings in patients, mostly suffering from heart ailments, from countries like Bangladesh, the UAE, Nepal, Sri Lanka and Malaysia to Bangalore. A by-pass surgery that costs Rs. 5 lakh in Malaysia costs only Rs. 90,000 in Bangalore. The Karnataka government, in association with the Confederation of Indian Industry (CII), is currently creating a blueprint for a competitive hospital infrastructure in the city. "Bangalore has the potential to become the world's third largest health care hub after Phoenix (Arizona) and Florida," says D.A. Prasanna, CEO, Wipro Health Care and Life Science. Prasanna heads the recently formed 50-member CII Committee for Health Care with trade body, government, academia and health care industry representatives. According to him, the panel is in the process of locating potential niches in health care. "All these will enhance medical infrastructure of the city to be on par with global standards."

Vishal Bali, Wockhardt President and Head, CII Task Force on Health, feels Bangalore definitely is the leading health care destination in the entire Asian sub-continent. "We have competitive technology, clinical expertise and a clear focus on patients' satisfaction." Wockhardt is the only hospital in the country to have a tie-up with the Harvard Medical School. "We are trying to create Bangalore as a health care hub through international partnerships and expertise sharing. We are trying to bring in global medical and clinical practices and expertise," Bali adds. Here's what Narayana Hrudayala founder Devi Shetty has to say: "The basic requirement for health care is super-specialty professionals, and Bangalore has a large pool of them." According to him, even reputed doctors from the US, Europe and West Asia are willing to relocate to Bangalore as the hospitals are capable of matching their salaries. Setting up hospital infrastructure in Bangalore is cost-effective, reasons Dr. Shetty. For instance, a hospital which costs Rs. 100 crore in Bangalore will cost Rs. 500 crore in Mumbai. Novo Nordisk India Managing Director Dr. Anil Kapur says Bangalore, which is already an IT hub, is fast becoming a biotechnology base. Though the biotech-based pharma industry is still in a nascent stage in the city, it can easily capitalize on the existing medical infrastructure to become a leading player in terms of patient-record systems, drug research and telemedicine. Dr. S. Anand Kumar, director, Research Foundation of AstraZeneca, says Bangalore had an excellent environment for drug discovery, but needs a marketing push.

Destination Bangalore

Some of the lead institutes and private hospitals in Bangalore with regular patients from abroad include: Hosmat, Recoup, Soukya, Manipal, Narayana Hrudalaya, NIMHANS, Wockhardt, Advanced fertility centre, Sagar Apollo, Kidwai Memorial Institute of Oncology, Sri Jayadeva Institute of Cardiology, St. John's Hospital, St. Martha's, Victoria Hospital and Sri Sathya Sai Institute of Higher Medical Sciences, Mallya Hospital, Manipal Hospital and The Bangalore Hospital.

Popular specializations for medical consultation, treatments and surgeries in Bangalore include Cardiology, Orthopedics, Nephrology, Neurology, Neurosurgery, Dentistry, Oncology, Infertility, Gynecology, Homeopathy, Ayurveda, Naturopathy, etc.

KOVAI MEDICAL CENTRE AND HOSPITAL LTD.

Spread over a campus of around 20 acres, Kovai Medical Center and Hospital Ltd. (KMCH) is a 400-bed multi-disciplinary super-specialty corporate hospital located in Coimbatore. The hospital is equipped with most modern equipments like CT Scanner, Angiography equipment, Operating Microscope, Mammography, Color Doppler, etc.

The hospital has over 30 Medical Departments and 11 Operation Theatres. The hospital is fully equipped and has developed expertise to conduct Super Specialty procedures like Coronary Bypass Surgeries, Coronary Angioplasty, Stent Implantation, Laparoscopic and Vascular Surgeries, Hip and Knee replacements, Kidney transplants, and complex Neuro-surgeries. The hospital is recognized to carry out Renal transplants, Corneal transplants and Heart transplants by Tamil Nadu Government.

Satellite Centres

The hospital has two satellite medical centers located at Ramnagar in Coimbatore and Perundurai, Distt. Erode. The satellite centre at Coimbatore is a 10 bed hospital with facilities like 24 hours Accident and Emergency Services, 24 hours pharmacy, Laboratory, X-Ray and ECG Services, Obstetrics and Gynecology, Pediatrics, Dermatology, General Consultation, Physiotherapy Centre and Dental Hospital.

The other satellite centre located at Perundurai is a 50 bed hospital with facilities like 24 hours Accident and Emergency Services, Laboratory, Radiology and pharmacy services, General Medicine, Chest Clinic, Obstetrics and Gynecology, Pediatrics, Dermatology, General Consultation, and Physiotherapy Centre.

Financials

The latest financials of the company are given as under:

(Rs. in Crores)

Particulars	*Qurt. Ended (Dec. 2006)*	*Qurt. Ended (Dec. 2005)*	*Qurt. Ended (% Var.)*	*YTD/ Latest Half (Dec. 2006)*	*YTD/ Latest Half (Dec. 2005)*	*YTD/ Latest Half (% Var.)*	*Year Ended (Mar. 2006)*	*Year Ended (Mar. 2005)*	*Year Ended (% Var.)*
Sales	18	13.31	35.2	48.5	37.7	28.6	51.18	40.55	26.2
Other Income	0.14	0.14	0	0.36	0.41	-12.2	0.58	0.56	3.6
PBIDT	4.4	2.97	48.1	11.15	8.15	36.8	9.9	5.96	66.1
Interest	0.21	0.23	-8.7	0.79	0.73	8.2	0.96	0.94	2.1
PBDT	4.19	2.74	52.9	10.36	7.42	39.6	8.94	5.02	78.1
Depreciation	0.85	0.78	9	2.57	2.33	10.3	3.07	2.69	14.1
PBT	3.34	1.96	70.4	7.79	5.09	53	5.87	2.33	151.9
Tax	1.11	0.26	326.9	2.53	0.51	396.1	1.16	0.19	510.5
Deferred Tax	0.35	0	-	0.3	0	0	0.83	0.98	-15.3
PAT	1.88	1.7	10.6	4.96	4.58	8.3	3.88	1.16	234.5

Source: Capitaline.

The company is scaling up its capacity through an expansion project and through acquisitions. The company is currently expanding its capacity by 200 beds at its existing campus at Coimbatore. The specialty block is under construction and is expected to start operations from June 2008. The expansion programme will also improve certain infrastructure facilities like captive power generation, centralized air-conditioning system, pneumatic pipe line system for transporting materials and a state of the art IT Infrastructure for managing the Hospital operations. The company is also making substantial investments to upgrade the diagnostic treatment facilities to cover specialty departments in the Hospital like Cardiology, General Surgery, Orthopedics, and Intensive Care, etc. The company has recently entered into a Memorandum of Understanding (MOU) with Idhayam Hospitals Erode Ltd. located at Erode to acquire 100% stake in the company. The agreed purchase consideration is Rs. 925 Lacs, which involves discharge of unsecured loans, one time settlement with the Lenders, Cost of Medical Equipments and payment to the shareholders. Idhayam Hospital has a 50-bedded Hospital at Erode, which is exclusively for Cardio-thoracic patients.

Kovai Medical owns a 400-bed hospital and two Satellite Centres located in Southern part of the country. The company is aggressively scaling up its capacity—both through organic and inorganic route. For the current FY, the expected revenues of the company are Rs. 70-72 crores with a PAT of Rs. 7.0 crores. With its existing market cap of Rs. 60 crores, the valuations of the company look attractive, when compared with the peer group.

The new hospital acquired by the company is capable of adding Rs. 8-10 crores to the topline of the company in a year. Therefore assuming a growth of 20% from the existing operations and addition from Idhayam Hospital, the company can target revenues of Rs. 90-95 crores in FY 07-08. Moreover, with the expansion at its existing campus in Coimbatore getting completed by June 08, one can look forward to substantially higher revenues in the future.

DR. VIVEK SAGGAR'S DENTAL CARE AND CURE CENTRE, LUDHIANA

The newest and fastest-growing area of medical tourism is a visit to the dentist, where costs are often not covered by basic insurance and by

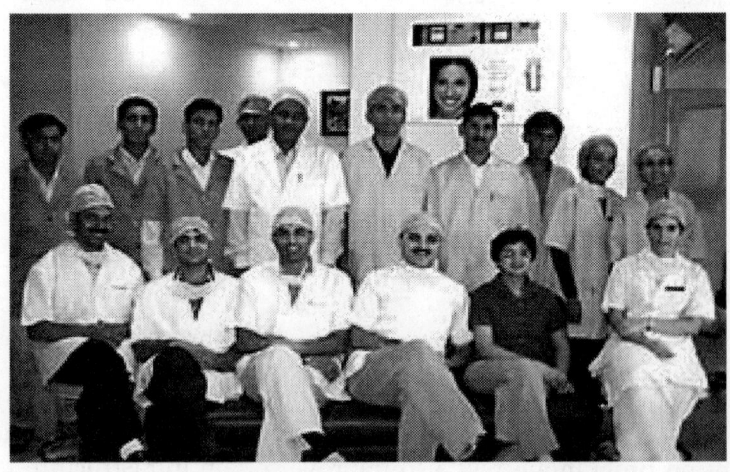

only some extended insurance policies. India, Thailand and Hungary attract patients who want to combine a filling, extraction or root canal with a vacation.

Dental Care and Cure Centre is, centrally located in Ludhiana, easily approachable from any part of Punjab by rail or road. It takes not more than two hours from any part of Punjab to reach this place. Theirs is a 6 chair operatory with an in-house dental lab, the Dental Caps, Crowns and Beyond Dental Lab, which has been designed on the European standards. The office has been designed to provide an environment of comfort that combines exceptional skill levels, a respectful approach to treatment, clinical and technical excellence with an individualized care approach by providing the most advanced, optimal dental care to the best of our ability. Theirs is a full service cosmetic and general dental office specializing in creating beautiful smiles. The in-house facility of Dental Caps, Crowns and Beyond . . . Dental Lab gives them the unmatched time advantage plus international quality control. For NRI's and foreigners they provide special care in the form of appointments at a short notice and the work is completed within the span of 3-5 days keeping in mind your tight schedule.

Advanced technology

- Smile Designing.
- Crown and Bridge Work.
- Tooth Whitening.
- Dental Implants (single tooth or entire set of teeth).
- Oral and Maxillofacial Surgery (third molar extractions, apicoectomy surgeries, management of mandible fractures).
- Geriatric Patient (partial and complete dentures, implant supported dentures, complete extractions under local anesthesia).
- Diagnostic and Preventive (cancer screening, occlusal splints, tooth desensitization).
- Care of the Child Patient (fluoride treatment, milk teeth as well as permanent teeth restorations, preventive orthodontics, fixed orthodontics, habit breaking appliances, sedation dentistry.

5

Flow of International Patients to Kerala: The Wellness Paradise

Kerala is probably the greenest place you will ever see. The coconut palms, the red tilted houses, the innumerable lakes and beaches will remain long lasting impressions to any visitor. The colourful festivals like ONAM and VISHU, various dances like Kathakali, Kaikottikali, Mohiniyattom and Koodiyattam, martial arts like Kalaripayattu and wildlife sanctuaries are the other attractions. Kerala is a very attractive tourist place in India. Location: Kerala is a narrow strip of land located on the south western edge of the Indian Sub-continent. It is sandwiched between the Western Ghats mountain range on the East and the Arabian Sea on the West.

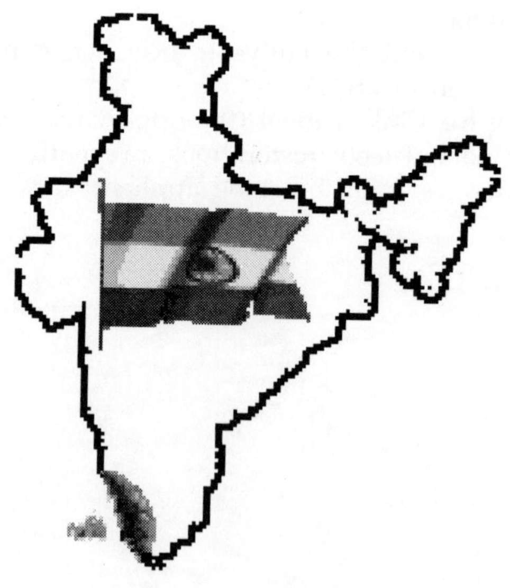

Area	38,863 sq km
Population	29,011,237 census 1991
Density of Population	749/sq km
Capital	Thiruvananthapuram (Trivandrum)
Language	Malayalam, Hindi, English
Time	GMT +5.30 hrs
Climate	Summer—February to May (Max. 33°C Min. 24°C) Monsoon—June to September (Max. 28°C Min. 22°C) Winter—October to September (Max. 32°C Min. 22°C)
Best Time To Visit	September to May

Geologist are of the view that Kerala was formed much later than the rest of the subcontinent. Submarine earth movement probably pushed up the land between the curves of the Western Ghats to form this wonderful land. It is possible that the earth inhabitants could have witnessed this geological event leading to the creation of the myths and legends concerning the birth of Kerala.

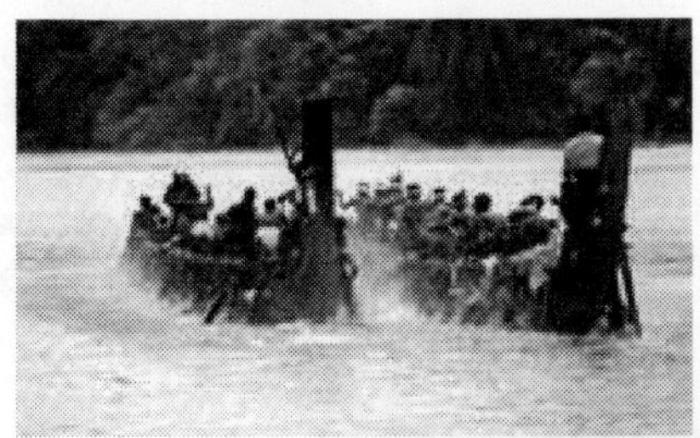

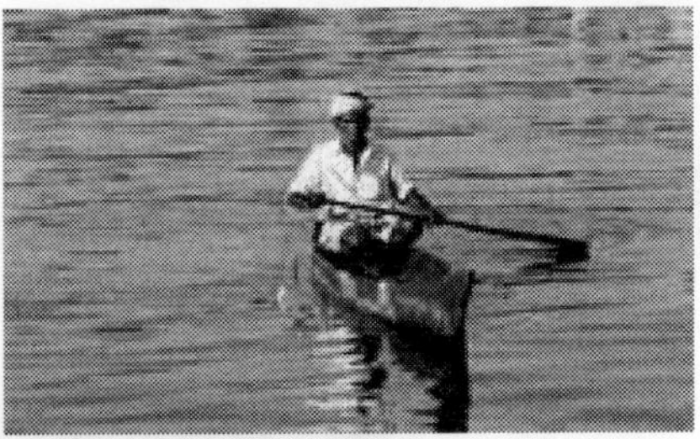

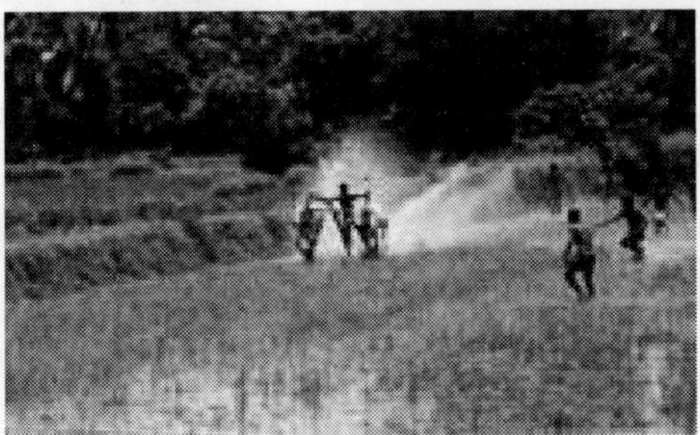

The interesting thing about the myths and legends of Kerala are that they are so strongly interlinked with scientific facts and history that it is very difficult to distinguish between fact and fiction.

The Pioneer State for International health tourists

Kerala, 'God's Own Country', has pioneered health and medical tourism in India. Kerala and Ayurveda have virtually become synonymous with each other. However, wide array of treatments and medication are also available in the other forms of medicine as well as in modern medical treatment. Ayurveda the 3000 year old system of medicine (recognized by World Health Organisation as a system of alternative medicine), is becoming very popular all over the world. Estimates have shown that by 2010, Kerala could witness a growth of more than one lakh medical tourists. The Government is aiming to make the state a global hub for medical tourism. The beautiful South Indian state of Kerala is becoming a very appealing tourism investment destination, particularly for Non-Resident Indians. However, Kerala is seeing some foreign investors as well that would like to invest in the state's tourism potential. Two million Keralites who work abroad, has huge allocation to India, which is estimated to be around Rs. 200 billion a year. The government of Kerala has come up with a new health tourism policy that promises investment opportunities for Non-Resident Keralites, which ensures steady returns in the long-run. See appendix 2 for more on the wellness centres in Kerala and other places in India.

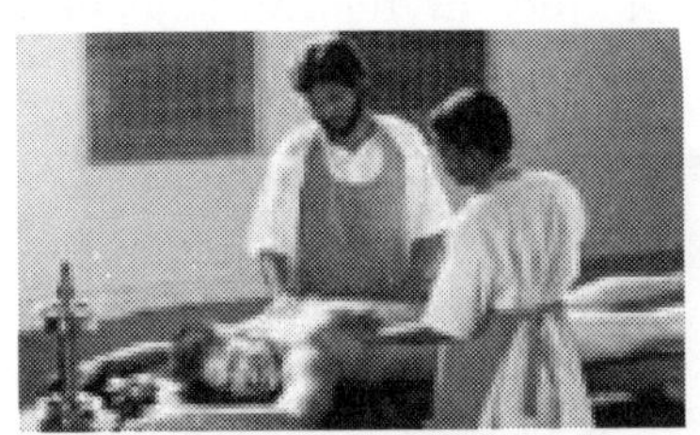

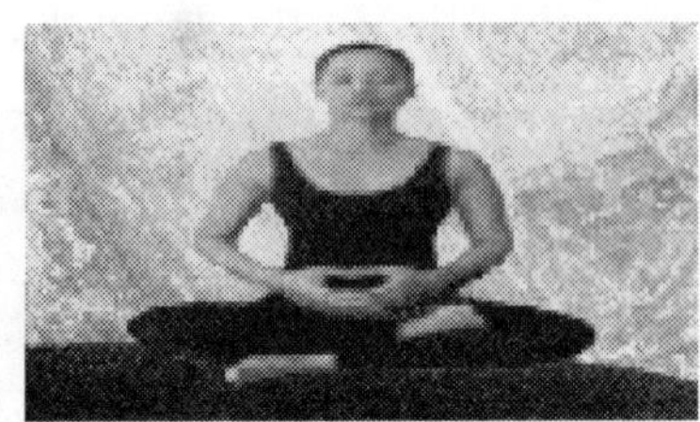

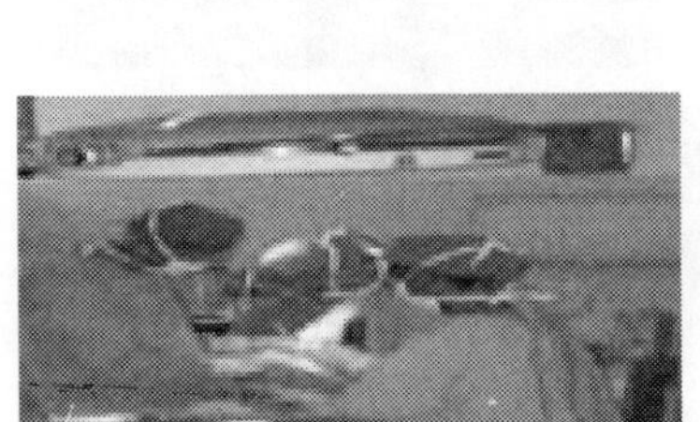

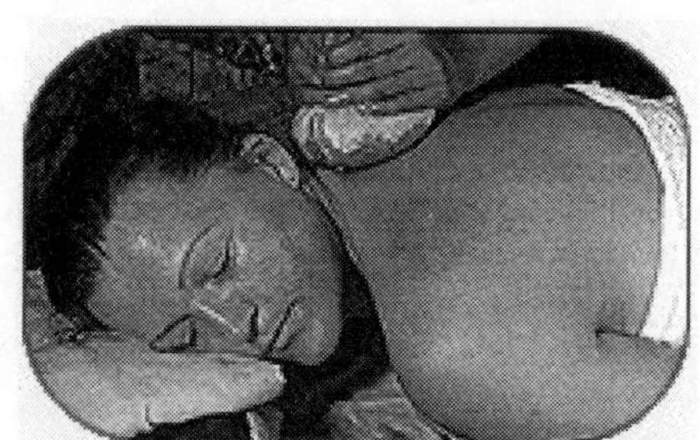

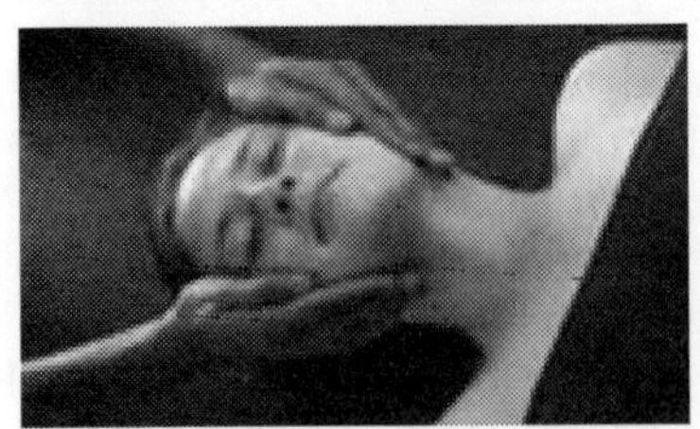

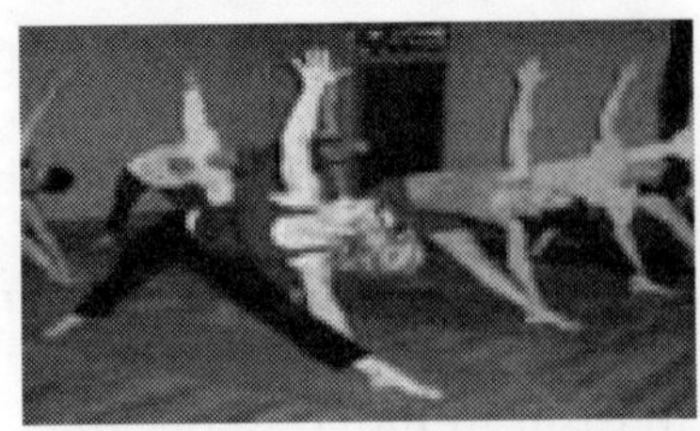

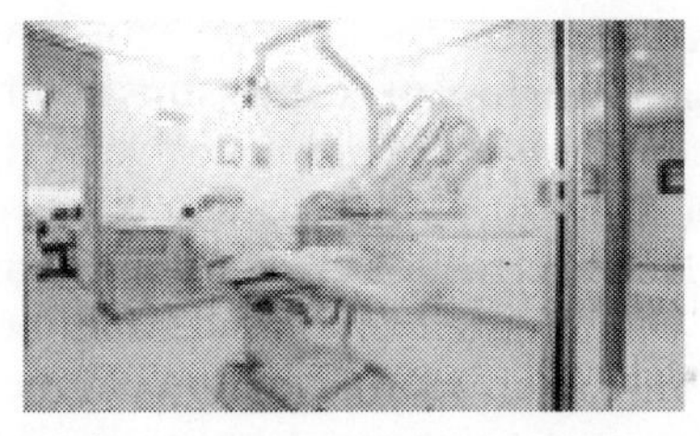

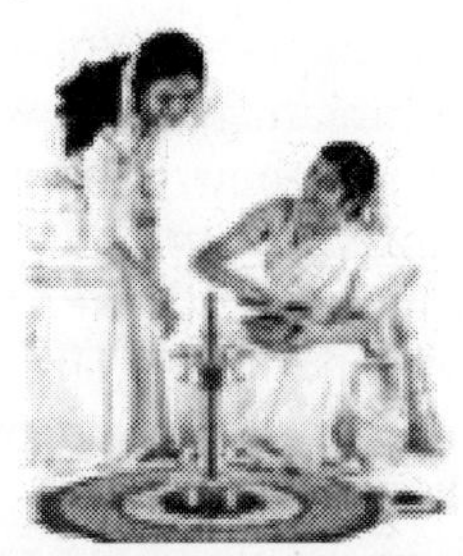

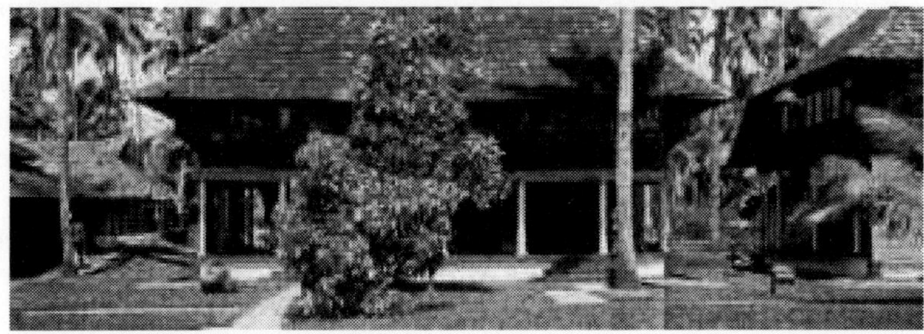

Traditional form of Indian medicine

Many people from the developed world come to India for the rejuvenation promised by yoga and ayurvedic massage. Ayurveda the traditional form of Indian medicine was developed by ancient sages whose astute observations led to the development of constitutional medicine. Traditional Chinese Medicine too has similar origins. Over the past 5000 years the Ayurvedic and Chinese traditions have developed sophisticated systems of medicines.

Benefits of Ayurveda

When alternative lifestyles and stressful schedules are talking points in the cosmopolitan circuits, Ayurveda, the art of ancient Indian healing cannot be far behind. The inability of modern medicine to allay all sicknesses and diseases has made an increasing number of people turn to Ayurveda, which has a cornucopia of ancient secret cures for stubborn diseases. Along with yoga, Ayurveda is the new balm for fevered souls. It uses natural herbs and their oils to treat ailments and ensure a healthy life. Most of the centres for Ayurveda, called Ayurveda Shalas, are in Kerala on the South Coast. This is beach country as well, so bring along your sunscreens and hats. In fact many westerners have made Ayurvedic spas their annual treat, combining a relaxing holiday with cleansing for their bodies.

The Massages: Oils and herbs

Say "massage" in the context of an Asian country, and the first thoughts that come flooding in are those of the exotic massage parlours of Pattaya. But with Ayurvedic be prepared to get some energetic flesh pounding from experts. While you soak in the herbs you can watch the beaches of Vizhinjam packed with boats out to sail in the sunset. From the beach you can see their lights strung out like pearls in a necklace from the coast. Look forward to being draped with pieces of linen, dipped in lukewarm herbal oils, all over the body by two to four trained therapists in a special rhythmic way. This goes on continuously for about 60 to 90 minutes per day for a period of 7 to 21 days, and is said to be an effective remedy for rheumatic diseases. It's supposed to be good for your nerves too and should pep up your overall energy levels as well. Ayurveda believes that the imbalance of fire, air and phlegm causes disease in the human body and tries to correct it majorly through cleaning and massage. Once the balance of humours is restored, the body copes better with external factors like pollution, strain and infections. The type of oil used for massage differs according to the ailment being treated. It is one of these: camphor, neem, mustard and castor. To these are added various powdered herbs, nuts and the bark of trees. The Ayurvedic practitioner may conduct the massage using the palm of the hand, poultices, and cloth.

YOGA; the Indian miracle cure

This ancient health and fitness practice provides both physical and mental therapy. It considers ageing as largely an artificial condition, caused mainly by autointoxication or self-poisoning. By keeping the body parts clean and well lubricated, cell deterioration can be greately reduced. To get the maximum benefits of yoga one has to follow three main guidelines, i.e. practice of asanas, pranayama and yoga nidra. With the regular practice of asanas, we control our cholesterol level, reduce weight, normalise blood pressure and improve cardiac performance. Asanas harmonize our mental energy flow by clearing any blockages in the subtle body, leading to mental equilibrium and calmness.

Pranayama

The practice of pranayama, the correct breathing technique, helps to manipulate our energies. Most of us breathe incorrectly. Pranayama is a technique where in it re-educates our breathing process, helps to release tensions and develop a relaxed state of mind. It balances our nervous system, reduces the need for sleep and encourages creative thinking. Increasing oxygen to our brain, improves mental clarity, alertness and physical well-being. Yoga nidra performed while lying on the back in the shavasana pose, it relaxes the physiological and psychological systems. This technique completely rejuvenates the body and mind, giving a sense of well-being. YOGA continues to be practiced in the traditional way in India and its gentle stretching and mental concentration exercises have been proven to have a beneficial effect on the body and mind. Each posture or asana exercises some of the muscles of the body and combinations of these asanas can provide you with a complete physical and mental workout routine. Asanas such as "Suryanamaskara," an invocation to the

Sun god can be the ideal way to start your day. Savasana while involves meditation while lying flat on ones back, can provide relief from stress and restore a sense of calm. Yoga is not merely a form of exercise or meditation but is a complete health giving system that will keep you fit as you travel on your journey through life.

Abhyanga

A synchronized full body massage performed by two therapists using specific herbal oils prescribed according to the body type. Improves eyesight, promotes sleep and gives a glow to the skin.

Shirodhara

Treatment for chronic headaches, insomnia, mental tension and cases of hysteria, hallucination and insanity. Lukewarm herbal oil is poured in a continuous stream on the forehead, while a gentle massage is simultaneously given, also on the forehead, for rejuvenating and revitalizing the body and mind. It relieves stress and strain-related problems, slows the aging process, improves memory, and is known to have a curative effect on paralysis and other neurological malfunctions. Herbal oils, medicated milk or buttermilk and decoctions are poured on the forehead/whole body in a special manner.

Oordhwanga Dhara (good for diseases of the eyes, ears and skin).

Choornaswedan

A vigorous massage, with a cloth bundle containing herbal powders. Induces profuse perspiration leading to relief of neurological disorders, rheumatism, arthritis and sports injuries.

Takra Dhara

Medicated buttermilk (takra) is poured in a stream (dhara) on the forehead to calm and give relief from conditions like insomnia, depression and other stress-related problems. (For those suffering from memory loss, severe headache or insanity).

Sarvanga Dhara (for both head and body)

Snehapanam—Treatment to alleviate Osteo-arthritis, leukaemia, etc.

Kashaya Vasti—This therapy is usually taken after a course of Sneha Vasti. A cleansing enema of honey, oil and herbs leads to nourishment and rebuilding of the Dhatus (body tissues), strengthens their respective functioning, restores and fortifies the body's immune system. Medicated ghee is given internally in a gradually increased quantity for specific periods.

Sirovasti—Treatment for dryness of nostrils, mouth and throat, severe headaches, facial paralysis and burning sensation in the head.

Lukewarm herbal oils are poured into a leather cap fitted on the head for specific durations as per physician's recommendation.

Kaval—Holding in the mouth and gargling with medicated oil/ decoction is highly beneficial for ear, nose, throat disorders, improves the voice and brings a glow to the face.

Pizhichil—Treatment for spondiliosis, rheumatic diseases like arthritis, paralysis, hemiplegia, nervous weaknesses and nervous disorders. A combination of two classical Ayurvedic treatments: Snehana (oliation) and Swedana (sudation). Pizhichil is considered to be the most natural way to purify different body systems, to protect from illnesses and build up immunity for a healthy life. Lukewarm herbal oil is applied with fresh linen all over the body by trained masseurs in a rhythmic manner for a period of 1 to 1½ hours daily for 7 to 21 days.

Udvarthanam—Treatment for diseases like hemiplegia, paralysis, obesity and certain rheumatic ailments. A deep, dry massage using herbal powders to stimulate hair follicles and tissue in order to break down the subcutaneous, stored fat. Slimming of the body is the significant effect. Therapeutic massage with herbal powders.

Marma Chikitsa—Treatment for musculo-skeletal ailments due to trauma or accidents. Treatment that works on the extremely sensitive vital points of the body (the 107 marmas). Gandusa—Retention of medicated oil/decoration in the mouth for several minutes. Lends a radiance to the face, improves lines and wrinkles, tones the skin and assists with any kind of mouth, voice or teeth disorders while cleansing the ear, nose and throat pathways.

Nasyam—Treatment for nasal ailments. The face, shoulders and chest are massaged with specific herbal oils, inducing perspiration. The medicine is measured out in the exact doze and poured into the nostrils while inhaling. A highly effective treatment for headaches, sinusitis and migraine. Inhalation of medicated herbal preparations, decoction oils, ghee, etc. to eliminate the morbid factors from the head and neck area.

Karnapooranam—Treatment for ear ailments. Medicated oils are applied to the ear for 5 to 10 minutes daily to clean as well as treat specific ailments.

Tharpanam—Preventing cataract and strengthening vision. Medicated ghee made with black gram powder, is smeared on the eyes. This has a cooling effect on irritated and stressed eyes. A treatment for the eyes effective in preventing cataract and strengthening the optic nerve.

Njavarakizhi

Treatment for wasting of muscles, rheumatism, sports injuries, pain in the joints, emaciation of the body or parts of the body and certain kinds of skin diseases. Massage with small linen bags filled with cooked Njavara rice. This procedure is highly rejuvenating, nourishing and prepares the body for the stress and strain of a busy lifestyle. The whole body is made to perspire by the external application of medicated rice packs in the form of boluses tied in muslin bags.

The ayurvedic physician will decide on a separate programme for every individual after evaluation. Short duration treatments for minor ailments like back pain, muscular pain, etc. with herbal steam bath, spinal bath and therapeutic massages will be provided only on the advice of the physician. Often women have female technicians for body massage and other health programmes. Some of the programmes are not suitable for the very aged, very young (under 7) infirm, heart patients and pregnant women.

The doctors are prescribing meditation as a way to lower blood pressure, improve exercise performance in people with angina, help asthmatics breathe easier, relieve insomnia and generally ease the everyday stresses of life. Meditation is a safe and simple way to balance a person's physical, emotional and mental states. The concept of meditation works on the principle that when the mind is calm and focused on the present. Neither is it reacting to memories from the past nor being preoccupied with plans for the future: two major sources of chronic stress known to impact health.

There are several techniques of meditation but they all have one thing in common—focus on quietening the busy mind. The concept is not to remove stimulation but rather to direct concentration to one healing element: one sound, one word, one image, or one's breath. The simplest form of meditation is to sit quietly and focus attention on the breath. Yoga and meditation practitioners believe that there is a direct correlation between one's breath one's state of the mind. For example, when a person is anxious, frightened, agitated or distracted, the breath will tend to be shallow, rapid and uneven. On the other hand, when the mind is calm focused and composed the breath will tend to be slow, deep and regular. As one focuses one's awareness on the breath, the mind becomes absorbed in the rhythm of inhalation and exhalation. As a result, breathing will become slower and deeper, and the mind will become more tranquil and aware. This helps to gain a more calm, clear and non-reactive state of mind. Studies show that after meditation, reactions are faster, creativity greater and comprehension broader. In addition, by silencing the mind, meditation can also put one in touch with the self, allowing the body's own inner wisdom to be heard.

Naturopathy

The nature cure movement was started in Germany by a farmer named by Vincent Priessnitz (1799-1851) but it gained momentum in India under the aegis of Mahatma Gandhi. He established a Bapu nature cure Hospital in Uruli Kanchan in Pune. Naturopathy believes that nature is the greatest healer and the body has the capacity to prevent itself from the diseases regain health. The treatment can include consultations on lifestyle and diet, recommendations of mantras medication, moxibustion (burning of herb mugwort), use of supplements and massage with specially formulated herbal oil, and occasionally, acupuncture. The practice of nature cure is based on the three principles; 1. Accumulation of morbid matter, 2. Abnormal composition of blood and lymph, and 3. Lowered vitality

The system of nature cure states that the basic cause of disease is not bacteria. Bacteria develop after the accumulation of morbid matter when a favourable atmosphere for their growth develops in the body. All diseases arise due to this morbid matter in the body, and if latitude is given for its removal, the body provides a cure. Nature cure takes into account the totality of factors responsible for diseases such as habits in living, working, sleeping, relaxing, sexual indulgence and considers the environmental factors involved, which on the whole disturbs the normal functioning of the body and leads it to a morbid, weak and toxic state. The five main modalities of treatment are air, water, heat, mud and space. The recent development of nature cure advocates the practice of drugless therapies like massage, electrotherapy, physiotherapy, acupuncture, acupressure and magneto therapy

Acupuncture and Acupressure

Acupuncture is based on an ancient Chinese theory. This theory states that life force flows through human body via fourteen invisible channels regulating the mental and physical processes. The 'puncture' in the word acupuncture, refers to the insertion of tiny needles in specific points on the surface of body. The use of this therapy has been widely successful in easing withdrawal from the addiction to drugs and alcohol, and is used in many detoxification clinics in the United States. Although it has been practised for many years as a method of traditional healing. Indians have only recently started to embrace this method. Acupressure deals with the human body and the flow of natural energy within the body. It is practiced with the use of only one tool, the human thumb. Pressure is applied on different pressure points on the body stimulates the corresponding glands of the body.

Gem therapy

Crystals, gems and minerals are solidified reflection of properties that are already within the human body. Gems and precious metals are used to balance planetary influences and to act directly on life forces. Having the capacity to both attract and dispel positive or negative energies, their healing properties are applied by wearing them in or having them in some way close to the body. The healing effect of gems can be experienced even by placing them in water overnight and drinking the water the next day, drinking water from vessels made of specific metals such as gold, silver or copper.

Precious stones and metals are also oxidized and purified in medicines in India. Called 'bhasma', these substances go deep into the body and can help in the healing of deep-seated illness or in rejuvenation. If gems are to be used for healing they should be purified. Immersing gems in salt water for two days purifies them. There power can also be enhanced by chanting sacred mantras over them. Gems are most effective when they weigh more than two carats and are worn in contact with skin. Some of the commonly worn stones include the:

- Topaz, which is said to help overcome fear.
- A yellow Sapphire is worn to enhance energy and vitality and is generally considered good for health.
- Opal is considered to have a positive influence on the wearer, promoting friendship, compassion, creativity and understanding.
- Precious stones like Diamond Sapphires Rubies and semi-precious stones like Lapis Lazuli, Coral, Beryl and Moonstone, have their own attributes and are recommended to correct various imbalances in the body.

Aromatherapy

Aromatherapy has been around for over 6000 years. In India and other ancient civilizations of the East, plant essences were used for their fragrance to purify the air. Agarbattis and dhoop (incense sticks) are still in use as they were in ancient times in India. The modern era of aromatherapy in 1930 when the French chemist Rene Maurice Gattefosse coined the term 'aromatherapy' for the therapeutic use of essential oils.

Our sense of smell works at a subconscious level. Olfactory nerves conduct smell sensations to a part of the brain, which also regulates and controls our moods, emotions, memory and learning. Studies with 'Briar wave frequency' have shown that smelling lavender increases alpha waves, which are associated with relaxation in the back of the head. Fragrance of jasmine increases beta waves, which are associated with a more alert state in the front of the head. Aromatherapy is particularly effective for stress, anxiety, and psychosomatic induced problems, muscular and rheumatic pains, digestive disorders and gynecological problems, such as PMS, menopausal complaints and postnatal depression.

Magnet therapy

The earliest mention of the magnet being used as a healing agent is in the Atharva Veda, the ancient Indian treatise on medicine and a part of one of the four Vedas. The ancient Egyptians were also familiar with the properties of magnetic forces, as they utilized it to preserve mummies. Their legendry queen, Cleopatra was said to have worn a tiny magnet on her forehead in order to preserve her charm. Dr. Samuel Hahneman, the father of homeopathy, was convinced of the magnet's healing powers and recommended its use. Magnetic therapy is very effective in drawing out pain and reliving stiffness.

The magnets influence the iron in the blood, thereby removing calcium, cholesterol and other deposits. It cleanses, purifies and ionizes the blood. The ionized blood flows easily, resulting in case in the activity of the heart and normalization of blood pressure. The secretion of hormones is also regulated and this improves the luster of the skin. Magnet of various shapes, sizes and strengths are used to regulate and strengthen the natural system and preserve the balance of magnetic field in the body. Two types of artificial magnets are used electromagnets and permanent magnets. For most treatments, disc shaped magnets of medium to high potency are generally used.

Chakra therapy

Energy healing is one of the most profound and fundamental alternative therapies in the field of alternative medicine and holistic health. It employs spiritual healing methods which expand the awareness of the energy healer and uses energy, colour and light healing techniques to catalyze healing in the patient's energy field (aura and chakra system)—helping the patient break free from afflictions and limitations of body, mind and spirit. It may provide enhanced quality of life for the patient, and facilitate spiritual growth. Energy healing is often a powerful spiritual path for the practitioner, as well.

The stress of everyday life takes a toll on your physical body, but also on your energy system. Some chakras are affected more than others, creating an imbalance in your aura, or energy field. Chakra meditation is a useful way to restore balance.

Those ancient Singing Bowls, found to be spiritually attuned to each Chakra, are allowed to dominate in this music, so affording the maximum stimulation to the chakra in question, i.e., it is possible to focus one's listening attention upon the bowl(s) in question in each piece whilst allowing them to convey teaching or whatever other form of spiritual communication to your Being.

REIKI

Allowing energy to flow through peoples and directing the excess energy either to ourselves or to others is the essence of REIKI. 'Re' means universal and 'Ki' means vital like force. Disease according to Reiki is caused by an energy imbalance, the depletion or congestion of energy. The treatment in this system of medicine consists of correcting imbalance. Reiki is similar to pranic healing; as it also uses Prana or energy to affect a cure but the technique of Reiki vary from pranic healing. Here the healer draws the prana or energy through his or her crown (chakra), and allows the energy to flow through the hands or the chakra. The healer or therapist is the energy channel

Homeopathy

Dr. Samnal Hahnemana sought to create a system of gentler healing. He began creating a new system using plants, minerals and animal substances, combining them into energetic compounds. The word 'Homeopathy' is derived from two Greek words, 'homeo' meaning similar, 'pathos', meaning suffering. Homeopathy simply means treating diseases with remedies, prescribed in minute quantity, which produce symptoms similar to the disease when taken by healthy people. It is based on the natural law of healing—'Similia Similibus Curarantur' which means "like is cured by like". For example, the effects of peeling an onion are very similar to acute cold. The remedy prepared from the red onion Allium cepa is used to treat that type cold

Homeopathy is concerned with the treatment of the whole person as an individual. Rather than the disease alone a homeopathy does not concentrate his therapy on, say arthritis or bronchitis or cancer. Rather he treats the mental, emotional and physical aspects of the patients. The physician's interest is not only to alleviate the patient's present symptoms but also his long-term well-being. Homeopathic medicines contain extremely small quantities of substance called potencies. These high dilutions not only enhance their curative properties, but also avoid undesirable side effects. Homeopathy has been serving humanity for over two centuries and has emerged as a time-tested therapy.

Rejuvenating Programmes: Rasayana Chikitsa—Rejuvenation Therapy

Tones up the skin and rejuvenates and strengthens all the tissues so as to achieve ideal health and longevity. Increases 'Ojas' (primary vitality) and improves 'Sattva' (mental clarity) and thereby increases the resistance of the body. Includes head and face massage with medicated oils and creams, body massage with herbal oil or powder by hand and foot, internal rejuvenating medicines and medicated steam bath. Herbal baths are also used.

Kayakalpa Chikitsa—Body Immunisation and Longevity Treatment

This therapy is a prime treatment for retarding the ageing process, arresting the degeneration of body cells and immunisation of the system. Includes intake of Rasayana (special Ayurvedic medicines and diet) and comprehensive body care programmes. Most effective if undertaken before the age of 50.

Sweda Karma—Body Sudation

Medicated steam baths eliminate impurities from the body, improve the tone and complexion of the skin, reduce fat and are recommended for certain rheumatic diseases, particularly for pain. Precious herbs and herbal leaves are boiled and the steam is passed over the entire body for 10 to 20 minutes daily. Hand massage with herbal oils or herbal powder improves blood circulation and tones up the muscles.

Beauty Care

Herbal face pack, herbal oil massage, intake of herbal tea, etc. improves complexion and beautifies the body.

Mental and Physical Well-being (Meditation and Yoga)

Mental and physical exercises meant to isolate the ego from the body and mind—designed to hone your concentration, improve health and help attain peace of mind through eight stages of training: Disciplined behaviour (yama), Self purification (niyama), Bodily postures such as the lotus position (asana), Control of breathing (pranayama), Control of the senses (pratyahara), Fixing of the mind on a chosen object (dharana), Meditation (dhyana) and Samadhi—a state of being where you experience absolute tranquillity and well-being.

Panchkarma

Panchkarma is the cornerstone of Ayurvedic treatment. While diet, lifestyle, and herbal supplements play roles in creating and maintaining health Panchkarma is the process, which gets to the root cause of the problem. There are several eliminative procedures in Panchkarma—This purification therapy aims at correcting the imbalance of the body's Doshas or bio energies (Vata, Pitta and Kapha) in order to maintain their inherent equilibrium and Ama, which forms as a result. Panchakarma therapy has three main stages: Poorvakarma, Pradhanakarma and Paschatkarma. Poorvakarma, the first stage, comprises essential preliminary procedures for preparing the body to unload stored toxins. The treatments help to loosen Ama (toxins) and move it out to the deep structures into the gastro-intestinal tract, where Panchakarma's cleaning therapies can then eliminate it.

Pradhanakarma is the second stage and includes the main cleansing therapies.

Paschatkarma is the final stage and describes the measures employed after the main treatment, such as diet, medicines and daily routine.

Vamana—therapeutic Vomiting—promotes elimination from the stomach and thoracic cavity—Administering herbal decoction to induce therapeutic vomiting. Very beneficial for Kapha imbalances such as asthma, cough, psoriasis and other skin disorders.

Virechana—puragation—promotes elimination from the small intestine—Administration of Virechak Aushdhi, a purgative, in milk or warm water. Alleviates excess Pitta in the body and helps treat dermatitis, chronic fever, heartburn and jaundice.

Vasti—therapeutic enema—works on the colon—An oil enema. The main seat of the Vata Doshi is Pakwashaya (large intestine), therefore Vasti is the main therapy for all Vata disorders such as constipation, neurological ailments, paralysis, flatulence, lower backache, gout and rheumatism

Unani

This ancient medical tradition, with its origin in the Mediterranean world was developed in the Middle East. The Unani system of medicine was founded on the principles propounded by Galen, a Greek practitioner. Unani system of medicine revolves around the fact that food is transformed by the natural warmth in the stomach into different substances. A part of these substances that are useful to the body are transported by the blood to different organs, while the waste is excreted. The main products of this process according to the Unani system were the four cardinal humours:

- Blood • Mucus • Yellow bile • Black bile

These humours were combined with the four primary qualities

- Warmth (or heat) • Cold • Moisture (or damp) • Dryness

This system of medicine states that if the four humours and the four primary qualities are all in a state of mutual equilibrium, man is healthy. It is the influence of external factors such as climate, age, profession and the customs that causes a dominance of one of the four humours observed in every human body. Both rules and noblemen from the beginning of the Muslim rule, built hospitals that followed the Unani system. During the reign of Akbar, there was a mass exodus of learned men from regions where Arabian medicine was taught.

Later when the English took over, these medicine practices lay neglected and forgotten. Towards the last quarter of the nineteenth century that a national reawakening aroused the interest of a few educate Indians to this system of medicine. Today various charitable organisations colleges throughout the country promote this form of medicine.

Siddha

This system of medical practice is associated with the Tamil speaking parts of India. The term Siddha is derived from Siddha, which means attainment of perfection. The origin of this system of medicine is associated with the desire of saints who relentlessly took efforts to attain salvation. These saints realised that a good physical body free from disease was required to attain eternal bliss. They evolved a system of medicine primarily for the healthy living and also for the elimination of disease. This traditional Tamil system was refined by Saivite saints called siddhars. It's also known as Agastya after it's famous exponent, sage Agastya.

Like all the traditional India medicines, siddha is based on body humours and other characteristics similar to those in Ayurveda. According to siddha system, the universe consists of 5 elements—earth, water, fire, air and ether that correspond to the five senses of the human body. A suitable proportion of these 5 elements in combination with each other produce a healthy person.

Mercury and sulphur play a major role in the therapeutics of this medical science and often, they are used in combination. Siddha medicine has an interesting way of categorizing drugs. On the basis of mutual interaction the drugs are called enemies or friends based on the compatibility with each other. The Siddha practitioner considers these aspects while administering the drugs. The diagnosis in siddha is based on findings from eight aspects: pulse, eyes, voice, touch, colour, tongue, faeces, and urine.

Tibetan

Two thousand years ago the indigenous people of Tibet had a traditional medical system, which was closely connected to their native spiritual system. They use an ancient form of medicine known as Gso-wa Rig-pa or the "knowledge of Healing" whose origins are believed to be based on the teachings of the Buddha. Tibetan medicine has existed in its present form for over one thousand years. Over the several centuries, medical knowledge was incorporated from the Indian Ayurveda, the Chinese system and the Greek medical systems. In addition, it also incorporated the buddhist thought. In Buddhist thought, all suffering and hence all illness, is caused by attachment, anger and ignorance, known as the "three interior poisons". The physical manifestation of the 3 poisons assume the form of three humours which are rlung (pronounced long), mkhris-pa and Bad-kan. In English these are generally translated as wind, bile, phlegm. When they are in harmony, they maintain well-being, but when they are disturbed or out of harmony, they are the cause of illness.

- Desire corresponds to disharmony of rlung (wind). Some symptoms of that are frothy urine, a rough and dry tongue or a 'jumpy' pulse.
- Hatred corresponds to disharmony of bile. Some symptoms are presence of thick or yellowish red urine, thick yellowish fur on the tongue or a 'full' pulse.
- Ignorance causes phlegm disorders. The urine in odorless, thin whitish and the pulse is "sluggish or heavy".

Furthermore Tibetans believe that karma (the law of cause and effect) from one's previous incarnations can also be responsible for our illnesses in our present experience.

Ignorance generates other negative states of the mind such as desire, hatred, jealousy and pride, which also contribute to our suffering. Understanding one's emotions is an essential part of the Buddhist journey to full awakening and freedom from unwanted conditions or all sorts. However, since most of us have very little ability to work with our emotional energies, medicines and other remedies are required. Treatment can include consultations on lifestyle and diet, recommendations of mantras and meditation, moxibustion (burning of the herb mugwort), the use of supplements and massage with specially formulated herbal oils and occasionally, acupuncture.

The ideal image of a healer in Tibetan medicine is that of "a man of noble character, capable of immediately making the right diagnosis of a patient's illness, without any examination or the least assistance" (Burang, p. 12). Needless to say, such physicians are quite rare. Consequently, before a physician acquires credibility, he must train at least twenty years in the tradition.

The Art of Living

The Art of Living Foundation is the largest non-governmental volunteer-based organisation in the world. The Foundation's service projects, programs on yoga, meditation and stress elimination have benefited over 20 million people from all walks of life. As a Non-Governmental Organisation, Art of Living Foundation works in special consultative status with the Economic and Social Council of the United Nations, participating in a variety of committees and activities relating to health, education, sustainable development and conflict resolution. Millions of people around the world have experienced physical and emotional healing from these the Art of Living programs, which help eliminate stress and create a sense of belonging. Sri Sri Ravi Shankar is the founder of the Art of Living Foundation

The Art of Living Course

Developed by H.H. Sri Sri Ravi Shankar, these courses offer simple and effective techniques for eliminating stress, resolving conflict thus improving health and living life with new joy and enthusiasm—A combination of the very best of ancient wisdom and modern science.

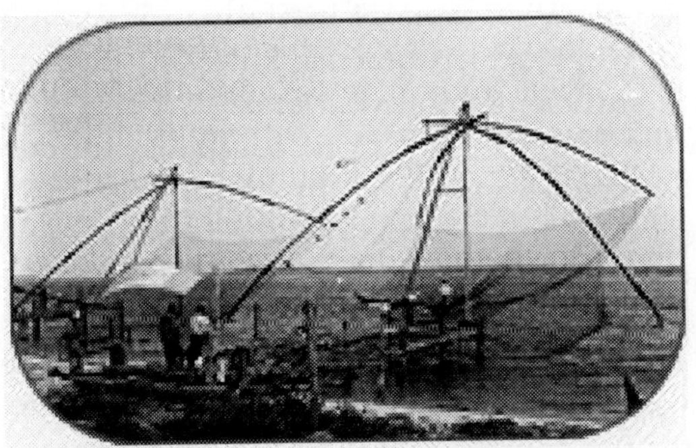

The Art of Living courses offer simple but effective techniques, which eliminate toxins, and stresses that accumulate in our systems over time. They are a unique way to harmonize and energize the Body, Breath, Mind, Emotions and Spirit.

The course is done in two parts

The first part is simple exercises aimed at relaxation, rejuvenation and improved circulation. The Course incorporates practical wisdom, ancient spiritual knowledge and health practices to increase the physical, mental, and emotional well-being of an individual. The Sudarshan Kriya is a powerful technique that purifies and rejuvenates both the mind and body. It is known to have beneficial effects on the physiology, nervous system, endocrine system and the immune system.

Part two of the course is about true relaxation. It's more about practice than learning. It includes a combination of:

"Silence" takes you deeper into yourself
"Sadhana" (Meditation), builds Energy
"Satsang" (Group Prayer), Supports and maintains it
"Seva" (Service), Energy is channelised into service for others

Sudarshan Kriya

The Sudarshan Kriya uses specific rhythms of breath to re-establish balance in life as it simultaneously floods the cells of the body with oxygen and energy. The Kriya links the breath to the mind-body system in a specific way, that rids the system of accumulated stress and toxins, releasing negative emotions and rejuvenating the body.

Reduce levels of stress Reduce cholesterol, Relieve anxiety and depression (mild, moderate and severe), Increase anti-oxidant protection, Enhanced brain function (increased mental focus and recovery from stressful stimuli), Enhance health and well-being. These simple, yet powerful breathing practices have a unique advantage over many other forms of treatment: they are free from unwanted side-effects, cut health care costs, and are easy to learn and practice in daily life.

Vipassana Meditation

The technique of Vipassana Meditation is taught at ten-day residential courses during which participants learn the basics of the method, and practice sufficiently to experience its beneficial results. There are no charges for the courses—not even to cover the cost of food and accommodation. All expenses are met by donations from people who, having completed a course and experienced the benefits of Vipassana, wish to give others the opportunity to also benefit.

A current schedule of 10-Day, free of cost courses is provided at each Centre for which it is available. To get the details of the dates available till 2005 please check http://www.dhamma.org/india.htm. After reviewing the Code of Discipline for the courses in Vipassana Meditation, you may make Application for a course at one of the Centres in India by contacting a Centre directly to obtain the current schedule of courses and then mailing or faxing the completed course application form.

APPENDIX I

LIST OF SELECTED HOSPITALS

Cardiology and Cardiac Surgery

Apollo Hospitals Enterprise Ltd.
Ali Towers, Ground Floor
No. 55, Greams Road
Chennai-600 006
Tel: 044-28291696/28294265
Fax: 044-28291407/28295706
www.apollohospital.com

ASIAN Heart Institute
G/N Block, Opp. ICICI Towers
Bandra-Kurla Complex
Bandra (East)
Mumbai-400 051 (India)
Tel: 022-56986666/26542088/56986585
Fax: 022-56986639/56986506
www.ahirc.com

BM Birla Heart Research Centre
1/1, National Library Avenue
Kolkata-700 027 (India)
Tel: 033-24567777/24567890
Fax: 033-24567000
www.birlaheart.com

Batra Hospital and Medical Research Centre
1, Tughlakabad Institutional Area
Mehrauli-Badarpur Road
New Delhi-110 062 (India)
Tel: 011-26057284
Fax: 011-26057284/29957661
www.batrahospitaldelhi.org

Breach Candy Hospital Trust
60-A, Bhulabhai Desai Road
Mumbai-400 026 (India)
Tel: 022-23671888/23672888/23667555
Fax: 022-23680750/23672666
www.breachcandyhospital.org

Care Hospital
Road No. 1, Banjara Hills
Hyderabad—500034 (India)
Tel: 040-55668888/23372424
Fax: 040-23327025/55625003
www.carehospitals.com

Escorts Heart Institute and Research Centre
Okhla Road
New Friends Colony
New Delhi-110 025 (India)
Tel: 011-26825000/26825001
Fax: 26825012/26825013
www.ehirc.com

Fortis Health Care Ltd.
Sector-62, Phase VIII
Mohali (Chandigarh)—160062 (Punjab) (India)
Tel: 0172-5096222
Fax: 0172-5096221
www.fortishealthcare.com

GNRC Heart Institute
Institute of Critical Care, Dispur
Guwahati-781006 (India)
Tel: 0361-2227700-04
Fax: 0361-2227711/2227715

G. Kuppuswamy Naidu Memorial Hospital
Post Box No. 6327
Pappanaickenpalayam
Coimbatore-641 037 (India)
Tel: 0422-2213501-07/2211000
Fax: 0422-2213509
www.gknmhospital.org

Jaslok Hospital and Research Centre
15, Dr. G. Deshmukh Marg
Mumbai-400 026 (India)
Tel: 022-56573333/56573313/56573321
Fax: 022-24950508/23520508
www.jaslokhospital.net

Kerala Institute of Medical Sciences (KIMS)
Anamukham, Post Box No. 1, Anayara P.O.
Kumarapuram Poonthi Road

Thiruvananthapuram-695 029 (Kerala)
Tel: 0471-2447575/2447676/: 98470-67687/98470-64166
Fax: 0471-2557169/2446535
www.kimskerala.com

KG Hospital and Post Graduate Medical Institute
No. 5, Government Arts College Road
Coimbatore-641 018
Tel: 0422-2212121-29/2218001-09
Fax: 0422-2211212
www.kghospital.org

Kovai Medical Center and Hospital Limited
P.B. No. 3209, Avanashi Road
Coimbatore-641 014 (Tamil Nadu) (India)
Tel: 0422-2627781/2627784-90
Fax: 0422-2627782
www.kmchonline.com

To Top

Lilavati Hospital and Research Centre
A-791, Bandra Reclamation
Bandra (West)
Mumbai-400 050 (India)
Tel: 022-26438281/26455891/26421111/26552222
Fax: 022-26451809/26407655
www.lilavatihospital.com

Max Devki Devi Heart and Vascular Institute
2 Press Enclave Road, Saket
New Delhi-110017 (India)
Tel: 011-26515858
Fax: 011-26565060
www.maxhealthcare.com

Manipal Hospital
98, Rustam Baugh
Airport Road
Bangalore-560 017 (India)
Tel: 080-25266646/25268901/25202269/25202271
www.manipalhospital.org

Mallya Hospital
No. 2, Vittal Mallya Road,
Bangalore-560001 (India)

Tel: 080-22277979
Fax: 080-22242326
www.mallyahospital.net

Narayana Hrudayalaya Institute of Cardiac Sciences
No. 258/A, Bommasandra Industrial Area
Anekal Taluk
Bangalore-560 099 (India)
Tel: 080-7835000-18
Fax: 080-7832648
www.hrudayalaya.com

P.D. Hinduja National Hospital and Medical Research Centre
Veer Savarkar Marg
Mahim
Mumbai-400 016 (India)
Tel: 022-24451515/24452222/24449199/24447718-19
Fax: 022-24449151
www.hindujahospital.com

Rabindranath Tagore International Institute of Cardiac Sciences
124, Mukundpur, EP Bypass
Near Santoshpur Connector
Kolkata-700099 (India)
Tel: 033-24363000/24363401-05
Fax: 033-24264204

Ruby General Hospital Limited
Kasba Golpark
EM Bypass
Kolkata-700 107
Tel: 033-24420291/24426091/24420857/24420887
Fax: 033-24426577
www.rubyhospital.com

Ruby Hall Clinic
40, Sassoon Road
Post Box No. 70
Pune-411 001 (India)
Tel: 020-26123391-92/56065368
Fax: 020-26124529
www.rubyhall.com

Rajinder Nagar
New Delhi-110 060 (India)
Tel: 25861463/25730501/25721800

Fax: 25864754/26257816
www.sgrh.com

Sri Ramachandra Medical College and Research Institute
No. 1, Ramachandra Nagar
Porur
Chennai-600 116.(India)
Tel: 044-24768403/24765997/24761549-50/24768027-29
Fax: 044-24767008/24765995
www.srmc.edu

The Bombay Hospital Trust
1402/03, Raheja Centre
Nariman Point
Mumbai-400 021 (India)
Tel: 022-22820240
Fax: 022-22875380/22079485
www.bombayhospital.com

Wockhardt Hospitals Limited
14, Cunningham Road
Bangalore-560 052 (India)
Tel: 080-51994444/22281146
Fax: 080-22281149
www.wockhardthospitals.com

Woodlands Medical Centre Limited
8/5, Alipore Road
Kolkata-700 027 (India)
Tel: 033-24567075-89
Fax: 033-24567090
www.woodlands-hosp.com

Westbank Hospital
Andul Road
Howrah-711 109
Tel: 033-26448673/26448888/26445516
Fax: 033-26448673
www.westbankhealth.org

Orthopedics—Joint Replacement

Apollo Hospitals Group
Indraprastha Apollo Hospitals
Sarita Vihar
Delhi-Mathura Road

New Delhi-110 044
Tel: 011-26925911/26825602
Fax: 011-26823629
www.apollohospitals.com

Batra Hospital and Medical Research Centre
1, Tughlakabad Institutional Area
Mehrauli Badarpur Road
New Delhi-110 062 (India)
Tel: 011-26057284
Fax: 011-26057284/29957661
www.batrahospitaldelhi.org

Breach Candy Hospital Trust
60-A, Bhulabhai Desai Road
Mumbai-400 026 (India)
Tel: 022-23671888/23672888/23667555
Fax: 022-23680750/23672666
www.breachcandyhospital.org

Escorts Hospital and Research Centre Limited
Neelam Bata Road
Faridabad-121001 (Haryana) (India)
Tel: 0129-2416096/2416097/2426590/5009999
Fax: 0129-2416260/2426586/5009973
www.ehirc.com

Fortis Health Care Limited
B-22, Sector-62
Noida—201301 (Uttar Pradesh) (India)
Tel: 0120-2400222/3945603-5
Fax: 0120-2402031
www.fortishealthcare.com

GNRC Heart Institute
Institute of Critical care
Dispur, Guwahati—781006 (India)
Tel: 0361-2227711/2227715

G Kuppuswamy Naidu Memorial Hospital
Post Box No. 6327
Pappanaickenpalayam
Coimbatore-641 037 (India)
Tel: 0422-2213501-07/2211000
Fax: 0422-2213509

Indian Spinal Injuries Centre
Sector—C, Opp. Police Station
Vasant Kunj
New Delhi-110070 (India)
Tel: 011-26898446/26898448
Fax: 011-26898810
www.isiconline.org

Jaslok Hospital and Research Centre
15, Dr. G. Deshmukh Marg
Mumbai-400026 (India)
Tel: 022-56573333/56573313/56573321
Fax: 022-24952508/23520508
www.jaslokhospital.net

Kerala Institute of Medical Sciences
Anamukham, Post Box No. 1, Anayara P.O.
Kumarapuram Poonthi Road
Thiruvananthapuram-695029 (Kerala) (India)
Tel: 0471-2447575/2447676/3041000
Fax: 0471-2557169/2446535
www.kimskerala.com

Kovai Medical Center and Hospital Limited
P.B. No. 3209, Avanashi Road
Coimbatore-641 014 (Tamil Nadu) (India)
Tel: 0422-2627781/2627784-90
Fax: 0422-2627782
www.kmchonline.com

KG Hospital and Post Graduate Medical Institute
No. 5, Government Arts College Road
Coimbatore-641 018
Tel: 0422-2212121-29/2218001-09
Fax: 0422-2211212
www.kghospital.org

Lilavati Hospital and Research Centre
A-791, Bandra Reclamation
Bandra (West)
Mumbai-400 050 (India)
Tel: 022-26438281/26455891/26421111/26552222
Fax: 022-26451809/26407655
www.lilavatihospital.com

Max Devki Devi Heart and Vascular Institute

2, Press Enclave Road, Saket
New Delhi-110017 (India)
Tel: 011-26515858
Fax: 011-26565060
www.maxhealthcare.com

Manipal Hospital
98, Rustam Baugh
Airport Road
Bangalore-560 017 (India)
Tel: 080-25266646/25268901/25202269/25202271
www.manipalhospital.org

Mallya Hospital
No. 2, Vittal Mallya Road,
Bangalore-560001 (India)
Tel: 080-22277979
Fax: 080-22242326
www.mallyahospital.net

P.D. Hinduja National Hospital and Medical Research Centre
Veer Savarkar Marg
Mahim
Mumbai-400 016 (India)
Tel: 022-24451515/24452222/24449199/24447718-19
Fax: 022-24449151
www.hindujahospital.com

Rockland Hospital
B-33-34, Qutab Institutional Area
New Delhi-110 016 (India)
Tel: 011-51688752-64/51222222
Fax: 51688765
www.rocklandhospital.com

Ruby General Hospital Limited
Kasba Golpark
EM Bypass
Kolkata-700 107
Tel: 033-24420291/24426091/24420857/24420887
Fax: 033-24426577
www.rubyhospital.com

Ruby Hall Clinic
40, Sassoon Road
Post Box No. 70

Pune-411 001
Tel: 020-26123391-92/56065368
Fax: 020-26124529
www.rubyhall.com

Sir Ganga Ram Hospital
Sir Ganga Ram Hospital Marg
Rajinder Nagar
New Delhi-110 060
Tel: 25861463/25730501/25721800
Fax: 25864754/26257816
www.sgrh.com

Sri Ramachandra Medical College and Research Institute
No. 1, Ramachandra Nagar
Porur
Chennai-600 116
Tel: 044-24768403/24765997/24761549-50/24768027-29
Fax: 044-24767008/24765995
www.srmc.edu

The Bombay Hospital Trust
1402/03, Raheja Centre
Nariman Point
Mumbai-400 021
Tel: 022-22820240
Fax: 022-22875380/22079485
www.bombayhospital.com

VIMHANS
No. 1, Institutional Area, Nehru Nagar
New Delhi-110065 (India)
Tel: 011-26310510/26310520
Fax: 011-26919916
www.vimhans.org

Wockhardt Hospitals Limited
Mulund Goregaon Link Road
Mumbai-400021 (India)
Tel: 022-55994444/5594400
Fax: 022-55994242
www.wockhardthospital.com

Woodlands Medical Centre Limited
8/5, Alipore Road
Kolkata-700 027 (India)

Tel: 033-24567075-89
Fax: 033-24567090
www.woodlands-hosp.com

Westbank Hospital
Andul Road
Howrah-711 109
Tel: 033-26448673/26448888/26445516
Fax: 033-26448673
www.westbankhealth.org

Minimally Invasive Surgery and Therapeutic Endoscopy

Apollo Hospitals Group
58, Canal Circular Road
Kolkata-700 054 (India)
Tel: +91-33-23585211-15
Fax: +91-33-23585218/23585198
www.apollohospitals.com

Batra Hospital and Medical Research Centre
1, Tughlakabad Institutional Area
Mehrauli-Badarpur Road
New Delhi-110 062 (India)
Tel: +91-11-26057284
Fax: +91-11-26057284/29957661
www.batrahospitaldelhi.org

Breach Candy Hospital Trust
60-A, Bhulabhai Desai Road
Mumbai-400 026 (India)
Tel: +91-22-23671888/23672888/23667555
Fax: +91-22-23680750/23672666
www.breachcandyhospital.org

Escorts Hospital
Neelam Bata Road
Faridabad-121 001 (Haryana) (India)
Tel: +91-129-2416096/2416097/2426590/5009999
Fax: +91-129-2416260/2426586/5009973
www.ehirc.com

Fortis Health Care Limited
B-22, Sector-62
Noida-201 301 (Uttar Pradesh) (India)
Tel: +91-120-2400222/3945603-5

Fax: +91-120-2402031
www.fortishealthcare.com

G Kuppuswamy Naidu Memorial Hospital
Post Box No. 6327
Pappanaickenpalayam
Coimbatore-641 037 (India)
Tel: +91-422-2213501-07/2211000
Fax: +91-422-2213509

Jaslok Hospital and Research Centre
15, Dr. G. Deshmukh Marg
Mumbai-400 026 (India)
Tel: +91-22-56573333/56573313/56573321
Fax: +91-22-24950508/23520508
www.jaslokhospital.net

Kovai Medical Center and Hospital Limited
P.B. No. 3209, Avanashi Road
Coimbatore-641 014 (Tamil Nadu) (India)
Tel: +91-422-2627781/2627784-90
Fax: +91-422-2627782
www.kmchonline.com

Manipal Hospital
98, Rustam Baugh
Airport Road
Bangalore-560 017 (India)
Tel: +91-80-25266646/25268901/25202269/25202271
www.manipalhospital.org

Max Devki Devi Heart and Vascular Institute
2, Press Enclave Road
Saket
New Delhi-110 017 (India)
Tel: +91-11-26515858
Fax: +91-11-26565060

P.D. Hinduja National Hospital and Medical Research Centre
Veer Savarkar Marg
Mahim
Mumbai-400 016 (India)
Tel: +91-22-24451515/24452222/24449199/24447718-19
Fax: +91-22-24449151
www.hindujahospital.com

Rockland Hospital
B-33-34, Qutab Institutional Area
New Delhi-110 016 (India)
Tel: +91-11-51688752-64/51222222
Fax: +91-11-51688765
www.rocklandhospital.com

Ruby General Hospital Limited
Kasba Golpark
E M Bypass
Kolkata-700 107 (India)
Tel: +91-33-24420291/24426091/24420857/24420887
Fax: +91-33-24426577

Ruby Hall Clinic
40, Sassoon Road
Post Box No. 70
Pune-411 001 (India)
Tel: +91-020-26123391-92/56065368
Fax: +91-020-26124529

Sir Ganga Ram Hospital
Sir Ganga Ram Hospital Marg
Rajinder Nagar
New Delhi-110 060 (India)
Tel: +91-11-25861463/25730501/25721800
Fax: +91-11-25864754/26257816
www.sgrh.com

Sri Ramachandra Medical College and Research Institute
No. 1, Ramachandra Nagar
Porur
Chennai-600 116 (India)
Tel: +91-44-24768403/24765997/24761549-50/24768027-29
Fax: +91-44-24767008/24765995
www.srmc.edu

The Bombay Hospital Trust
1402/03, Raheja Centre
Nariman Point
Mumbai-400 021 (India)
Tel: +91-22-22820240
Fax: +91-22-22875380/22079485

Tata Memorial Hospital
Dr. E. Borges Road, Parel,
Mumbai-400012 (India)
Tel: 022-24177000/24146750
Fax: 022-241469937
www.tatamemorialcentre.com

Wockhardt Hospitals
Mulund Goregaon Link Road
Mumbai-400 078 (India)
Tel: +91-22-55994444/55994400
Fax: +91-22-55994242
www.wockhardthospitals.com

Woodlands Medical Centre Limited
8/5, Alipore Road
Kolkata-700 027 (India)
Tel: +91-33-24567075-89
Fax: +91-33-24567090
www.woodlands-hosp.com

Westbank Hospital
Andul Road
Howrah-711 109 (India)
Tel: +91-33-26448673/26448888/26445516
Fax: +91-33-26448673

Oncology

Apollo Hospitals Group
Jubilee Hills
Hyderabad-500 033 (India)
Tel: +91-40-23608850/23607777
Fax: +91-40-23608050
www.apollohospitals.com

Batra Hospital and Medical Research Centre
1, Tughlakabad Institutional Area
Mehrauli-Badarpur Road
New Delhi-110 062 (India)
Tel: +91-11-26057284
Fax: +91-11-26057284/29957661
www.batrahospitaldelhi.org

Fortis Health Care Limited
Plot No. 7, Block 22

W.E.A. Karol Bagh
New Delhi-110 005 (India)
Tel: +91-11-25815145-7/25716781
Fax: +91-11-25745267/25815148
www.fortishealthcare.com

G Kuppuswamy Naidu Memorial Hospital
Post Box No. 6327
Pappanaickenpalayam
Coimbatore-641 037 (India)
Tel: +91-422-2213501-07/2211000
Fax: +91-422-2213509

Jaslok Hospital and Research Centre
15, Dr. G. Deshmukh Marg
Mumbai-400 026 (India)
Tel: +91-22-56573333/56573313/56573321
Fax: +91-22-24950508/23520508
www.jaslokhospital.net

KG Hospital
No. 5, Government Arts College Road
Coimbatore-641 018 (India)
Tel: +91-422-2212121-29/2218001-09
Fax: +91-422-2211212
www.kghospital.com

Lilavati Hospital and Research Centre
A-791, Bandra Reclamation
Bandra (West)
Mumbai-400 050 (India)
Tel: +91-22-26438281/26455891/26421111/26552222
Fax: +91-22-26451809/26407655
www.lilavatihospital.com

Manipal Hospital
98, Rustam Baugh
Airport Road
Bangalore-560 017 (India)
Tel: +91-80-25266646/25268901/25202269/25202271
www.manipalhospital.org

Mallya Hospital
No. 2, Vittal Mallya Road
Bangalore-560 001 (India)
Tel: +91-80-22277979

Fax: +91-80-22242326
www.mallyahospital.net

P.D. Hinduja National Hospital and Medical Research Centre
Veer Savarkar Marg
Mahim
Mumbai-400 016 (India)
Tel: +91-22-24451515/24452222/24449199/24447718-19
Fax: +91-22-24449151
www.hindujahospital.com

Rajiv Gandhi Cancer Institute and Research Centre
Sector-V
Rohini
New Delhi-110 085 (India)
Tel: +91-11-27051011-32
Fax: +91-11-27051037
www.rgci.org

Rockland Hospital
B-33-34, Qutab Institutional Area
New Delhi-110 016 (India)
Tel: +91-11-51688752-64/51222222
Fax: +91-11-51688765
www.rocklandhospital.com

Ruby General Hospital Limited
Kasba Golpark
EM Bypass
Kolkata-700 107 (India)
Tel: +91-33-24420291/24426091/24420857/24420887
Fax: +91-33-24426577

Ruby Hall Clinic
40, Sassoon Road
Post Box No. 70
Pune-411 001 (India)
Tel: +91-020-26123391-92/56065368
Fax: +91-020-26124529

Sir Ganga Ram Hospital
Sir Ganga Ram Hospital Marg
Rajinder Nagar
New Delhi-110 060 (India)
Tel: +91-11-25861463/25730501/25721800
Fax: +91-11-25864754/26257816
www.sgrh.com

The Bombay Hospital Trust
1402/03, Raheja Centre
Nariman Point
Mumbai-400 021 (India)
Tel: +91-22-22820240
Fax: +91-22-22875380/22079485
www.bombayhospital.com

Wockhardt Hospitals
Mulund-Goregaon Link Road
Mumbai-400 078 (India)
Tel: +91-22-55994444/55994400
Fax: +91-22-55994242
www.wockhardthospitals.com

Woodlands Medical Centre Limited
8/5, Alipore Road
Kolkata-700 027 (India)
Tel: +91-33-24567075-89
Fax: +91-33-24567090
www.woodland-hosp.com

Westbank Hospital
Andul Road
Howrah-711 109 (India)
Tel: +91-33-26448673/26448888/26445516
Fax: +91-33-26448673
www.westbankhealth.org

Cosmetology

The Cosmetic Surgery Institute
169, St. Andrew's Road
Opp. Macronells Roof Garden
Bandra (W)
Mumbai-400 050
Tel: 022-26405578/26456045
Fax: 022-26557990
Email: cosmodoc1@yahoo.co.in
www.csisite.com

Holistic Health Care

Soukya International Holistic Health Centre
Soukya Road
Samethanahalli

Whitefield Road
Bangalore-560 067
Tel: 080-7945001/04
Fax: 080-7945010
www.soukya.com

Arya Vaidya Sala
Vaidyaratnam PS Varier's
Arya Vaidyasala, Kottakal
Kerala-676503 (India)
Tel: 0483-2742216-19/2742561-64
Fax: 0483-2742210/2742572
www.aryavaidyasala.com

Sir Ganga Ram Hospital
Sir Ganga Ram Hospital Marg
Rajinder Nagar
New Delhi-110 060 (India)
Tel: +91-11-25861463/25730501/25721800
Fax: +91-11-25864754/26257816
www.sgrh.com

The Bombay Hospital Trust
1402/03, Raheja Centre
Nariman Point
Mumbai-400 021 (India)
Tel: +91-22-22820240
Fax: +91-22-22875380/22079485

Sri Ramachandra Medical College and Research Institute
No. 1, Ramachandra Nagar
Porur
Chennai-600 116 (India)
Tel: +91-44-24768403/24765997/24761549-50/24768027-29
Fax: +91-44-24767008/24765995
www.srmc.edu

Woodlands Medical Centre Limited
8/5, Alipore Road
Kolkata-700 027 (India)
Tel: +91-33-24567075-89
Fax: +91-33-24567090
www.woodland-hosp.com

Westbank Hospital
Andul Road

Howrah-711 109 (India)
Tel: +91-33-26448673/26448888/26445516
Fax: +91-33-26448673
www.westbankhealth.org

A non-exhaustive list of high-level hospitals welcoming medical tourists

All India Institute of Medical Science, Delhi

AIIMS' contribution in the fields of medical education, research and specialized treatment is widely acknowledged.

Apollo Heart Hospital, Delhi

Have eight state-of-the-art cath labs. Plain balloon angioplasty, directional coronary arthectomy, rotablatory coronary artery stenting.

B.M. Birla Heart Research Centre

A specialized hospital dedicated exclusively to the diagnosis, treatment and research related to cardiovascular diseases. It has established itself as India's most advanced heart center.

Christian Medical College, Vellore

Occupies a prominent placeamong medical institutions in India and in the world as a 1,700-bed multicampus complex that is a vital, diverse, interdenominational community.

Tata Memorial Hospital

Located at Dr. Ernest Borges Marg, Parel, in the Central District of Mumbai, a short taxi ride from the local stations, the hospital has private and deluxe rooms.

Apollo Cancer Hospital, Chennai

The first hospital in the country to be awarded the ISO 9002 certificate.

Indraprastha Medical Corporation

India's first corporate hospital and the third largest corporate hospital outside the USA.

Institute of Cardiovascular Diseases

Has gained a reputation for being one of the most advanced centers in the world.

Sahaj Dental Clinic—A Complete Dental Care. Offering a great oppurtunity to experience Mystic India with World Class Dental Treatment. Where you Save and Enjoy, both.

Medical Tourism India—The India Health Tourism Directory.

Medical Tourism India—Healing Opportunities in India... Don't forget that Medical Treatment in USA equals to A tour to India +. Medical Treatment + Savings.

Inspiration Kerala—One of the leading professional Kerala tour operator and travel agent in Kerala, South India, offering Kerala tour packages, honeymoon packages, ayurveda packages, backwater cruises and also wide range of travel and tourism-related services.

Advent Medical Services—A leading medical service provider based in India with accomplished and distinguished physicians and surgeons with vast experience in medical field.

GaramChai—Medical Tourism in India.

MediTours—Medical Tourism at your service. Kerala has been described by National Geographic as one of the must see places in the world. Meditours has tied up with some of the major hospitals.

IndianMediCare—Prerana Health Care Services. A managed care service organisation providing affordable and innovative services towards health care requirements.

Hinduja Hospital—Indian National Hospital and Medical esearch Centre.

MediEscapes India—Indian Medical Tourism operator which offers world class medical and health treatments combined with leisure holiday packages in India.

Care and Cure Medi-Tours—Offers comprehensive services to facilitate ailing patients in neighbouring countries to utilize the specialized treatment being provided in the specialty hospitals in Chennai (India) for a reasonable fee.

Howard's Heart—The story of Howard Staab, 53 years old, who has to treat a flailing mitral valve in urgence and required a surgery as soon as possible to replace the mitral valve with NO medical insurance.

Incredible India—General Tourism Information in India.

Doctors At Distance—Quality Health Care at Affordable Cost.

Medorama—Health Care and Leisure in India, the Medorama way.

Randhawa Hospital—The oldest non invasive cardiac center in North India. Hundreds of patients have avoided heart Byepass Surgery in the last 10 years and are leading active, healthy lives!

Longfield Management—World Class Economical Health Care.

Express Health Care management—India's First Newspaper for the Health Care Business.

Dr. Agarwal Vasans Eye Hospital—one of the leading eye hospitals in Tamilnadu with state of art facilities for comprehensive eye care. Lead by world renowned Ophthalmic surgeons Dr. Amar Agarwal.

India Full Circles Tours—Health Holiday Tours.

Swagatam Tours—Medical Tours in India.

KG Hospital—Medical tourism in India.

Appendix 2

A typical Ayurvedic Center in Kerala offers following facilities to visitor planning to visit India for Medical Tourism:

1. Review of your old Medical Records and past/present medication by our Doctors (preferably prior to your arrival in India) to determine the true state of your health. Modern methods are used to evaluate your Blood Reports based on Internationally accepted Standards of Optimum Values corresponding to perfect health. Consultation Cost is US $70.00 per person.
2. Root cause investigation and Root Cause diagnosis of all your chronic medical problems based on your Medical History and present symptoms.
3. Complete Detoxification and Rejuvenation of Colon, Kidneys, Liver, Lungs, Blood (preferably 4 to 8 weeks prior to your arrival in India) by means of a user friendly. Do It Yourself Kits which comprises of Safe Natural Herbal/Dietary Supplements. Each Program lasts approximately 4 weeks. Cost US $ 99.00 each for Detoxification and Rejuvenation Kit respectively.
4. On your arrival in India the following is carried out:
   (a) Evaluation of your Cardiac function and Ragland Postural Measurements to determine the state of your Cardiac Health/Adrenal Function. Check up for missed Heart Beats.
   (b) Complete Body Scanning on a special Microprocessor Controlled Electronic Machine to determine—Weight, Fat Mass, Bone Mass, Hydration Level/Water Retention, Average Calorie intake and Metabolic Age of the Body.
   (c) Measurement of Body pH to determine the level of acidity in your Blood.
   (d) Evaluation of your present diet pattern and recommendations for any changes if required. Cost of above Consultation lasting approximately 1 hour is US $100.00 per person.
5. Next day a complete evaluation of your Health by a Comprehensive Health Check Up Program. Time required: approximately 1 day. The following Tests are conducted:
   (a) Laboratory Tests—Complete Blood Count, ESR, Urine/Stool Examination
   (b) Tests for Diabetes—Fasting and Post Breakfast Blood Sugar
   (c) Tests for Kidney Function—BUN, Uric Acid, Creatinine, Serum Sodium, Potassium, Chlorides and Phosphorous

(d) Tests for Cholesterol/Lipids—Cholesterol, HDL, Triglycerides, Ratios, LDL Cholesterol, VLDL Cholesterol, Cholesterol/HDL Cholesterol Ratio
(e) Tests for Liver Function—Bilirubin, SGPT (ALT), SGOT (AST), Gamma GT (GGTP), Alkaline Phosphatase, Total Proteins (Albumin and Globulin)
(f) Special Tests—Serum Calcium, Acid Phosphatase, HBsAg
(g) Tests for Heart Disease—Risk Factor Review, ECG, Stress Test (Tread Mill)
(h) Sonography—Abdominal Organs, Prostate Scan for Males, Ovaries/Uterus Scan for Females
(i) X-Ray Chest
(j) Eye Check-up—Fundoscopy, Tonometry, Refraction Error By Opthalmologist
(k) Women's Check-up—Gynaecological Exam, PAP Smear Test
(l) Spirometry—Lung Function Test
(m) Dental Check-up—Dental And Oral Cancer Check-up

Complete Reports are available within 2 to 3 days. Cost US $ 200.00 per person.

Optional Tests which can be done simultaneously on the same day:

(a) EEG
(b) 2D Echo (Digital)
(c) Color Doppler (Digital)
(d) CT Scan
(e) Wide Open MRI
(f) PFT, Audiometry
(g) Mamography for Females
(h) PSA for Males
(i) Thyroid Free T3, Free T4, Ultrasensitive TSH
(j) HIV Test ELISA
(k) 2D Echo Color Doppler for Heart
(l) Glycosylated Hemoglobin for Diabetes

Optional Tests are at an additional cost not mentioned above.

6. Additional Blood Tests to evaluate Hormonal and Nutritional Imbalance and Heavy Metal Toxins. Time required: 1 day. Cost can vary from US $100 to US $500.00 maximum depending on the number of Blood Tests relevant and chosen as per each person's requirements and desire during Consultation. Blood sample is collected from your Hotel Room and Reports are normally available within 3 to 5 days. Heavy Metal Toxin Reports normally require 10 days.
7. Additional Blood Tests for:

(a) Cardiac Risk Profile—US $120.00
(Homocysteine, Lp(a), D-dimer, hsCRP, LDL, direct Apolipoproteins, A1(b)
(b) Cardiac Injury Profile—US $140.00
(Includes CK-MB, FABP, Glycogen Phosphorylase, Myoglobin, Troponin-l
(c) Diabetes Risk Profile—US $100.00
CBC, FBS, PPBS, Cholesterol, Triglycerides, Creatinine, Electrolytes, Urine routine, Insulin antibody, Microalbumin, Insulin, C-peptide, HbA1c)
(d) Infertility Profile (Male)—US $100.00
(e) Infertility Profile (Female)—US $90.00

Can be carried out simultaneously with the above Test with no further expenditure of time. Additional Cost: as shown above.

Once all the Reports are ready and gone through by our Panel of Doctors, a further 1 hour Consultation is offered to suggest ways and means to correct and improve upon the deficiencies in these Reports in a short 8 to 12 weeks time. We also offer Root Cause Investigation, Diagnosis and Treatment for all Chronic Health Challenges. All "Mission Impossible" of Medical Science are welcome. Cost US $100.00 per hour per person.

During this Consultation, Future Goals for a Perfect Health and Body are defined and an action plan is custom designed in conjunction with each person's requirement for ways and means to achieve the same. An action plan is drawn up for achieving a State of Perfect Health and Perfect Body in the near future.

The Center will draw up a Protocol of Treatment and an easy to follow Daily Calendar to guide you for a Safe Natural Treatment using only Herbs and Dietary Supplements. No Drugs or Chemicals are used to help you overcome or reduce the severity of any Chronic Health Challenge. Follow up weekly support by E-mail and Telephone is offered for implementation during your stay in India and for continuation upon your return back to your country. Cost typically varies from US $100.00 to $1,000.00 depending upon the severity of the Chronic Ailments involved and the response of each person concerned.

A Do It Yourself user friendly Detoxification/Rejuvenation Kit is offered for your use after returning back to your country. This comprises of a safe Natural Herbal/Dietary Supplements to be taken orally for improving the functioning of your Colon, Kidneys, Liver, Lungs, Blood and overhauling your entire body to make it run at peak efficiency. This leaves a Healthy Goal on your face which your friends can't help noticing.

Reservation in 4 to 5 Star Hotel/Service Apartment in Mumbai (Bombay), India. Sight seeing/shoping in Mumbai during your stay here.

4 to 10 day trips can be arranged to neighbouring towns and cities of your choice—Udaipur, Jaipur, Agra (Taj Mahal), New Delhi.

Relaxation Herbal Body Massages are offered for the treatment of Body Aches, Pains and other problems.

Stay in Ayurvedic Health Resorts in Kerala

Consultation/Treatment with reputed Doctors for all kinds of Cosmetic work/Plastic Surgery, Dental and Eye (Lasik) Treatment can be arranged. Visit to Optomerist for Eye Glasses can be arranged.

Consultation with Cardiologist for Angiography, Angioplasty and By Pass Surgery can also be arranged.

The Center has Protocol to boost the Immunity of AIDS, Hepatitis and Herpes Patients and to improve the quality of their life and longevity.

General Information for Tourists

Cost of Air Travel from the West Coast to Mumbai, India is roughly US $ 1400.00 to US $1800.00 per person traveling by Economy Class via the Atlantic on British Airways, Air France, Swiss Airlines, Lufthansa with transit stop in London, Paris, Zurich and Frankfurt respectively. With a quick connection—wait typically 2 to 3 hours.

Cost of Air Travel from the West Coast to Mumbai via the Pacific with transit stop in Hong Kong, Singapore, Seoul is roughly US $ 1200.00 to $1600.00 on Singapore Airlines, Cathy Pacific and Korean Airlines.

Cost of Hotel Rooms in Mumbai (Bombay) as approximately as follows:

4 Star Hotels—$125 to $200 per night for Double Occupancy

5 Star Hotels—$250.00 to $450.00 per night for Double Occupancy

The Government of India provides Tourist Visa of short duration and a special Medical Tourism Visa (M) of longer duration (up to 1 year) for persons and Visa (MX) for their accompanying spouse coming to India for Medical Treatment.

List of some Centres of Ayurveda and Wellness

KAIRALI AYURVEDIC HEALTH RESORT PVT. LTD.
(Health Centre and Corporate Office)
120 Andheri Modh, Mehrauli
New Delhi-110 030.
Ph: 011-26802106/26804879
Fax.: 011-26680875/2680
E-mail: kairaliresort@vsnl.com

Kairali Ayurvedic Health Resort
PO-Olassery, Kodumbu,
Palakkad Dist., 678551
Kerala, India.
Tel: 0091-4923-222553, 222623, 224402, 224403, 224404
Fax: 0091-4923-222732
E-mail: kairlpgt@md3.vsnl.net.in
Waterscapes Resort
Kumarakom
Ph: 0481-2525861

Kairali Ayurvedic Health Spa
C-30, Rockland, Panchsheel Enclave
New Delhi-110 017, India
Tel: 0091-11-26491803, 26491804

Kairali Ayurvedic Health Spa
2/40, Central Market
West Punjabi Bagh
New Delhi.
Ph: 011-25160175/76

Kairali Ayurvedic Health Spa
367, Rajita Villa,
6th Road, Chembur
Mumbai-400 071
Ph: 022-25294477/99
E-mail: kairali01@vsnl.net
Khajuraho

Kairali Ayurvedic Health Centre
Opposite Khajuraho Airport,
Khajuraho-471 505
Madhya Pradesh, India
Ph: 07686-272219/274757
Email: kairali274@sancharnet.in

Art of Living International Headquarters—Asia
21st km, Kanakapura Road
Udayapura
Bangalore-560082
India
Tel: 91-80-28432273
91-80-28432274
E-mail: ashram@artofliving.org
Website: http://www.artofliving.org

Vipassana International Academy
Dhamma Giri; P.O. Box 6;
Igatpuri 422 403
District Nasik; Maharashtra; India
Ph: [91](02553) 244076, 244086
Fax: [91](02553) 244176
E-Mail: info@giri.dhamma.org

Nashik Vipassana Kendra
Dhamma Nasika; Opp. Water Filtration Plant,

Shivaji Nagar, Satpur, Nashik-422 222; Maharashtra, India
Ph: [91](0253) 561-6242
E-Mail: info@nasika.dhamma.org

Deccan Vipassana Research Centre
Dhammalaya; Near Majle Bus Stand; Hatkangale,
Kolhapur-416 109; Maharashtra; India
Ph: [91](0232) 483-316.
City Office: "Khushbu"; 6, Shivaji Park;
Kolhapur-416 001; Maharashtra; India
Ph: [91](0231) 651-146; Fax: [91](0231) 658-519

Nagpur Vipassana Centre

Dhamma Naga; Village Mahurjhari, Near Nagpur-Kalmeshwar Road; Nagpur, Maharashtra, India.

or

c/o Mr. Goverdhandas Kela; Central Engineering Corporation, Abhyankar Road, Sitabuldi; Near Anand Bhandar, Nagpur-440 012, Maharashtra, India.

Off: [91](0712) 524-685; Fax: [91](0712) 522-291; Res: [91](0712) 532-798.

or

Kalyanmitra Charitable Trust; Abhyankar Smaraka Trust Building;
Abhyankar Road; Dhantoli, Nagpur-440 012; Maharashtra; India
Ph: [91](0712)522-169
E-Mail: dhamma_ngp@sancharnet.in
Khandesh Vipassana Centre

Dhamma Sarovara; Survey No. 166; Near Dedargaon Water Purification Plant; At Post Tikhi, Dhule; Maharashtra; India

or

c/o Sri Prakash Borse; 12 Tulsiram Nagar; Deopur, Dhule-424 002; Maharashtra; India.

Ph: [91](0256) 222-741; Office: 222-614.

Pune City Vipassana Centre Dhammaananda; Pune City Vipassana Samiti, Dadawadi, Opp. Nehru Stadium, Near Anand Mangal Karyalaya, Pune-411 002; Maharashtra, India.

Ph: [91](020) 446-8903; 446-4243.
E-Mail: info@ananda.dhamma.org

Pune Riverside Vipassana Centre

Dhamma Punna; Pune Riverside Vipassana Samiti, 2, Vinay Chambers, Vetal Chowk, 971, Senapati Bapat Road, Pune-411 016; Maharashtra, India.

Ph: [91](0212) 355-472; Fax: [91](0212) 680-558.
E-Mail: mukti@giaspn01.vsnl.net.in

Ajanta International Vipassana Centre

Dhamma Ajanta; 11, Ashok Vihar Society; Opp. MIDC Office; Station Road, Aurangabad-431 005, Maharashtra; India.

Ph: [91](0240) 334-532; 332-324; 484-445.

GUJRAT CENTRES

Dhamma Sindhu; Village: Bada, District: Kutch, Gujarat, India-370 475
Ph: [91](2834) 273-303; Fax:[91](2834)224-267 and [91](2834)222-811; Res.: [91](2834)273-304
E-Mail:info@sindhu.dhamma.org

City Contact: Ishwarlal C. Shah, K.T. Shah Road, Mandvi, Kutch Gujarat, India, 370 465.

Ph: [91](2834) 223-076 (cloth-shop); 223-406 (Res); Fax: [91](2834) 224-267; 222-811

Ahmedabad Vipassana Centre

Dhamma Pitha; c/o Sri S.S. Choudhary; 1, Patel Society; Opposite Office of Police Commissioner; Ahmedabad-380 004; Gujarat; India

Ph: [91](079) 562-4631; 562-4253; 342-2473; Fax: [91](079) 212-2016.

Rajkot Vipassana Centre
Dhamma Kota; c/o Rajesh Mehta; Bhabah Guest House;
Panchnath Road; Rajkot; Gujarat-360 001; India
Ph: [91](0281) 34789/32187

Mehsana Vipassana Centre

Dhamma Divakara; c/o Mr. Upendra Patel; 18, Shraddha Complex, 2nd Floor; Mehsana, Gujarat-384 001; India

Office Ph: [91](02762) 254 634; Res. Ph: [91](02762) 253 315.

NORTHERN INDIA

Vipassana Centre

Dhamma Thali; P.O. Box 208; (Sisodiarani Baug-Galtaji Road); Jaipur-302 001; Rajasthan; India

Ph: [91](0141) 268-0220, 268-0311; Fax: [91](0141) 561-283.

E-Mail: info@thali.dhamma.org

Delhi Vipassana Centre

Dhamma Sota; Vipassana Sadhana Sansthan; Hemkunt Towers, 16th Floor; 98 Nehru Place; New Delhi-110 019; India.

Ph: [91](011) 645-2772; Fax: [91](011) 647-0658.

Kammaspur Vipassana Centre

Dhamma Patthana; Off Delhi-Ambala National Highway, Haryana; India

For additional information and registration please contact:

Delhi Vipassana Centre
Dhamma Sota; Vipassana Sadhana Sansthan; Hemkunt Towers, 16th Floor; 98 Nehru Place; New Delhi-110 019; India.
Ph: [91](011) 645-2772; Fax: [91](011) 647-0658

Karnal Vipassana Centre
Dhamma Karunika; Near Sainik School; Kunjpura, Karnal-132 001; Haryana; India For additional information please contact:
Mr. Brij Mohan Verma
5, Shakti Colony, Near SBI; Karnal; Haryana; India
Ph: [91](0184) 225 0543; Fax: [91](0184) 225 7543.
E-Mail: bmverma_universe@yahoo.com
Dehradun Vipassana Centre
Dhamma Salila; c/o Mr. T.S. Bhandari; 16, Tagore Villa; Chakrata Road; Dehradun 248 001; Uttaranchal; India
Ph: [91](0135) 2715189 or 2754880; Fax: [91](0135) 2715580.
E-Mail: assorep@nde.vsnl.net.in
Himachal Vipassana Centre
Dhamma Sikhara;
MacLeodganj; Dharamsala 176 219; Dist. Kangra; Himachal Pradesh; India;
Ph: [91](1892) 21-309;
Email: info@sikhara.dhamma.org
Website: http://www.sikhara.dhamma.org

Sarnath Vipassana Centre
Dhamma Cakkaa; c/o Mr. Parmanand Maheshwari; "Mangalam",
C27/273, Indian Press Colony; Madhalla; Varanasi; Uttar Pradesh-221 002; India
Ph: [91](054) 246-644; 344-713.

Jetvan Vipassana Meditation Centre
Dhamma Suvatthi; Katra By-Pass; Sravasti; Uttar Pradesh-271 845, India
Tel: [91](05252) 265-439.

Kushinagar Vipassana Centre
Dhamma Vimutti; c/o Dr. V. D. Modi; Arogya Mandir; Gorakhpur; Uttar Pradesh-273 003; India
Ph: [91](0551) 335 805/336 469.

Lucknow Vipassana Centre
Dhamma Lakkhana; Asti Road; Bakshi ka Talab, Lucknow; Uttar Pradesh; India.

Ph: [91](0522) 250 8525.
E-Mail: dhammalakkhan@rediffmail.com
For additional information please contact:
Mr. Pankaj Jain
A-302, Sterling Appts., 9 University Road; Lucknow, U.P.; India
Ph: [91](0522) 278 2795.

Hoshiarpur Vipassana Centre
Dhamma Dhaja; Punjab Vipassana Trust; Anand Public School; Anandgadh village; Post Melawali; Dist. Hoshiarpur-146110; Punjab, India.
Tel: 01882-272333, 240202.
E-Mail: dhammadhaja@yahoo.com

CENTRAL INDIA
Balaghat Vipassana Centre
Dhamma Kanana; Bank of Wainganga; P.O. Garra; Balaghat.
or
c/o Sri Haridas Meshram; G-8, Bagh Colony; Civil Line
Balaghat-481 001; Madhya Pradesh; India.
Ph: [91](076) 322-473; Res. 322-554.

Durg Vipassana Centre
Dhamma Ketu; Village Thanod; via Anjora, District Durg; Chaattisgarh, Madhya Pradesh-491 001; India
Ph: (0788) 241-1813.
Contact:
Mr. Sureshchandra Kathane, B-269, Street 5, Smritinagar, P.O. Nehru Nagar, Bhilai-490 020, M.P.; India.
Ph: (0788) 232-1539 (Res.).

Bophal Vipassana Centre
Dhamma Pala; c/o Mr. Ashok Kela; Vipassana Samiti, E-1/182, Arera Colony; Bophal; Madhya Pradesh; India
Ph: [91](0755) 563 113; 557-761; 557-762; Fax: [91](0755) 564 520.
E-Mail: info@pala.dhamma.org

EASTERN INDIA
Calcutta Vipassana Centre
Dhamma Ganga; Bara Mandir Ghat; Harishchandra Dutta Road; Panihati (Sodepur); Dt. 24 Paraganas; West Bengal-743 176; India.
Ph: [91](033) 553 2855.
or
City Office: 9, Bonfield Lane; Calcutta-700 001; India.
Ph: [91](033) 242-1767, 242-8043;
Fax: c/o Mr. M.K. Badani [91](033) 225-5174.

Vaishali Vipassana Centre
Dhamma Licchavi; Atardah (Lalitkunj), Muzaffarpur, Bihar-842 001; India
or
c/o Rajkumar Goenka; Parijat, Marwari Bazar; Samastipur; Bihar; India
Ph: [91](0621) 243-403; 243-206.

Bodh Gaya Vipassana Centre
Dhamma Bodhi; Gaya-Dhoba Road; Near Magadh University; Bodhgaya 824 231; Bihar; India
Office:
Shanti Dham; Kankarbagh Road; Patna-800 020; Bihar; India.
Ph and Fax: [91](0612) 352-874;[91](0631)400-437.

Baracakia Vipassana Centre
Dhamma Upavana; c/o Mr. Ishwarchandra Sinha; Khabhada Road; Muzaffarpur-842 001, Bihar, India
Ph: [91](0621) 244-975.

SOUTHERN INDIA
Vipassana International Meditation Centre
Dhamma Khetta; 12.6 km. Nagarjun Sagar Road; Kusum Nagar, Vanasthali Puram; Hyderabad-500 070; Andhra Pradesh; India
Ph: [91](040) 402-0290; 402-1746; 473-2569; Fax: [91](040) 461-3941.
E-Mail: info@khetta.dhamma.org
For additional information about Vipassana activities in the Hyderabad area visit the http://www.khetta.dhamma.org/

Nizamabad Vipassana Meditation Centre
Dhamma Nijjhana; Indhur, Post Pocharam, Yedpalli Mandal;
District Nizamabad; Andhra Pradesh-503 186; India
Ph: [91](08462) 273433
E-Mail:dhammanijjhana@yahoo.com

Vijayarayai Vipassana Centre
Dhamma Vijaya; Vijayarayai, Pedavegi Mandal (Post); District West Godavari, Andhra Pradesh-534 475; India.
Ph: [91](08812) 225522

Vipassana Meditation Centre, Dhamma Setu, 533, Pazhan Thandalam Road, Thiruneermalai Via, Thirumudivakkam Chennai-600 044, India
Ph: 44-24780953
Email Id: info@setu.dhamma.org
Website: www.setu.dhamma.org

Bangalore Vipassana Centre

Dhamma Sumana; c/o Bharat Silks; No. 185, Above Patel Roadways, 4th cross; Lalbagh Road; Bangalore; Karnataka-560 027; India.

Ph: [91](080) 2224330; Fax: [91](080) 221-5776

E-Mail:silksb@vsnl.com

or

Shri Chotmal Goenka. Ph: [91](080) 6637173

Shri Jyoti Prakash. Ph: [91](080) 6761646

Ayurvedic Therapies are found in:

Thiruvananthapuram--Shivananda Asharam—www.journeytoindia .com

Kerala—Taj Tamara—www.ashextourism.com

Agra; Mussoorie—Sansha healthspa—www.jaypeehotels.com

Conoor—Natural health Farm—www.ayurveda.org

Mysore—Indus Valley Ayurvdic centre and spa-www.ayurindus.com

Travelog—Ayurvda Beach Resort—www.Incredible India.com

Neemrana Hotels—Ayurvedic Rejuvnation www.neemrana.com

Kairali Centres—Kerala; Delhi; Mumbai—www.kairali.com

Rishikesh—Ananda Spa—http://www.anandaspa.com/

Haryana—Yorks Health Resort, Nolta—www.saitravels22.com\ Yorks.html

Appendix 3

GLOBALIZATION AND MEDICAL TOURISM

I. Identification

1. Issue

Globalization has caused many countries to reevaluate their economical strengths and weaknesses, as well as reassess what products or services in which nations can benefit. One such product and service that has emerged over the past decade is medical tourism. Medical tourism involves the practice of citizens exercising their personal health care choices in less restrictive areas. It is the traveling by candidate service recipients from one institution, jurisdiction or country where treatment is not available to another institution, jurisdiction or country where they can obtain the kind of medical procedures and innovative treatments they desire. Despite the less restrictive policies that encourage this business, these services often can also be offered as a lower-cost and more-timely option.

Because of the nature of this practice and its policies, this phenomenon has only occurred in certain, specific areas around the world. These regions and nations have attractive policies in place and have implemented unique marketing strategies that encourage the medical tourism business. This industry has demonstrated significant impact on these nations's economic health. Unfortunately, other nations, like the United States, have not been as successful in attracting the medical tourism business. Therefore, the issue is to more thoroughly understand, through the analysis of other country's experiences, policies and marketing strategies, why the United States should take advantage of the opportunity to further participate in this emerging industry.

2. Description

Medical tourism is a universal term that encompasses several specialty markets. Included in these specialty markets are health tourism, reproductive tourism, suicide tourism, as well as other niche business opportunities. Tourism, in the sense of this emerging market, is basically traveling from a place where treatment is not available, because of the prevailing rules, to a place where it is available. These rules are not necessarily laws but may also be the personal and moral convictions of the health care provider, institutional policy guidelines, and recommendations by committees. Thus, policy, in some fashion, is the driver of this industry.

Medical tourism is also the most common practice carried out all over world. However there are other specialty markets within medical tourism that are also emerging as significant businesses. Health tourism is travel in a recuperative climate with natural therapeutic resources. The health tourism business is more specifically known for offering yoga, massage, traditional ayurvedic medicine and spa resorts. Reproductive tourism is the practice of consumers exercising their personal reproductive choices in less restrictive areas by traveling to another jurisdiction or country where the desired medically assisted reproduction procedures and treatments can be obtained. Suicide tourism is a very small branch of medical tourism yet its presence is still notable. This practice, much more so than the others, is tightly structured by policy.

Once consumers commit to travel for their desired medical treatment, often consumers will also take the opportunity to be a tourist in the visiting country and enjoy what it has to offer. Thus, consumers may combine their holiday and medical care into one venture. Medical tourism is comprised of three basic aspects: hospital/health services, hotels and travel/leisure. Thus, with attractive policies and/or the correct marketing strategies, this emerging industry can have significant opportunity for economic growth and infrastructure development for participating nations.

3. Related Cases

As noted, medical tourism is the universal practice with numerous specialty markets within this business. Because this in an emerging industry, extensive research for any particular country or on any individual branch of medical tourism, its policies and marketing strategies are not available. Therefore, all areas comprising medical tourism for many of the participating geographical regions or nations will be addressed. In summary, this case study will address a broad overview of the industry.

II. Policy Impacts

5. Social

The policy behind medical tourism has two distinct functions. In the case of those countries benefiting from medical tourism, standing policy allows for the nation to promote this business to consumers who are willing to travel and have the ability to pay. In essence, policy allows consumers new and different options for their health care needs. Medical tourism policy offers consumers choices. Secondly, this policy can also be enacted to protect the nation and its consumers. In the health care field, ensuring necessary and quality service is of the utmost importance. Therefore, policy, in the medical tourism sense, protects the rights of its participants while also giving consumers more opportunity and choices in their health care.

6. Environmental

While medical tourism focuses on fulfilling health care choices, traveling to a different country or state is also necessary. This is the basic premise behind medical tourism. Thus, by traveling to another geographical area, it is promoting tourism to location. Tourism is being used as a means for providing capital for development and preservation of these geographical areas.

7. Economic

Medical tourism has had significant economic impacts on particular geographical regions and nations. The goal of this industry is to provide economic stimulus to the geographical areas, often developing nations. The objective of this business is to increase jobs, income, and quality of life of the participating nations of medical tourism. This business also promotes infrastructure development to support the industry.

8. Other

Since this is an emerging, competitive industry, countries seek education, advanced skills and training to benefit from this profitable business. Therefore, medical tourism, and the policies around it, has encouraged participants to receive continued education and training. Additionally, this business also requires the use of advanced technology, and this, in turn, encourages participating countries to gain more exposure to these various technologies.

9. Suggested Interventions

While there are several specialty markets of medical tourism that are very controversial, specifically reproductive and suicide tourism, countries are reconsidering and/or analyzing their standing policies. There are consumers who take advantage of these opportunities, as well as opposition from non-market groups who have forced possible policy reform. Thus, these nations must continue to analyze and revise their policies in order to protect the practice of medical tourism and its consumers.

III. Legal Clusters

10. Disclosure and Status/Policy Issue

While there is no main policy issue, policy, or less restrictive policy, is the backbone of this industry. Most often, consumers are willing to travel to receive medical procedures in a geographical location that maintains policies that are less prohibitive than their current location's policies. There are other factors, too, that encourage medical tourism, like time and money. However, if policy is not in place to encourage this business, regions or countries would not be able to participate and benefit from this industry. Additionally, because of their particular standing policies, nations are better able to market themselves to new consumers globally.

11. Forum and Scope/Existing Policy Framework

International: The concept of medical tourism is primarily to encourage travel by consumers globally. Therefore, most countries enact a policy framework that is attractive to worldwide consumers on the basis that if they are willing to travel and pay the necessary fee, consumers are able to receive the health care practice they desire.

National: Medical tourism does not require a consumer to have to cross national borders. Often, medical tourism is evident from state to state or jurisdiction to jurisdiction. In this case, policy encourages consumers to travel from one area to another area where policy is more attractive or less restrictive. This type of medical tourism that markets this practice is more often seen in the specialty market of reproductive tourism.

Regional: Although countries do not tend to formulate policies based on regional expectations, there are certain geographical areas that do benefit more from the medical tourism industry. Southeast Asia has marketed itself as the primary geographical area to cater to medical tourism consumers. Since this has become a competitive business, countries in this geographical area continue to analyze and reform their policies to encourage this practice and rise above their competitors. Additionally, as this industry continues to emerge, this similar phenomenon is becoming more apparent in the European Union as well.

12. Decision Breadth/Stakeholders/Policy Actors

Policy is often shaped by numerous actors. The government plays are large role in outlining medical tourism policy in its nation. However, there are other actors that can affect policy. Health Care providers, institutions, special committees, advisory boards, associations, as well as numerous other players, can all impact policy guidelines.

On the tourism aspect of this industry, there are also other actors that can also influence policy. Businesses, recreational organisations, as well other associations and groups can impact policy guidelines that encourage medical tourism.

13. Legal Standing/Legal Regulatory Framework/Suggested Policy Interventions

Although there is no documented legal regulatory framework for the medical tourism industry, there is always a legal liability concern when dealing with the health care industry. The health care industry is a much regulated business entwined with liability issues. Therefore, countries enact policies that address this concern on an individual basis. Because some countries are willing to take on more risk with health care liability, they have been able to emerge as leaders in this industry. Other countries, like the United States, have not been able to benefit as greatly from medical tourism because of increased legal liability and policy.

IV. Trade Clusters

14. Type of Measure

Research states that the economic profit that the medical tourism industry contributes to the nation's gross domestic product (GDP) is the measure of success. This financial revenue can be calculated by health care earnings, as well as the profits from tourism related activities. Besides the monetary value that is calculated, countries can measure the affects of this industry by the increase in number of tourists, as well as the number of new jobs. Together, countries are able to determine the many influences that the medical tourism industry has on its economy.

15. Relation of Trade Measure to Environmental/Tourism Impacts

Directly Related to Product: The revenue generated from the consumers traveling to the country for their health care needs will go towards building the nation's health care system and tourism infrastructure.

Indirectly Related to Product: Because medical tourism crosses many different types of business sectors, the revenue generated will also indirectly support these other sectors indirectly as well. While this practice will primarily benefit the health care and lodging industries, the service and recreational industries will also profit from this business.

Not Related to Product: The result of the medical tourism industry is far-reaching. Not only will it benefit many different business sectors directly and indirectly, medical tourism can provide an increase in a nation's overall economic health. Revenue generation will increase the GDP. This resultant growth will encourage development of the nation's infrastructure and its people's quality of life.

Related to Process: Revenue generation from this business will hopefully encourage the further development of the infrastructure that is required to carry out the medical tourism product. Development of the health care system, as well as the travel and tourism infrastructure, will benefit the nation and its people on the whole.

16. Trade Product Identification/Trade and Services

The medical tourism product generally provides numerous types of services. First and foremost, medical tourism is providing a consumer with the health care service that they need or desire. In addition, this type of business also offers the consumer the lodging services that they require to participate in this process. Often consumers will also take part in some leisure, recreational or sightseeing activities while visiting the country. Therefore, the tourism industry may also be providing a service to these consumers as well.

17. Economic Data

The medical tourism industry can be a product for any country. However, numerous nations have significantly benefited from this business more than others. The country's that have demonstrated the most significant gains are noted below.

- o Medical tourism has contributed approximately $25 million per year to Cuba's economic status.

- India has seen a 27 percent increase in tourists while medical tourism, itself, has demonstrated a 20 percent growth. Additionally, India has attracted 150,000 medical tourists in 2003. By 2012, medical tourism is expected to bring an additional $1.1-2.2 billion in annual revenue.
- In 2002, Thailand treated more than 600,000 tourists that generated approximately $503 million in revenues.
- In 2000, Singapore attracted more than 150,000 tourists for medical care which added 0.19 percent to its GDP. By 2012, this island is expected to treat more than 1 million tourists. This figure will complement a 3 percent market share for health care services, generate some $3 billion in revenue, add 1 percent to the GDP and lead to some 13,000 new jobs

18. Impact of Trade Restriction

Because the basis of this industry requires consumers to travel for their health care needs, trade restrictions on travel would impact its capabilities. Among the two most problematic restrictions would be on visa issuing and International Travel Bans to specific regions or countries. Thus, if the consumers are unable to travel to the desired country, the product and service cannot be sold.

19. Industry Sector

As suggested previously, the primary industry sector for medical tourism includes: the health care industry, as well as the international travel and tourism industry. The secondary industry sectors would include: service, information technology and communication industries.

20. Exporters and Importers

In the medical tourism industry, the export is the consumer. Because the consumer comes into the country for their health care needs, they provide foreign currency to the economy. In the end, they leave the country with the desired medical care. It is the hope that there are no real imports and that all of the goods and services are provided domestically.

V. Macro/Environment Cluster/Tourism Policy Clusters

21. Environmental Problem Type/Environmental Aspects

Although the main focus of the medical tourism product is the health care service provided, countries are also encouraging consumers to be tourists. As a tourist, they are enjoying the beauty and recreation of the area. The hope is that some of the revenues from these activities will go into developing the environmental infrastructure, as well as conservation and preservation.

22. Resource Impact and Effect

This type of practice does not really require any substantial amount of environmental resources. Therefore, there are no major impacts or effects of the medical tourism business on a nation's environmental resources.

23. Urgency and Policy Review

On the whole, medical tourism is still in an emergent state. Therefore, this practice has not necessitated any type of real urgency. However, most of the countries participating in this business have launched a global advertising and marketing campaign to varying extents. Each country has unique marketing strategies that target specific markets. Additionally, because each country seeks growth, each has their own unique policies that allow for the attraction of these consumer markets.

24. Substitutes and Alternative Policies

The most common alternative to receiving health care in one's desired country is obtaining one's health care needs in a competitive country. Therefore, countries attempt to make their policies as attractive and simplified as possible to attract the consumer. If not, consumers may find a different country with less restrictive policies to provide them their desired care.

VI. Other Factors

25. Culture

Because this industry is carried out in many different countries around the world with various languages and practices, culture can play a significant role in this business. Nations must be cognizant of culture when marketing to specific target markets. Additionally, consumers must appreciate culture and traditions that may affect their foreign health care experience. Because many of the countries providing this service are developing countries, culture can be very different and varied. All participants in this business must understand and appreciate that culture can play a significant role in the medical tourism process.

26.Trans-boundary Issues

For medical tourism on a whole, overwhelming trans-boundary issues are not present. However, there are two specific markets within medical tourism, reproductive and suicide tourism, which do present trans-boundary challenges. With reproductive tourism, often consumers travel to another jurisdiction to receive a service that cannot be provided at home. Abortions and decisions surrounding *in vitro* fertilization can be two specific practices that can present challenges to the consumer. This is true for suicide tourism as well. There are issues surrounding the rights of the individual accompanying the consumer. Some countries view this as assistance, which often is prohibited. Therefore, although medical tourism does not present too many trans-boundary issues, specific markets can present challenges and should be more closely analyzed.

27. Rights

For the most part, medical tourism is not affected by one's rights. However, when dealing with reproductive and suicide tourism, a consumer's rights must be considered. Consumers have rights. However, they may be affected by receiving treatment in a foreign country or upon returning to their home country. Consumers must consider their rights, and they make seek treatment in alternative locations if a different area's policies better serve a patient's rights. This could be true for practices or procedures such as abortions, in vitro fertilization, as well as euthanasia. Thus, consumer's rights may play a part in decisions made for the medical tourism product.

28. Policy Implications

Many nations around the world, particularly developing countries, have taken advantage of the benefits of medical tourism. This emerging industry can provide significant economic stimulus for a nation's revenue growth and financial health. It can also stimulate infrastructure development and improve the quality of life of the nation's people. However, nations must position themselves correctly to reap this profit.

Countries must establish attractive policies that encourage medical tourism practice in their country as well as attract consumers to participate in this phenomenon. Nation's often demonstrate less restrictive policies than its neighbours and competitors.

Once a nation has policies in place, they must correctly market themselves. Countries use different and unique marketing strategies, such as lower-cost, more-timely, higher-quality, to promote their services to their target market. Thus, this industry has demonstrated significant impact on the nation's economic health, however less-restrictive and attractive policies must be in place first. Countries must also market themselves properly to continually enjoy the benefits of this emerging business.

Appendix 4

DR. JASON YAP INTERVIEW—SINGAPORE TOURISM BOARD, FRIDAY, AUGUST 17, 2007

Q and A with Dr. Jason C.H. Yap, Director, Health Care Services, Singapore Tourism Board. Dr. Yap is a public health physician with nearly two decades in health care services and currently part of the SingaporeMedicine multi-agency initiative to promote and streamline services offered by Singapore's health care providers to international medical travelers.

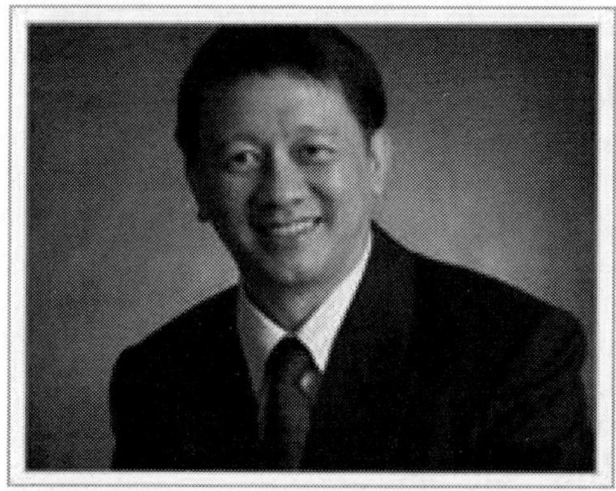

Dr. Yap is highly suited to be the public face of Singapore's medical tourism not only because of his background which includes stints as the IT Director for the National Health Care Group and before that with Singapore's Ministry of Health, but also because he sees himself as a product of Singapore's medical travel facilities, considering that his mother traveled from Malaysia to Singapore specifically for his birth.

Question: Dr. Yap, you are the Director of Health Care Services with the Singapore Tourism Board. I hope that is correct. So are your duties, and those of your office, tilted more towards health care or tourism? Or are you specifically handling medical tourism?

Dr. Yap: Yes, the designation is correct.

First and foremost, STB's focus goes beyond mere "medical tourism". We prefer to call it Medical Travel. While many do go on "medical holidays" where health care offerings are combined with leisure activities, a great many others travel solely for health care. Therefore, what STB takes care of are medical travelers.

Unlike our major competitors, Singapore has an unusual reason for being in the medical travel industry. While the revenue from international patients is naturally welcome in a country that has had to rely on international trade for its national survival, the reality is that Singapore would make more money investing its resources in other directions. However, the national imperative to make and maintain Singapore as an international medical hub arises from the need to look after its own citizens and residents.

Through the decades of strong economic growth, Singapore has invested in its own health care system and created one of the best health care systems in the world. Singapore sent its doctors overseas to train in the best international centers. These doctors eventually return to upgrade and improve local health care services to be on par with where they had trained. All the major health care networks are JCI-accredited and Singapore accounts for some one-third of all JCI-accredited health care facilities in Asia.

However, with a small population of only 4.5 million residents, Singapore finds it increasingly difficult to sustain the many sub-specialties, to maintain the many high-end services and to afford the technology. Thus, the effort to draw international patients is to maintain a critical mass of patients. Ironically, and unlike other countries, Singapore seeks foreign patients in order to serve local patients.

The Singapore Tourism Board (STB) plays an instrumental role to develop and maintain Singapore as a medical hub, not only for international patients, but for medical conferences and training, health care consultancy, regional and international headquarters of health care organisations, manufacturing of pharmaceuticals and medical devices, etc. STB's main role is in international marketing and the development of people-oriented services for medical travelers.

Question: What advantages does Singapore hold, for a medical tourist, as compared to countries like Thailand or India?

Dr. Yap: There are several reasons why medical travelers choose Singapore as their choice health care destination.

The first and foremost reason is simply that, it is Singapore. Singapore is known for its excellence, efficiency and effectiveness. Having the best international airport, the best airline, and the busiest port in the world, these accolades are evidence of Singapore's world-class standards and achievements.

The clinical services in Singapore emphasize excellence, safety and trustworthiness, with internationally accredited facilities and renowned physicians trained in the best centers in the world. In 2000, the World Health Organisation ranked Singapore's health care system as the sixth best in the world and the best in Asia, and Singapore accounts for one-third of all JCI-accredited facilities in Asia. Beyond international certifications, the quality of health care is also seen in published clinical indicators. Many health care institutions in Singapore publish their success rates on their corporate websites, and these rates are comparable to, if not exceeding, international standards.

Singapore is a true multi-faceted regional medical hub, not only for patients' services but also as a meeting place for medical professionals for conferences and training, as a base for health care consultancy and operations management, and as the centre for research and clinical trials.

Cost is an important consideration for many international patients. For instance, an angioplasty costs approximately US$57,000-83,000 for an uninsured patient in the United States, whereas in Singapore, it costs only US $13,000, similar to the costs at other major Asian medical travel destinations. So even after factoring in travel and accommodation expenses of the patient and their accompanying persons, the cost savings are still considerable. On top of the affordability, patients in Singapore are assured of world-class treatment and high clinical outcomes.

Finally, Singapore is an international city which welcomes people of all cultures. The Singapore Changi International Airport is connected to some 180 cities in the world, making it highly accessible. Transport and accessibility within the country is equally easy and convenient. English is the first language of education and business. The people in Singapore enjoy high security and low crime. As Singapore is a multi-racial and multi-culturally accommodating city, patients of all race and creed will not find it difficult to meet people in Singapore who speak their language or share their religion.

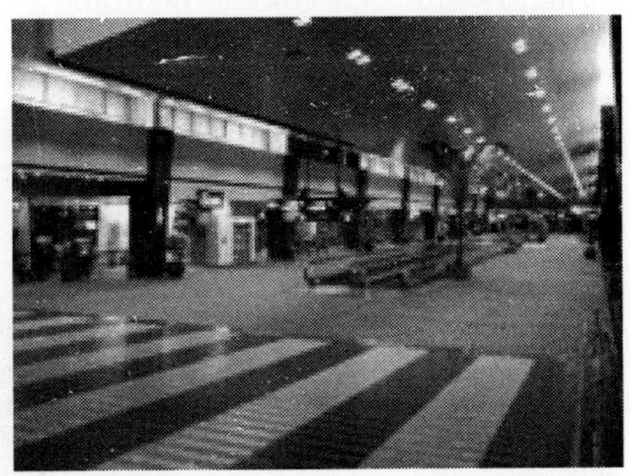

Ultimately, the medical traveler seeks peace of mind. They do not want to go where there are uncertainties about the quality of care or the safety of the blood, rumors of wars and bombs, government or social unrest, natural disasters, or any concerns about safety for themselves and their families. Singapore is one destination where medical travelers will have no such fears, where they can enjoy peace of mind when their health really matters.

Question: Approximately how many international patients does Singapore receive annually, from which parts of the world, and what are the most sought after treatments by these patients? How much growth is Singapore expecting in this area in the next year and beyond?

Dr. Yap: Based on exit surveys conducted of international patients, out of the nearly 10 million visitors to Singapore in 2006, approximately 410,000 or four percent travelled specifically for health care. These patients did not come alone. Approximately 89,000 persons accompanied them on their visits. Another 56,000 received health care incidentally when on visits for other purposes. In total, some 555,000 international visitors to Singapore in 2006 were involved in some aspect of medical travel.

The majority of our medical travelers come from the established markets of Indonesia, Malaysia and Brunei, but the list of countries that patients now come from have gone up tremendously in the past half-decade. Singapore continues to be a favoured destination for our established markets. Readers Digest in a 25,000-reader survey found that their readers ranked Singapore only after USA as most favoured health care destination, even ahead of Europe. Consider how the number of health care visitors grew from 320,000 in 2004 to 410,000 in 2006, a 28% increase. Some of that increase is accounted by gradual increases in numbers from the relatively stable, established markets, but the remainder is from the rapidly growing markets in ASEAN, the Middle East, South Asia, Russia, etc.

Singapore offers a wide spectrum of health care services ranging from health screening and cosmetic surgery to complex specialty care such as ophthalmology, orthopedic surgery, cardiology, cardiothoracic surgery, obstetrics and gynecology, neurology, neurosurgery and oncology amongst others.

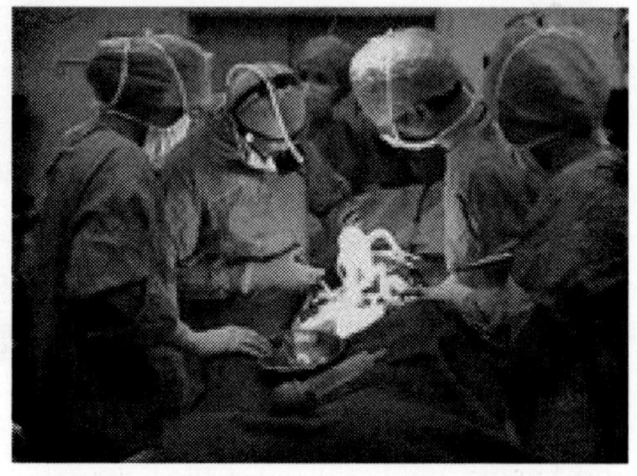

Categorically, international patients come to Singapore for four main types of health care. They come for essential health care where the care is not available in their own country, affordable health care where the care is available but not affordable, quality health care where the care available locally is or is perceived to be of inferior quality, and premium health care where traveling for health care is seen as a luxury and adds prestige to the traveling person.

The most significant reason for patients coming to Singapore from the surrounding regions such as Indonesia, Malaysia, Indo-China and India, is for quality health care. Many also come for essential health care, in particular, complex heart, brain, lung, liver and orthopedic surgeries, organ transplantations, as well as cancer care where their home countries just do not have a similarly high level of medical sophistication, whereas patients from the United Kingdom come to Singapore to avoid long waiting times for surgeries like hip replacements.

For visitors from the United States who usually come to Singapore for orthopedic surgeries and cardiology, the biggest motivation is the cost savings for high quality health care, as patients can receive US-standard health care from JCI-accredited health care facilities and internationally known doctors at a fifth of the price back home or less.

In total, some 555,000 international visitors to Singapore in 2006 were involved in some aspect of medical travel. Thus, medical travel is a very big market. Singapore hopes to attract at least 1 million medical travelers to Singapore every year starting from 2012.

Question: The Singapore Government seems to be much more involved in promoting medical tourism and getting the various agencies to coordinate in order to provide a better experience for visiting patients. Is this a conscious effort, or is it just the way you do things?

Dr. Yap: While many other countries and regions announce their plans to "go into medical tourism", Singapore has been quietly doing it all along. The "Whole of Government" approach to supporting Singapore's international medical travel industry is evident in the SingaporeMedicine initiative.

SingaporeMedicine is a multi-agency government-industry partnership to develop and maintain Singapore as a medical hub and international patient destination. It is led by the Ministry of Health, and supported by three government agencies: the Economic Development Board which develops industry capabilities, the International Enterprise Singapore which fosters regionalization by Singapore's local health care players, and the Singapore Tourism Board which manages international marketing and associated people-oriented services.

The government agencies work with the local and international health care and medical travel industries to ensure that patients are well taken care of. Where there are issues affecting other government agencies (e.g. visas), there is a government-wide consensus and effort to balance the different needs to achieve the best solutions.

Most important of all, as mentioned in Q1, the main motivation behind the government supporting medical travel is that Singapore needs to have patient volumes to maintain the clinical sub-specialty expertise, and to gain economies of scale for its technology.

So yes, it is a conscious effort by the government to ultimately provide and sustain the level of clinical expertise and medical care that Singaporeans have since become used to.

Question: We recently interviewed Dr. Milica Bookman, who is doing research on the effect of medical tourism on developing countries. Not to say that Singapore is a developing country, but is medical tourism having any effect on health care you offer to your own citizens? If so, could you elaborate on that?

Dr. Yap: As emphasized in Q1, Singapore needs foreign patients in order to serve its own patients.

Question: Please tell us a bit more about Singapore medicine (Singaporemedicine.com), its mission and activities.

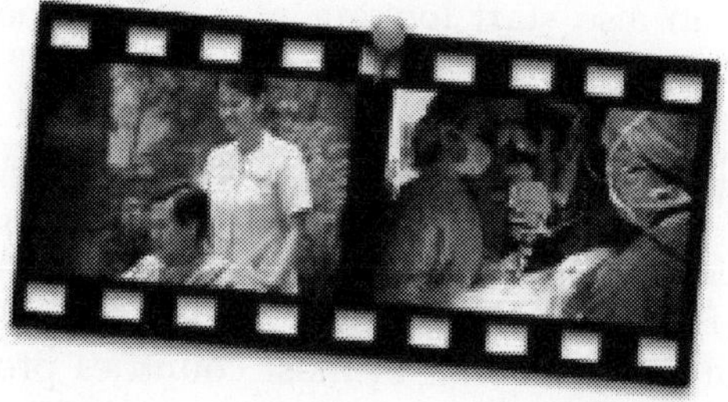

Dr. Yap: Activities undertaken by Singapore-Medicine partners include: Media familiarization trips for international journalists.

Participation in health care conferences and tradeshows in key and emerging overseas markets such as Indonesia, Malaysia, India, Bangladesh, the Middle East, Russia, and more recently, the United States.

Intensified market development, business development and product development programmes by the Singapore health care providers through the support of SingaporeMedicine.

SingaporeMedicine is also working closely with medical institutions to improve international patient support through the provision of international patient liaison services, translation and interpretation services as well as foreign language signages to meet the diverse needs of foreign patients.

Question: We're seeing some employers and insurers showing interest in medical tourism in the U.S. What do you think about medical tourism as an industry? What's the potential? What changes do you see in the near future?

Dr. Yap: The Medical Tourism market is currently valued at US$20 billion annually. Some of these dollars is perhaps hype but the market is obviously significant whatever the actual numbers. These numbers are expected to double by 2010.

The world has flattened for many industries like manufacturing and software engineering, where many companies have gone to China and India respectively. We expect to see the flattening of the world (as in Thomas Friedman's book) finally reach the health care world. Today people in many countries and regions find that the health care in their own locality is not accessible, affordable, adequate or acceptable. With the relative ease and low costs of travel today, patients will travel in search of better health care.

The medical travel industry has grown in several waves. Initially, there was the local/proximate movements of people to nearby countries for better health care, for example, Singapore has been serving the peoples of Indonesia, Malaysia, Brunei and the rest of the ASEAN region long before the term "medical tourism" was ever coined. The people started moving farther afield when they found that they, as consumers, had the ability to choose, which was when individual, often uninsured, Americans started looking to Asia for lower cost health care.

The next wave is waiting, when corporate entities realise that, just they can source worldwide for manpower and means of production, they can also start looking overseas for health care for their manpower. When corporations, for example in the US and the developed world, started sending their staff around the world for the best and the most affordable health care, then truly the world would be flat indeed.

Question: The main worry about medical tourism is that there's no legal recourse in case things go wrong when you opt for surgery abroad. There is realistically very little chance of a successful and timely malpractice suit in most countries promoting medical tourism. What is the status of Singapore, in this regard?

Dr. Yap: Patients travelling for health care should by and large be seeking reliable and safe health care, and legal proceedings should ideally be a low probability event. Given the excellent clinical outcomes and assured quality of health care in Singapore, the chances of patients having to seek legal recourse are significantly lower as compared to other health care destinations. However, medicine being what it is, it is not possible to rule out completely the possibility of mishaps and other untoward events. Legal suits related to health care services delivered in Singapore would generally be contested in Singaporean law courts. The legal system in Singapore is well known for its impartiality and reliability. In 2004, the Political and Economic Risks Consultancy (PERC) rated Singapore's judicial system as the best in Asia, ahead of Hong Kong and Japan. It also ranked Singapore as the top in consistency of application of laws. In addition, Singapore's legal system has been praised by the International Monetary Fund and the Economic Intelligence Unit. Therefore, the medical traveler can be assured of fairness in the rare event that legal action is appropriate.

That was Dr. Jason Yap, Director, Health Care Services, STB. The main advantage Singapore has is that things work efficiently, and on time. A medical tourist in Singapore gets the same, if not better, level of care, at a fraction of the price, has legal recourse which is fair and quick, and best of all, you have the option of recuperating with a great post surgical vacation in Singapore. And an indicator of their efficiency is the fact that the SingaporeMedicine website can be accessed in five languages—English, Chinese, Arabic, Indonesian and Vietnamese. That shows how consumer-friendly they are, and how far they are willing to go to attract and satisfy medical tourists. Stay tuned for more interviews.

Thursday, August 16, 2007

Bargain Surgery Abroad

"The Chaophya hospital is one of five hospitals in Thailand and in Singapore offering stem cell therapy for end-stage heart disease. Thailand is also a destination for medical tourists with a very different agenda from those of Dr. Supachai's patients: it is one of the world's leading centers for sex reassignment surgery. The boom in medical tourism in recent years has spawned the growth of a new travel market, with specialized agencies ready to serve their clients' clinical and travel needs, whether they're Americans seeking cosmetic surgery, or Canadians who don't want to wait up to a year for a government-funded hip replacement."

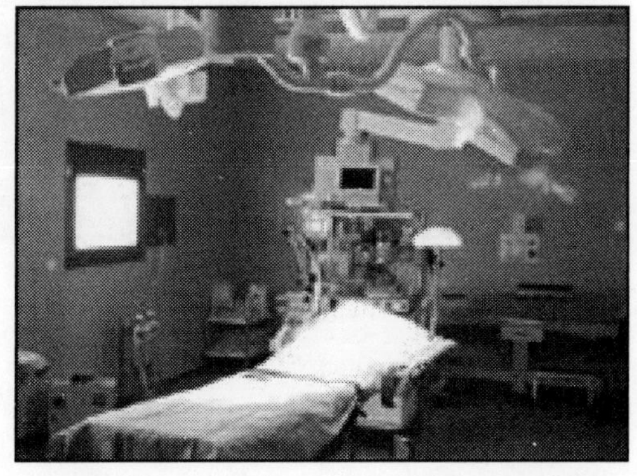

Medical tourism is an increasingly attractive option for any kind of medical treatment or surgery which is not immediately available or is unaffordable locally. And unless employers and health plans start considering medical tourism as an option, the slow bleed of patients going abroad, without any kind of safety net will continue.

Dentists in eastern Europe were the first to attract British patients for teeth whitening and other cosmetic work. But now plastic surgeons are following suit-offering bargain breast implants and other procedures."

Richard Slater lives at a nursing home in Mexico, comfortably settled into his own cottage surrounded by purple bougainvillea and pomegranate trees....He gets 24-hour nursing care and three meals a day, cooked in a homey kitchen and served in a sun-washed dining room. For this, Slater pays just $550 a month, less than one-tenth of the going rate back home in Las Vegas. For an additional $140 a year, he gets complete medical coverage from the Mexican government, including all his medicine and insulin for his diabetes. "This would all cost me a fortune in the United States," said Slater, a 65-year-old retired headwaiter. "I'm real happy with the place." Um...Maybe the Mexicans should build a border fence to prevent all those seniors from the United States sneaking across the border into Mexico, trying to escape the squalor and poverty at home and enjoy the good times in Mexico....

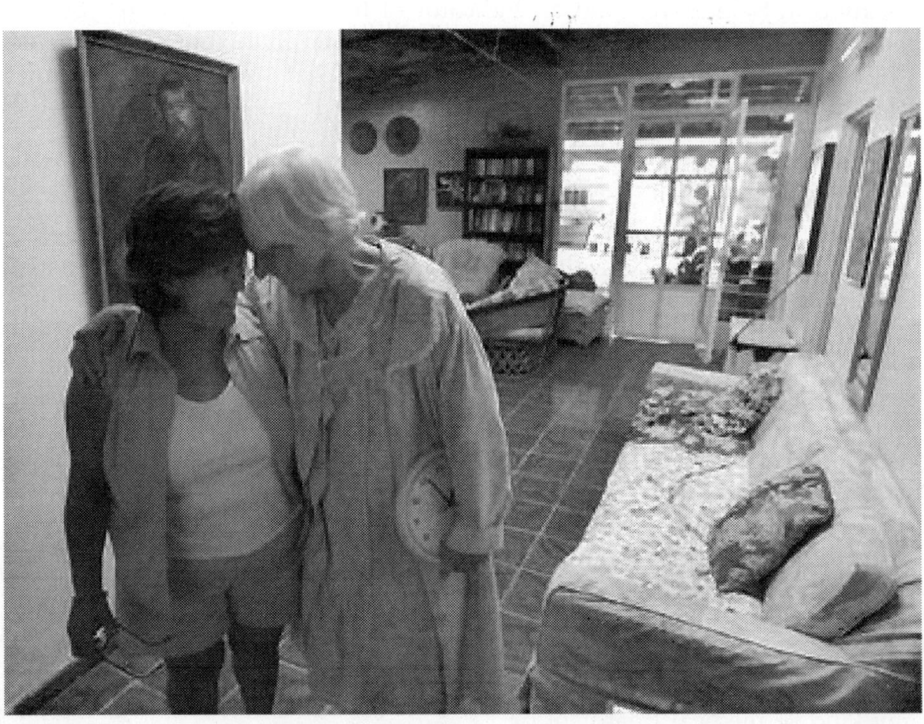

Appendix 5

CASE STUDY OF SOME INDIAN HOSPITALS

A. L.V. PRASAD EYE INSTITUTE, HYDERABAD

The mission of L.V. Prasad Eye Institute is to provide excellent eye care with equity. We believe that the second component of our mission, equity, is measurable and we have done well all these years. Excellence, on the other hand is a continuous path and we constantly strive to tread firmly along it as we improve ourselves. Excellence in patient care is not merely excellence in clinical outcomes, but total patient care is not merely excellence in clinical outcomes, but total patient satisfaction. This necessarily means that all employees involved in patient care understand the importance of the role played by them, and have a sense of ownership and price. As an organisation grows in size and scale, these core values can become somewhat blurred. With the support of our newly restructured leadership, we are working towards improving total quantity in our patient care services.

The real measure of everything we do is its impact on patient's lives. Medical and surgical interventions here are based on the latest know how tempered with compassion and a concern for the real contexts that patients come from and must go back to. Whether it is helping a student realize his ambitions or taking a family from despair to hope, or making a young man feel good about himself again, our clinicians are clear about one thing—they do not treat eyes, they treat people.

Patient care is the focal point of LVPEI's activities and we continue to get patients from all over India and many other countries. The number of patients from abroad has increased, especially from the Middle East (Oman, UAE, Madagascar) and the African continent. Our tiered payment structure cross subsidizes eye care costs for people of all levels, while we continue to provide quality eye care at no cost to the less privileged.

While striving to serve the needs of the especially vulnerable sections—children, the elderly, and the rural poor—we proactively develop new and better approaches for treatment and management of eye diseases. Similarly, each of our subsequently areas kept pace with global advances through continual upgradation of knowledge, skills and infrastructure and our investments for these always go hand in hand. Large volumes of Corneal Transplants, Comprehensive Ocular Oncology Services, an extensive network of ROP (retinopathy of prematurity) care, increasing demands for all sub-specialities characterized the year.

The Ramayamma International Eye Bank addresses the problem of corneal blindness by enhancing the country eye banking systems through training, research, capacity building and advocacy, while continuing to act as a national monitor for all eye banks.

L.V. Prasad Eye Institute, Bhubaneswar

The Bhubaneswar L.V. Prasad Eye Institute Began functioning the very next day after its inauguration on July 4, 2006. On the first day over 50 patients registered and underwent detailed eye examinations. The operating rooms opened for surgeries in the month of October after a rigorous critical inspection. LVPEI will serve as a tertiary care centre for the state of Orissa and the neigbouring states in eastern India.

Performance statistics

Services	*Paying*	*Non-paying*	*Total*
Outpatient visits (8 months)	12,412	4,181	16,593
Surgical procedures (4 months)	796	469	1265

Events

Bhubaneswar Eye meet

The Bhubaneswar eye meet was held at Bhubaneswar LVPEI under the aegins of the Orissa State Ophthalmological Society on January 13-14, 2007. It was attended by 89 opthalmologists from various parts of Orissa. Dr. Suryasnata Rath was the organizing secretary and the meeting covered various sub-sepecialities of ophthalmology. The guest faculty included Dr. G. Chandrasekhar and Dr. Virender S. Sangwan from LVPEI, Hyderabad; Dr. J. Biswas from Sankara Nethralaya, Chennai; and Dr. Kim Ramasamy and Dr. Usha Kim from Aravind Eye hospital, Madurai.

School eye screening

Seventeen teachers and two pharmacists from the school of Kalinga Institute of Social sciences (KISS), Bhubaneswar were trained for the school eye screening program. The training was conducted by the staff B-LVPEI, who included Mr. Bikash Chandra Malhotra, Dr. Sanghamitra Dash, Dr. Srikantha Sahu, Mr. Mukesh Singh, Mr. A. Jeevan Rao, Mr. Shyam Sunder Nayak and Ms. Sujata Mishra.

Community screening program

At the behest of Mr. A.K. Bhandari, Zonal Manager, Bank of India, Bhubaneswar, the first community eye screening program was organized by B-LVPEI on March 18, 2007. A total of 100 patients were examined, of which 14 were counseled for further check up, 10 were prescribed medication, 25 were advised to change their spectacles; 23 were advised to continue using their spectacles, and 19 were advised to use spectacles.

L.V. Prasad Eye Institute, Visakhapatnam

The L.V. Prasad Eye Institute, Visakhapatnam commenced patient care activities on July 7th 2006. On the first day over 100 patients registered and underwent detailed eye examination. The operating room complex was operational from the month of November after a rigorous inspection. LVPEI, Visakhapatnam serves as a tertiary care centre for the northern part of Andhra Pradesh State and the neighbouring areas in eastern India.

Performance Statistices

Services	*Paying*	*Non-paying*	*Total*
Outpatient visits (8 months)	9,977	4,229	14,206
Surgical procedures (4 months)	431	271	702

Analysis of surgical procedures (%)

Cataract Surgery	386
Corneal procedures	88
Retina Surgery	103
Glaucoma Surgery	14
IOAB*	111

In addition, 45 children were examined and treated under anesthesia (EUA).

Note: The No. of surgical procedures (1096) is greater than the No. of eyes (728) as multiple procedures were done on some eyes.

Rob Ohlson Centre for Sight Enhancement and Rehabilitation for the Blind

October 2006—March 2007

Low vision care during the year	
New patients	38
Follow up patients	8
Total	46

Optical Devices Prescribed	
Spectacles	8
Bifocals	12
Magnifiers	11
Telescopes	17

Age wise Analysis of Patients (%)	
Birth to 15 yrs.	25
16 to 45 yrs.	25
46 to 60 yrs.	5
61 to above	6

Non-OpticalDevices Prescribed)	
Reading Stand	9
Reading lamp	13
Typo scope	2
Approach magnification	38
Light control devices	12
Closed circuit television	1

Rehabilitation Services	
Counseling	118
*Special skills training	27

L.V. Prasad Eye Instiute, Hyderabad

Hospital Performance Statistics

Services	*Paying*	*Non-paying*	*Total*
Outpatient visits	129665	55011	184676
Surgical procedures	12753	10103	22856

Patients from all over the world and across India

International			*National*	
Afghanistan	Nigeria	Andhra Pradesh	Karnataka	Punjab
Australia	Oman	Assam	Kerala	Rajasthan
Bangladesh	Pakistan	Bihar	Madhya Pradesh	Sikkim
Bhutan	Philippines	Chandigarh	Maharashtra	Tamil Nadu
Botswana	Singapore	Chattisgarh	Manipur	Tripura
Canada	Spain	Goa	Meghalaya	Uttar Pradesh
Guyana	Tanzania	Gujarat	Mizoram	Uttaran-chal
Kenya	Uganda	Haryana	Nagaland	West Bengal
Malawi	UAE	Himachal	New Delhi	
Mauritius	UK	Pradesh	Jammu and Kashmir Orissa	
Madagascar	USA	Jharkhand		
Pondicherry	Nepal	Zimbabwe		
New Zealand				

Cataract	10,879
Corneal transplants	882
Glaucoma surgeries	879
Plastic surgeries	2,028
Squint surgeries	585
Retina vitreous	3669
Lasers	251
Corneal surgeries	2946
Other surgeries	737

In addition, 2724 children were examined and treated under anaesthesia (EUA).

Jasti V. Ramayamma Children Eye Care Centre

Performance Statistics

Retinoapthy of Prematurity (ROP) Program

Since 1998, L.V. Prasad Eye institute ROP screening program has helped identify and ROP in scores of pre-term babies. The low rate of ROP Surgeries and higher number of prophylactic lasers reflects the success of the screening program.

Babies screened	989 (676 in NICU*s)
Laser sessions	159 (23 in NICUs)
Pediatric retinal surgeries	489
ROP surgeries	18

ROP Public Education Forum: A Public Education Forum on ROP was held on Octorber 14, 2006, to increase awareness about retinopathy of prematurity. The program was held with support from Mr. Ramesh Prasad, CEO, PRASADS IMAX.

Appraisal and audit: Sight Savers International, UK, conducted an evaluation of our Sight Savers funded ROP treatment and training grant project in November 2006. Experience gained from this project will be utilized to plan ROP training programs in India and other countries, especially in the context of the VISION 2020. The Right to Sight initiative, which has identified ROP as an important cause of preventable blindness among children.

Ramayamma International Eye Bank

L.V. Prasad Eye Institute, Hyderabad

My grandmother lived a long and happy life, and it seemed right to help someone else have the opportunity to have a similarly fulfilled life by donating her eyes. We were aware that due to her advanced age (96) the corneas may not be a graft quality, but at least they could be used for research, which too was an important cause to support.

Programs under the ORBIS—ESI-LVPEI project

Under the ORBIS—ESI-LVPEI project training was provided to 11 eye bank technicians, 2 eye donation counselors, 14 ophthalmologists and 2 eye bank managers.

The 8th zonal workshop on eye banking was held in collaboration with Sri Sankaradeva Nethralaya, Guwahati, on May 6, 2006; there were 72 participants including the faculty. The 9th zonal workshop was held at lions NAB eye hospital, Miraj, Sangli, on July 22, 2006. in collaboration with Lions Parasmal Kocheta Eye Bank. There were 152 participants, including the faculty.

RIEB is conducting a study in collaboration with Bristol Eye bank, UK and Eye sight international, Canada, under the ORBIS—ESI-LVPEI project to explore the possibility of increasing the donor pool. In the study, the issue of safety of corneas received from septicemic and ventilator dependent donor for transplantation will be scientifically addressed employed the organ culture technique. Corneas procured from 62 donors were investigated.

Eye Donation Fortnight: The 21st National Eye Donation Fortnight (EDF) was observed from August 25-September 8, 2006, posters and publicity material was placed and distributed at various hospitals in Hyderabad; slides were also screened at cinema theatres to spread the message of eye donation.

Record Eye Donations: Mr. A. Raghu, eye donation counselor, motivated 32 people for eye donation between January 26 and February 25, 2007. This was the highest number of eye donations received through counseling by an individual in one month in Andhra Pradesh.

Vision Rehabilitation Centres

The Rehabilitation Centres at L.V. Prasad Eye Institute, apart from providing low vision and rehabilitative services through hospital and community based programs, are engaged in research aimed at identifying barriers to the provision and uptake of low vision services, and designing new products and processes that enhance service delivery to persons with severe vision impairment. The two rehabilitation centres are the Meera and L.B. Deshpande Centre for Sight Enhancement and the Dr. P.R.K. Prasad Centre for Rehabilitation of Blind and Visually Impaired, both of which work together to develop a comprehensive rehabilitation plan for persons with vision Impairment.

During the year 101 ophthalmologists and optometrists participated in the low vision awareness program, conducted by LVPEI, and 8 optometrists underwent a short term (3 months) course in low vision care. Overall the centres have trained 415 opthalmologists, optometrists, and special educators through the low vision awareness program and 46 optometrists in the short term course.

Meera and L.B. Deshpande Centre for Sight Enhancement

Low vision care during the year		*Optical devices prescribed*	
New patients	1467	Spectacles	312
Follow-up patients	618	Bifocals	139
Total	2085	Magnifiers	401
		Telescopes	127
		Non-optical devices prescribed	
		Reading stand	70
		Reading lamp	65

Typoscope	—
Approach magnification	1398
Light control devices	85
Closed-circuit television	—

Birth—15 years	587
16—45 years	450
46—60 years	254
61 and above	176

Dr. PRK Prasad Centre for Rehabilitation of Blind and Visually Impaired

Children's Centre	1461
Adults Centre	2374

Rehabilitation Services

Counselling	3768
Special Skills Training	869
Instruction in use of	
• Assistive devices (computers)	208
• Low vision devices	784
Environmental modification	2260
Educational guidance	1034
Vocational guidance	317
Supportive services	3316
Referral to other services	280
Follow-up	1404

EDUCATION CENTRE

Training has now taken on a new dimension at LVPEI, with the Education Centre offering a wide variety of programs apart from the traditional subspecialty fellowships and observerships. Drawing from our engagement in the field, both within India and globally, we have developed programs that are increasingly attracting professionals from across regions, specializations and levels of eye care service delivery. The uniqueness of our programs is their relevance to the world of practice and to addressing the gap in human resources in eye care in underserved areas both in India and abroad.

Our Education Centre's recognized capability to provide comprehensive indepth training programs attracts ophthalmologists and other eye care professionals from across India and the world. This year we had participants from Australia, China, Malaysia, Nepal, Nigeria, Pakistan, United Kingdom, USA, Vietnam and Zambia, as well as from all over India. Our training programs cover eye care personnel at all levels—front office, counselors, ophthalmic nursing assistants, administrators, vision technicians, optometrists and ophthalmologists. The Education Centre also coordinates the training of candidates for LVPEI's rural secondary and primary care centres.

As part of our collaboration with ORBIS international we have initiated and launched the Pediatric Opthalmology Learning and Training Center program (POLTC) in October 2006 to address issues related to childhood blindness in India and South East Asia. The main objective of the 3½ year project is to train 5 pediatric eye care teams from across India.

This year too eminent guest faculty visited the institute and shared their experiences and perceptions with the faculty and staff. This exposure to a great wealth of knowledge from around the world is a great boon to out group.

Ophthalmology Training Program

Cornea and Anterior Segment (15 months)

Dr. Syed Maaz Mohiuddin	Hyderabad, Andhra Pradesh
Dr. Aneeta Jabbar	Kozhikode, Kerala
Dr. Sunita Chourasia	Ghaziabad, Uttar Pradesh
Dr. Vu Thi Tue Khanh	Hanoi, Vietnam
Dr. Aditi Biyani	Mumbai, Maharashtra
Dr. Meghna K. Chandrakar	Mumbai, Maharashtra

Cornea and Anterior Segment (3 months)

Dr. Thang Diep Huu	Ho Chi Minh, Vietnam
Dr. Rupa Jain	Salatwada, Vadodara
Dr. Sunil Kumar Thangaraj	Visakhapatnam, Andhra Pradesh
Dr. Rushit H. Sheth	Rajkot, Gujarat
Dr. Manish R. Kadam	Vadodara, Gujarat
Dr. Md Saifullah	Dhaka, Bangladesh

Glaucoma (15 months)

Dr. Debasis Chakraborti	Kolkata, West Bengal
Dr. K.P. Narendra	Sringeri, Karnataka

Glaucoma (3 months)

Dr. Trang Thanh Nghiep	Ho Chi Minh, Vietnam
Dr. Vinita Ramnani	Bairagarh, Bhopal
Dr. Indra Man Maharjan	Pokhara, Nepal
Dr. Chanda Shahani	Kutch, Gujarat
Dr. Elizabeth Varghese	Kothamangalam, Kerala

Dr. Debabrat Haldarthe	Kolkata, West Bengal

Retina Vitreous (15 months)

Dr. Saumil Sharad Sheth	Mumbai, Maharashtra
Dr. Tariq Reza Ali	Dhaka, Bangladesh
Dr. Sushma Raja	Hyderabad, Andhra Pradesh

Retina Vitreous (3 months)

Dr. R.S. Vinay Kumar	Mahaboobnagar, Andhra Pradesh
Dr. Oluleye Tunji Sunday	Ibadan, Nigeria
Dr. Sana Ullah Jan	Peshawar, Pakistan
Dr. Srinivasulu	Dharamavaram, Andhra Pradesh
Dr. Velaldanda Raghu	Karimnagar, Andhra Pradesh

Comprehensive Opthalmology (3 years)

Dr. Partha Pratim Pal	Agartala, Tripura
Dr. Manjunath D. Patil	Solapur, Maharashtra
Dr. Manish Malhotra	New Delhi
Dr. Prashant Gupta	Aligarh, Uttar Pradesh
Dr. Prateek Teotia	Mumbai, Maharashtra
Dr. Bhavleen Kaur	Chandigarh
Dr. Jayasudha	Gulbarga, Karnataka

Comprehensive Opthalmology (1 year)

Dr. V. Ravi Kumar	Visakhapatnam, Andhra Pradesh

Comprehensive Opthalmology (3 months)

Dr. Alok Pratap Singh	Gorakhpur, Uttar Pradesh
Dr. Ch. Manimala	Tanuku, Andhra Pradesh

Pediatric Opthalmology (15 months)

Dr. Siddarth Kesarwani	New Delhi
Dr. Manish Shyamkul	Mumbai, Maharashtra

Pediatric Opthalmology (3 months)

Dr. Mahesh	Guntur, Andhra Pradesh
Dr. Dupe Popoola	Ilorin, Nigeria

Opthalmic Plastic Surgery, Orbit and Ocular Oncology (15 months)

Dr. Vikas Menon	Amritsar, Punjab
Dr. Sima Das	New Delhi

Opthalmic Plastic Surgery, Orbit and Oncology (3 months)

Dr. Rahul Deshpande	Pune, Maharashtra
Dr. Maj B.V. Rao	Hyderabad, Andhra Pradesh

Retina Laser (1 month)

Dr. Praful Gangashnakar Nakar	Dhule, Maharashtra
Dr. Arul Malar	Chennai, Tamilnadu
Dr. Jasprit Singh Hans	Patiala, Punjab
Dr. Renu Dhasmana	Dehradun, Uttaranchal
Dr. Sonia Nankani	Mumbai, Maharashtra
Dr. Challa Jagannath	Tirupati, Andhra Pradesh
Dr. Naseem Hussain	Hyderabad, Andhra Pradesh
Dr. Brijesh Panwar	Hissar, Haryana
Dr. Manoj Khatri	Chennai, Tamilnadu

Phacoemulsification (1 month)

Dr. Rajeeta Rani Jaiswal	Hyderabad, Andhra Pradesh
Dr. Kavitha Patil	Narkatpaly, Andhra Pradesh
Dr. R.C. Mishra	Dhanbad, Jharkhand
Dr. P.B. Dhagat	Chandrapur, Maharashtra
Dr. Raman Mehta	Kolkata, West Bengal
Dr. (Cap) Chandra Prakash Patel	Berhampur, West Bengal
Dr. Ashok Kumar	Hazaribagh, Jharkhand
Dr. Chinmoyee Deka	Dimapur, Nagaland
Dr. Ch. Chandrasekhar	Markapur, Andhra Pradesh
Dr. Saima Jalal	Rochester, USA
Dr. Mamata Choudhury	Hyderabad, Andhra Pradesh

Retinopathy of Prematurity (1 month)

Dr. G.V. Narendra	Vijayawada, Andhra Pradesh
Dr. Sudhindra	Kolar, Karnataka
Dr. Dhiraj Jaiswal	Nagpur, Maharashtra
Dr. Rooshitha B Singh	Nagercoil, Tamilnadu

EYE RESEARCH

Prof. Brien Holden Eye Research Centre

The Hyderabad Eye Research Foundation (HERF) administers both basic and clinical research at L.V. Prasad Eye Institute (LVPEI). It continues to compete and receive grants from all over the world to conduct cutting edge research on the eye. The Prof. Brien Holden Eye Research Centre (BHERC) investigates the causes and treatment strategies through its various components, namely the Jhaveri Microbiology Centre, the Saroja A. Rao Immunology Laboratory, the Kallam Anji Reddy Molecular Genetics Laboratory, the Ophthalmic Pathology Laboratory, the Sudhakar and Sreekanth Ravi Stem Cell Biology Laboratory, and the clinical research laboratories. Each of these components has been named after its donor, in recognition of their generous donations.

Support and recognition

Research at LVPEI has concentrated on molecular genetics of inherited eye diseases, devising molecular diagnostics for early detection, microbiology of eye infections, biochemical features of cataract, and stem cell technology for reconstruction of the damaged ocular outer surface. Support for these projects have come from competitive grants received from the Department of Biotechnology (DBT), Department of Science and Technology (DST), Council of Scientific and Industrial Research (ICMR)—all from India, as well as the National Eye Institute (NEI, National Institutes of Health), USA. Thanks to the recently finalized US-India eye research collaboration, several joint research projects have been initiated at HERF, in collaboration with researchers in the US. Likewise, HERF is one of the four pillars of the multinational research and development group called Vision CRC (operating from Sydney, Australia) and conducts research on its behalf on the genetics of myopia, as well as a series of clinical studies such as on antibacterial contact lenses, corneal onlays, etc.

The institute is recognized as an external research centre by the University of Hyderabad, Hyderabad; Birla Institute of Technology and Science (BITS), Pilani; and the University of New South Wales, Sydney, Australia. This enables research scholars from LVPEI to register with, and obtain their Ph.D. degrees from these universities. Collaborative research has also been forged with national laboratories such as the Centre for Cellular and Molecular Biology (CCMB), Centre for DNA Fingerprinting and Diagnostics (CDFD) and University of Hyderabad—all in Hyderabad, and the Indian Institute of Science, Bangalore. The agreements allow researchers at LVPEI to access state-of-the-art equipment and sophisticated facilities at these centres.

Clinical Research

LVPEI's multidisciplinary clinical research is of international standards and is sponsored by Indian funding agencies and multinational companies from USA and France. The group conducts not only intramural clinical research, but also participates in multicentre clinical trials.

Clinical research has also pursued the study of the suitability of using extended wear contact lenses. This involves recruitment of volunteers and monitoring comfort levels and related factors upon the use of contact lenses over a period of time. Another area of study was the efficiency, pharmacodynamics and related features of ophthalmic drugs and antibiotics. Many of the studies are conducted in collaboration with leading pharmaceutical companies.

Translational Research Centre

The year 2006-07 has been a special one for the research groups of the Institute. A welcome addition has been Dr. Yashoda Ghanekar, who has joined us with special expertise in cellular and molecular biology, adding greater strength to our stem cell research efforts. The plans for setting up a translational research centre in eye diseases (TRACER) are fast bearing fruit. Grant applications sent to the Champalimaud Foundation, Portugal, and to the Department of Biotechnology, Government of India, have passed the first round and we have submitted the detailed proposals. When they are approved, we would we able to put up a cGMP type facility for our stem cell research and therapy.

In the mean while, we have been able to obtain competitive research grant funding from just about every national agency. Research work by our group of 7 basic and 25 clinical colleagues, and 23 research fellows and associates, has been very productive, both in basic and clinical areas. We published 90 papers in peer-reviewed journals.

Now that our younger siblings at Bhubaneswar and Visakhapatnam are fully functional, we expect an enlarged activity profile and research progress in the coming years.

Awards and Honors

Among the major awards this year, we are delighted that our colleagues Virender Sangwan was awarded the Bhatnagar Prize in Medical Sciences for the year 2006, and Dr. Gullapalli N. Ro received the International Blindness Prevention Award in 2006. Two research students completed their research under Dr. Savitri Sharma, and were awarded the Ph.D. degree. These are Drs. Joveeta Joseph and Aparna Duggirala, and we congratulate them.

Origin and migration of diseases-associated mutations in primary congenital glaucoma

Primary congenital glaucoma (PCG) is a severely blinding disorder in children with a prevalence of 1 in 3300 live births in Andhra Pradesh. It is an autosomal recessive disorder manifested by two copies of the mutant allele in the children; parents are usually asymptomatic carriers. The cytochrome P450 gene (CYP1B1) happens to be a major culprit as defects in this gene (mutations) account for a varied proportion of primary congenital glaucoma cases worldwide.

The glaucoma research group at the Institute (Dr. Subharata Chakrabarti, Ms Kiranpreet Kaur and Dr. Inderjeet Kaur from the research wing and Drs Anil Mandal, Rajul Parikh and Ravi Thomas from the clinical services) has been working on the genetics of PCG for the last several years. They wanted to address a rather unusual question—why are the mutation spectrums in CYP1B1 in PCG patients similar even across different countries? Dr. Chakrabarti, in collaboration with Prof. Partha P. Majumder, a renowned geneticist at the Indian Statistical Institute, Kolkata, addressed this issue with the help of genetic signatures (haplotypes) in CYP1B1 in PCG patients and unaffected normal control patients. These were analyzed in conjunction with data available from other populations along with ancestral great apes like chimpanzees.

The team observed that common mutations in CYP1B1 associated with PCG occurred on a uniform haplotype background among Indian patients that were completely distinct from the most frequent haplotype found among unaffected Indian control patients. Globally, there was a strong clustering of mutations by geographical and haplotype backgrounds. Together with the data of chimpanzees, and of normal controls from India and other global regions, it was possible to reconstruct the evolution of these mutations on different haplotype backgrounds.

The presence of predominant CYP1B1 mutations on specific haplotypes, irrespective of geographical regions, is indicative of common founders and population movements. Some of these observations could be correlated with the ancient population movements from Saudi Arabia to India, immigration of the Roma gypsies from India to northern and central Asia and so forth. These results are useful for predictive testing of PCG and call for similar studies on PCG mutations that are not associated with CYP1B1.

The detailed results of the study were published in the *Journal Investigate Opthalmology and Visual Sciences* (January 2006 issue) and also cited in the directory of the Online Mendelian Inheritance in Man (OMIM).

Visualization of *in situ* aggregation of two cataract-associated human g-Crystallin mutants in human lens epithelial cells

Investigators: Venu Talla, D Balasubramanian, in collaboration with N Srinivasan of IISC, Bangalore, Support: DST.

Gamma crystallins are part of the structural proteins constituting the human eye lens. Mutations in them are associated with congenital cataract in infants. We have cloned and expressed two such mutant human g-crystallins, namely W157X gD-crystalline and W157X human gC-crystalline, each associated with autosomal dominant congenital cataract. We transfected their cDNAs individually into human lens epithelial cells, in order to check whether they form scattering particles in situ. We then studies the structural features of the expressed proteins, so as to understand the molecular phenotype of this form of cataract. Transfection of GFP—tagged wild type cDNAs into several cell lines did not lead to any marked changes, while similar transfection of the mutants led to the visualization of scattering bodies and self-aggregates. Turning to the properties of the expressed proteins, the mutant molecules showed a thousand-fold reduction in solubility than the wild type. They showed subtle structural changes—a more open structure, and a greater degree of surface hydrophobicity, in comparison to the wild type molecules. They also displayed less structural stability towards thermal and chemical denaturants. Molecular modeling studies confirmed these features. The deletion of 17 residues in the carboxy-terminus of human gC- and gD-crystallins is seen to expose the side chains of several hydrophobic residues in the sequence to the solvent, causing the molecule to selt-aggregate. This feature appears to be reflected *in situ,* upon introduction of the mutants in human lens epithelial cells. These results are consistent with the observed cataract.

A glaucoma-associated mutant of optineurin selectively induces death of retinal ganglion cells, which is inhibited by antioxidants

Investigators: Madhavi Latha Chalasani, D Balasubramanian, in collaboration with Vegesna Radha, Vijay Gupta and Ghanshyam Swarup (CCMB) and Neeraj Agarwal (Univ. North Texas). Support: DST.

Certain missense mutation in the coding region of the optineurin gene (OPTN) are associated with normal tension glaucoma as well as POAG. While the function of the optineurin protein is yet to be elucidated, its most common mutation, E50K, is associated with a severe phenotype. In the present study we have explored some of the functional characteristic of optineurin and its mutants, in particular E50K. The E50K mutant was seen to selectively induce the death of rat retinal ganglion cells (RGC-5) but not of the other cell lines tested (Cos-1, HeLa and IMR-32). Neither the other mutants nor WT optineurin were seen to do so. This cell death was seen to require capases, and inhibited by Bcl-2. it was also inhibited by a variety of anti-oxidants and the free redical scavenger enzyme MnSOD. While expression of wild type and E50K mutant suppressed cell death induced by TNF-a in HeLa cells, they were seen to potentiate such cell death in RGC-5 cells. The E50K mutant ofoptineurin has thus acquired the ability to induce cell death selectively in retinal ganglion cells. This cell death is mediated by oxidative stress, since it is inhibited by antioxidants and by MnSOD. Our findings thus raise the possibility of the use of antioxidants for delaying or controlling some forms of glaucoma.

Molecular studies on hereditary congenital cataract

Investigators: Chitra Kannabiran, GP Surya Prakash, Ramesh Kekunnaya, Sushma Tejwani, BSR Murthy.

Support: HERF

Cataract is opacity of the eye's lens and can be hereditary. Hereditary cataracts are mostly congenital or developmental in type, appearing in infancy or childhood. They are inherited as autosomal dominant, autosomal recessive and X-linked diseases. The study aimed at indentifying genes causing hereditary cataracts in Indian families. Patients with bilateral familial cataract with no associated developmental, systemic or ocular disorders and their family members were part of the study. A detailed ophthalmic evaluation was done to screen affected individuals for disease-causing alterations in genes known to cause hereditary cataract. The genes selected for screening were those encoding various crystalline proteins, which are the major structural proteins in the lens, and also connexins or gap junction proteins that maintain intercellular transport of molecules within the lens. Eight genes were screended in 40 patients. An insertion of a single base in the connexin-50 gene (GJA8) was found in tow affected siblings in a family with recessive cataract. This mutation is expected to lead to truncated protein and is the first association of a connexin gene with recessive cataract in humans. Screening of the families for several other genes is in progress.

Mutational screening of SLC4A11 gene in autosomal recessive congenital hereditary endothelial dystrophy

Investigators: Chitra Kannabiran, Afla Sultana, Prashant Garg, BSR Murthy, and Geeta K. Vemuganti. Support: HERF

Congenital hereditary endothelial dystrophy (CHED) is a hereditary corneal disorder in which patients develop corneal opacities leading to loss of vision at birth or early in life. CHED involves a defect in the corneal endothelium, which normally functions as a pump, removing excess water from the cornea, thus maintaining it in a transparent state. Due to accumulation of water within the cornea, there is corneal edema and a bluish-white opacification resembling "ground glass."

Our earlier studies on autosomal recessive CHED had led to the gene underlying this disorder being indentified as SLC4A11, a gene coding for a transporter protein that probably functions in transport of anions across the cells. We screened a larger group of patients with recessive CHED to determine mutations in SLCA1A11 in CHED. Forty-two families (49 afected and 73 unaffected members) affected with recessive CHED underwent ophthalmic evaluation as well as mutational screening. The corneal buttons of these patients were evaluated by histopathology. Twenty-seven different mutations were indentified in 35 unrelated families, of which 19 are not previously reported. These comprised 13 missense, five nonsense, seven deletions, one splice site mutation. Examination of this mutation data with clinical and histopathologic features of the patients did not revel any studies establish the high degree of mutational heterogeneity in autosomal recessive CHED in Indian patients.

Evaluation of tear film proteinases in the pathogenesis of human fungal keratitis

Investigators: Joveeta Joseph, Usha Gopinathan, Prashant Garg, Geeta K. Vemuganti, D. Balasubramanian, Savitri Sharma. Support: CSIR.

The study is aimed at determining whether matrix metaqlloproteinase activity in tears of patients with mycotic keratitis will affect the disease course. The test group included 5 eye each with active or healed fungal keratitis and control group included 10 normal eyes. Tears were collected by Schirmer's strips, eluted using extraction buffer and analyzed by gelation zymography. Proforms of MMP-2 and MMP-9 were detected in patients with healed ulcers. Evaluation of MMP activity in the tears might help understand diseases progression in fungal keratitis.

Detection of biofilms forming capability of ocular isolates of coagulase negative staphylococci and effect of biofilm inhibitors

Investigators: Aparna Duggirala, Dorairajan Balasubramanian, Savitri Sharma. Support: HERF.

This study compares the methods used to assey biofilm formation and the efficiency of biofilm inhibitors in coagulase negative staphylococci (CoNS) isolated from human eyes with or without infection. It also studies the synergy of biofilm inhibitors on the action of gatifloxacin on the growth of fluoroquinolone resistant strains of CoNS. The test group included CoNS isolates . Biofilm formation was monitored by PCR for the ica AB gene and by phenotypic asseys.

Our results showed that phenotypic methods differentiated pathogenic CoNS from non-pathogenic. Quercetin and EGCG appear best biofilm inhibitors. They also appear to act in synergy with gatifloxacin in inhibiting the growth.

Phenotypic and genotypic characterization of limbal stem cells cultivated limbal epithelial cells, and persistence of these characteristics after clinical transplantation

Investigatiors: Virender Singh Sangwan, Geeta K. Vemuganti, D. Balasubramanian, Annes Fatima, M. Lakshmi Soundarya. Support: DBT.

During this year, 103 cases of limbal stem cell deficiency were treated with cultivated limbal epithelial transplanatation. Of these 101 were autologous cultivated limbal epithelial transplants while 2 were co-cultures of limbus and conjunctiva. Of these 101 were autologous, while 2 were allogenic. No complications have been seen in these cases; all the patients are doing well.

The mean of these patients was 22 years, including 33 children. The etiology was mostly chemical burns; firecracker burns, blask injuries, stevens Johnson syndrome, etc.

Cultivation and characterization of oral mucosal epithelium for regenerating ocular surface in patients with bilateral limbal stem cell deficiency

Investigators: Yashoda Ghanekar, Soundarya Laxmi Madhira, Anirban Bhaduri, Virender S. Sangwan, Geeta K. Vemuganti. Support: DBT, HERF.

This study is aimed at reconstructing the ocular surface in patients with bilateral limbal stem cell deficiency using autologous oral epithelial cells. Ocular surface reconstruction in these patients is currently performed using allogenous limbal cells. However, problems such as lack of suitable allogenous limbal tissue and need for life long use of immunosuppressants have prompted research or appropriate autologous substitute. Cultivated oral mucosal epithelium has been proposed as an alternative for ocular surface reconstruction in these patients.

In this study, -we have been successful in establishing healthy, contamination free and feeder cell free cultures from oral mucosa with a success rate of 40%. The tissue was harvested from healthy volunteers after informed consent and was cultured as an explant using de epithelialized amniotic membrane. The cultures were confluent within 3-4 weeks, underwent stratification to form 2-3 layers of epithelial cells and were devoid of goblet cells. RT-PCR and immunohistochemical analyses showed that the cultures expressed markers such as cytokeratins K3, K15 a enolase, connexin 42 that are also expressed by cultivated limbal epithelial cells. The cultures also expressed p75, a stem cell market for oral epithelial cells, and p. 69, a market for limbal stem cells. Electron microscopy studies show that these cells adhere well to the basement membrance and also from intercellular gap junctions and tight junctions. The studies indicate that cultured oral mucosal epithelial cells are morphologically and phenotypically similar to cultured limbal epithelial. The project will now go into the clinical phase, where cultivated autologous oral mucosal epithelial cells will be transplanted into patients with bilateral limbal stem cell deficiency.

Isolation of bone marrow stromal cells and attempts to transdifferentiate them into neuroretinal cells

Investigators: Geeta K. Vemuganti, T. Das, D. Balasubramanian, K. Purushottam Reddy. Support: DBT.

During this year we tried two methods of differentiation for retinal photoreceptor lineage: using retinal pigment epithelium 65 (RPE65) cell line conditioned media and also co-culture standardizations in this regard are in progress. The molecular characterization of BMSCs differentiated into neuronal lineage by RT-PCR and western blotting is in progress. We are now standardizing the isolation protocol of murine stromal cells. Dr. Shalesh Kaushal of the University of Florida is helping us with the electrophysiology experiments in animal models.

Evaluation and characterization of cancer stem cells in retinoblastoma tumor

Investigators: Geeta K. Vemuganti, Chitra Kannabiran, Santosh Honavar, Ramesh Murthy, Balla Sagar, Support: ICMR.

It is believed that some tumor cells in retinoblastoma could probably contribute to chemoresistance, recurrence and metasatic potential of retinoblastoma. This subset of cells may have stem cell like properties and could be evaluated by clonal culture, presence of specific markers and by invitro assays. We believe this will improve our knowledge on the pathobiology of tumor progression, resistance, metastasis and be useful in designing effective and targeted therapies.

The primary cultures from retinoblastoma are in progress. We also initiated work on Y79 retinoblastoma cell lines, and initiated clonal assays in these cells lines. An interesting observation was made while evaluating the putative stem cells in about 50 cases of Ocular surface squamous neoplasis (OSSN). The differential expression in invasive and *in situ* lesions raises a possibility that they play an important role in proliferation and differentiation.

Variants in the 10q26 gene cluster exhibit enhanced risk of age-related macular degeneration along with complement factor H in Indian patients

Investigators: Inderjeet Kaur, Subhabrata Chakrabarti, Yashoda Ghanekar, Saritha Katta, Avid Hussain, Nazimul Hussain, Raja Narayanan, Annie Mathai, Subhadra Jalali, Rajiv K. Reddy, K. Ramesh, Ajit B. Majji. Support: HERF.

AMD is a late onset complex disorder with multifactorial etiologies. Both genetic and environemental factors play a role in the disease pathogenesis. AMD is the third leading causes of blindness in the elderly. Familial aggregation, segregation studies and linkage analysis have provided both qualitative and quantitative evidence on the genetic basis in AMD.

Earlier, in a cohort of AMD cases in India, we had conformed the association of the Tyr402His SNP in the Complement factor H gene (CFH) and AMD through LD and haplotype analysis.

As of now, we have screened 250 patients with age-related macular degeneration and 250 normal age matched controls for SNPs in five candidate genes namely, complement factor H, apolipoprotein E, LOC387715, HTRA1 and Toll like receptor 4 genes. AMD cases had a higher frequency of the risk alleles [LOC387715 (rs 10490924) ($p = 4.47 \times 10^{-13}$), HTRA1 (rs 11200638) ($p = 3.53 \times 10^{-6}$) and rs 2672598 ($p = 4.88 \times 10^{-8}$) and also exhibited higher disease odds in the corresponding risk genotypes. The "G–C–T–A–C" was the risk haplotypes ($p = 4.66 \times 10^{-13}$), while the "G–C–G–G–T" haplotype was protective ($p = 7.40 \times 10^{-4}$). The additive effect of the CFH risk genotypes exhibited a PAR of 69.5% with LOC387715 (OR = 8.83, 95%Cl, 5.49–14.21) and 71.3% with HTRA1 (OR = 7.67, 95% Cl, 4.47–13.18). These associations underscore their significant involvement in AMD susceptibility and may be useful for predictive testing.

Fork head transcriptional factor gene (Fox 12) mutations in Indian patients with Blepharophimosis ptosis epicanthus inversus syndrome

Investigators: Inderjeet Kaur, Avid Hussain, Milind Naik, Santosh G. Honavar. Support: HERF.

Blepharophimosis ptosis epicanthus inversus syndrome is an autosomal dominant rare eye disorder, and is of two types: the purpose of the study is to screen mutations in the FOXL2 gene in Indian BPES cases so as to understand the diseases pathogenesis. Four mutations and two variants in heterozygous state were identified in four families and one sporadic case, including two hot sport duplications two frame shift mutation and two variants the variant g.738C> T was also identified in 13/60 (21.6%) normal individuals in the present study. Interestingly, in our study all the mutations identified localize to the downstream forkhead region of gene. The presence of mutations in the FOXL2 gene in all the six BPES families supports its role in the development of BPES in Indian patients.

B. COLUMBIA ASIA MEDICAL CENTERS

Malaysia

Columbia Asia Medical Center, Seremban, a Multispecialty hospital near Kuala Lumpur.

Columbia asia medical centre, Miri a multi speciality hospital in east Malaysia.

Columbia Asia Medical Center, Shah Alam, a nursing and rehabilitation center near Kuala Lumpur.

Vietnam

Columbia Asia Medical Centre, Gia Dinh, a multispecialty hospital in Saigon.

Columbia Asia Saigon International Clinic, a multispecialty clinic in Saigon.

India

Columbia Asia Medical Centre, Hebbal, a multispecialty hospital in Bangalore.

Anesthesiology
Cosmetic dermatology
Dental care
Dermatology
Ear, Nose and Throat
Gastroenterology
General surgery
Internal medicine
Maxillo facial surgery
Medical oncology
Nephrology
Neurology
Neurosurgery
Non-invasive cardiology

Obstetrics and gynecology
Ophthalmology
Orthopedics surgery
Pediatrics
Pediatric surgery
Psychiatry
Surgical oncology
Urology
Vascular surgery

Features and facilities

90 beds
24 hour emergency room
24 hour laboratory services
24 hour pharmacy
24 hour radiology
5 operating rooms
Day surgery center
Dedicated labour and delivery suites
Dialysis center
Dietectics
Endoscopy suite
Intensive care unit
Minimal access (laparoscopic) surgery
Nursery and special care baby unit
Outpatient specialist clinics
Preventive health screening
Physiotherapy

The Columbia Asia difference

Plasma TVs to aid the queuing system and scheduling.

Unique proprietary software with electronic medicians record system.

Centralized medical gas systems.

Operating theatres designed to conform to ASHRA (America society of heating, refrigeration and air conditioning) standards.

Spacious icu and 4 bedded and 5 bedded rooms.

Delivery suites.

Day care centre.

CME (continuing medical education) training for our nurses and doctors.

State of the art medical equipment and international standard infrastructure.

A contemporary and patient-friendly design allows easy access to all departments.

High level of expertise and trained professionals.

Ensuring specialized care and attention with the best technology, infrastructure and expertise are the essential components of effective health care. At Columbia Asia, we take great efforts in understanding and providing sophisticated medical care by bringing together the very best of technology and specialists.

The Columbia Asia advantage

Affordable health care, services, targeting the growing middle income groups of India.

State of the art medical equipment and international standard infrastructure.

International standards for medical, nursing and operating protocols.

Unique proprietary operating software and electronic medical records systems.

A team of nationally and internationally qualified doctors.

A contemporary and patient friendly design allows easy access to all departments.

Advanced health care with a human touch

At Columbia Asia, technology and service walk hand in hand with you for a better life and a brighter tomorrow.

Columbia Asia provides multi specialty health care facilities including outpatient and inpatient services. The facilities here incorporate our professional and internationally proven health care systems that are modern, effective and yet affordable.

Birth Record

Name of the Doctor: ______________________________
Date of Birth: ______________________________
Time of Birth: ________________ Sex Male/Female ______
Delivery: Normal/Vacuum/Forceps/Caesarean
Neonatal Status:
Birth Weight: ____________________ Length: ________
Head Circumference:________________ Blood Group: ______
Remarks: ______________________________
____
Name of the Child: ______________________________

Name of Mother: ______________ Name of Father: ______________
Mother's Blood Group ________ Father's Blood Group ____________
Details of Siblings ____
____
Home Address ____
____

Immunization Record

Age	*Vaccine*	*Due on*	*Given on*	*Make*	*Batch*	*Remarks*
Birth	BCG					
	Oral Polio Vaccine – 1st dose					
	Hepatitis B Vaccine – 1st dose					
6 weeks	DPT—1st dose					
	Oral Polio Vaccine – 2nd dose					
	Hepatitis B Vaccine – 2nd dose					
10 weeks	DPT – 2nd dose					
	Oral Polio Vaccine – 3rd dose					
14 weeks	DPT—3rd dose					
	Oral Polio Vaccine – 4th dose					
6-9 months	Oral Polio Vaccine – 5th dose					
	Hepatitis B Vaccine – 3rd dose					
9 months	Measles Vaccine					
15-18 months	MMR (Measles, Mumps, Rubella)					
	DPT – 1st booster dose					
	Oral Polio Vaccine – 6th dose					
5 years	DPT – 2nd booster dose					
	Oral Polio Vaccine – 7th dose					
10 years	TT (Tetanus) – 3rd booster dose					
	Hepatitis B Vaccine booster dose					
15-16 years	TT (Tetanus) – 4th booster dose					
	Optional Vaccines*					
	Typhoid Vaccine					
	Haemophilus influenza type b					

* Typhoid and haemophilus influenza type b vaccines are optional as recommended by the Indian Academy of Pediatrics. Consult your doctor.

Parent's to note

The suggested schedule may be modified by your Doctor as per the need.

Immunization can be given in the presence of a minor illness.

After the immunization, reactions are usually mild.

Prior to immunization, inform your Doctor if the child has had any significant reactions to the last done.

BCG

A nodule appears 3-4 weeks after BCG vaccination. It may soften or ulcerate in 2-4 weeks. No application of fomentation is necessary. It heals, leaving a scar, indicating effective vaccination.

DPT

There may be mild fever and pain, redness and swelling at the site of the injection. A small painless lump may remain for a few weeks. For fever and pain, paracetamol syrup/tablet may be given. The dose can be repeated every 4-6 hours if required. Please consult your Doctor for any reaction.

Measles/MMR

A few children get fever 4 to 10 days after the vaccination. Paracetamol syrup/tablet may be given if required.

C. RAMACHANDRAN HOSPITAL AND MEDICAL CENTRE, CHENNAI

Sri Ramachandra Medical Center (SRMC) is a tertiary, care multispecialty university hospital. The medical center was founded as a teaching hospital of Sri Ramachandra Medical College and Research Institute in 1985 with the intention of translating the experience and expertise in medical education into tangible affordable health care for the community. Today SRMC is a leader in health care delivery in South India providing cutting edge state of the art care for over 3000 patients who walk through its portals daily and many more who seek remote health care through its connectivity and telemedicine services.

SRMC is located in Porur right at the intersection of the busy Chennai Bangalore expressway and the Chingelpet Chennai Toll way. It is 8 K.M. from the International airport and 12 km from the heart of the city. It is easily accessible with good motorable roads and a slew of public transport options.

The Medical Center is situated in a sprawling 175 acre University township that is lush green throughout the year. The Medical Center itself is a 8 storey building with over two million square feet of built up area and 1,640 beds. The physical facilities have been designed aesthetically with great attention to accessibility, safety and adequate privacy for patients. For the discerning patient, suites that overlook the beautiful lake are available.

The emphasis is on a clean, healthy, soothingly calm environment that hastens healing.

With over 1,640 beds, SRMC is the largest single health care facility in Chennai. Rooms are designed aesthetically and with particular emphasis on patient safety and privacy. Elegantly designed suites and deluxe rooms adorn the seventh floor overlooking the scenic campus and are available for patients who value luxury. Budget accommodation ranges from shared cubicles to single rooms all under one roof.

SRI RAMACHANDRA UNIVERSITY AND MEDICAL CENTRE

Started in 1985 as a teaching hospital attached to the Sri Ramachandra Medical College and Research Institute, the Sri Ramachandra Medical Centre today has emerged as a superspecialty hospital offering world class tertiary care services. In addition to providing basic health care facilities for the community in the rural and semi-urban neighbourhood, the hospital attracts a large number of patients from many parts of the country and from abroad for advanced diagnostic procedures and management of complex medical and surgical problems. Some of the important features of the services provided at Sri Ramachandra Medical Centre include the following:

Highly specialized health care facilities

Sri Ramachandra Medical Centre ensures that clinicians working here possess the highest level of professional skills and competence in addition to their teaching ability. Whether they are physicians, surgeons or interventionists, they are sure to accomplish the best results to the patient even in the most complex and challenging situations. The professional development programs frequently conducted in the campus and the other professional conferences, seminars and workshops our faculty participate in many other centers in India and abroad keep them abreast with contemporary issues in clinical practice and help them have their technical skills.

Some of the areas where such highly specialized care is offered include:

- Surgery for coronary arterial disease and for complex congenital heart diseases,
- Surgical treatment for head injuries and complex congenital vascular anomalies of the brain,
- Advanced Orthopedic surgery that includes total joint replacement, corrective surgery for spinal deformities, arthroscopic surgery and treatment of sports injuries,
- Kidney transplant operations and dialysis services,
- Interventional procedures for coronary and cerebrovascular conditions such as angioplasty, stenting,
- Laparoscopic surgery,
- Plastic and reconstructive surgery including microvascular procedures and corrective surgery for congenital defects like cleft lip and palate,

- Diagnosis and treatment of infertility,
- Bone marrow transplant,
- Advanced neonatal care,
- Specialized ENT procedures like cochlear implant,
- Specialized methods of diagnosis, treatment and rehabilitation for patients with speech and hearing defects, and
- It is important to add that these procedures are offered free of charge to a large number of patients who cannot afford such treatment.

Evidence-based care

In focusing on the provision of advanced health care services, the clinical faculty and staff at Sri Ramachandra are trained in evidence-based practices. What this means to the patient is that in selecting the diagnostic and management option, they ensure that the patient gets the most optimum method as accepted by contemporary clinical studies and research of the highest international standards. The patients and their families are given opportunities to discuss this in detail with the clinical staff.

Nationwide reach

The Telemedicine services at Sri Ramachandra University developed with help from Indian Space Research Organisation (ISRO) allows health care measures to be taken to the farthest village in the country. Sri Ramachandra Medical Centre is able to provide clinical consultation for patients as far away as Assam, Guwahati, Imphal and Port Blair in Andaman and Nicobar.

Research

As the Sri Ramachandra Medical Center is an integral part of Sri Ramachandra University committed to education and research in addition to health care, a great deal of emphasis is placed on measures to identify major health problems in the community and develop appropriate strategies for their management. With this in mind, the University has established its own state of the art research facility that includes a Central Research Facility covering an area of 40,000 sq ft and equipped with all modern amenities and a modern animal house. These efforts have attracted a large number of faculty and research scholars to pursue meaningful research activities involving several vital areas. These include:

- Cell biology and tissue engineering.
- Epidemiological studies on the relation of lifestyles and cardiovascular risk factors.
- Characterization and standardization of herbal remedies.
- Molecular genetics and chromosomal studies.
- Environmental engineering and occupational health.
- Stem cell research.

Innovative steps in education

In the last 22 years, Sri Ramachandra University has been able to develop and put into practice several innovative ideas in health care education. These include:

- Excellent curricula for undergraduate and post-graduate education in several disciplines that meet or exceed the expectations of the various apex bodies like the Medical Council of India, the Dental Council and the Nursing Council of India.
- The integrated curriculum that our faculty has developed for the MBBS program has caught the imagination of several other medical colleges and has won the appreciation of faculty and students alike.
- The University continues its policy of introducing innovative courses that are relevant to the rapidly evolving health care scenario in our country. The fact that a significant number of graduates from such programs are readily accepted for employment by several national and global agencies is testimony to the quality of these programmes.

Global recognition

Several global and international agencies have recognized the great potential of Sri Ramachandra University and medical Centre as a centre of excellence and have accorded recognition and come forward to establish alliance with the institution:

- In 1997, Harvard Medical International entered into a long standing academic alliance with Sri Ramachandra. SRU is the only institution in this category to be recognized by HMI in India. The alliance has facilitated holding of several educational and faculty development programmes in addition to allowing visits by Ramachandra students, faculty and leadership to Harvard university and hospital.
- The World Health Organisation has recognized Sri Ramachandra University as a collaborating centre for research in Occupational and environmental health. Ramachandra is one of the four WHO collaborating centres in South Asia.
- The Royal College of Physicians (UK) has recently has communicated its decision to conduct the MRCP (UK) Part II clinical examinations in the Clinical Skills Centre in SRU.
- The University of Wisconsin in USA has come forward to develop collaborative programmes in Nursing Education. Many faculty from the College of Nursing have participated in leadership training programmes in USA under this arrangement.

FOCUS OF EXCELLENCE

Working against the pandemic of obesity and diabetes, Sri Ramachandra Medical Centre's diabetes and endocrine programme focuses on providing a multidisciplinary approach to prevention and treatment of the twin banes of urban life. The endocrine centre also has expertise in thyroid disease, osteoporosis disorders of growth and reproduction and Women's Health.

SRMC has the most modern interventional radiology facility in South Asia. Without need for surgery, radiologists can "coil" aneurysms, fix broken vertebrae and open up closed blood vessels. with the help of highly sophisticated technology and tremendous skill.

Sri Ramachandra Medical Centre for Assisted Reproductive Technology (SMART). SMART provides state-of-the-art care for couples who have difficulty in having children. With modern technology and expert medical specialists in gynecology, endocrinology and andrology, the infertility center helps couples walk through a traumatic phase in their lives with care and empathy. The Centre is having the state-of-the-art Infrastructure with latest equipment manned by experienced and dedicated reproductive medicine specialists. Embryologists and other paramedical staff including facility for counseling supported by well established human genetics department for counseling and Pre-Implantation Genetic Diagnosis. We have facility for IUI, IVF, ICSI, TESA-ICSI and frozen embryo transfer facilities and our results were comparable to any other well established art centers in the world.

The department of orthopaedics specializes in joint replacement surgeries. Arthroscopic procedures provide a minimally invasive diagnostic and therapeutic approach to joint problems. The center also focuses on sports medicine.

- Total knee replacement surgery
- Total hip replacement surgery
- Total shoulder replacement surgery
- Limb lengthening
- Spinal surgery
- Multiple fracture management

Through a small incision and sophisticated laparoscopic techniques the surgeon at SRMC can operate on almost any organ without much disturbance to surrounding tissues. Because of small incisions high technology and great attention to sterile techniques, long hospitalizations and convalescences have become a thing of the past. Many patients can come in the morning, have their surgery and go back home the same evening to sleep in their own beds.

The neuro-care center focuses on care of patients with problems with circulation of the brain, epilepsy, disorders of sleep and movement. The neurosurgical team is one of the few in the country with expertise in treating aneurysms and malformations of the blood vessels of the brain. Care of patients with brain tumors and complex epilepsy are other important areas of focus.

SRMC is one of the pioneers in transplantation services in this region. Backed by a world-class nephrology and dialysis service, the transplant team is one of the few in the country to routinely do cadaveric kidney transplants. SRMC also has expertise in corneal, cardiac and liver transplantations. The urology department operates a Quality Management System, which complies with the requirements of BS EN ISO 9001: 2000.

Lithotripsy is a convenient, non-invasive technique that literally pulverizes renal stones. With the help of the lithotripter, the urologist is able to treat stones without need for prolonged hospitalization and complicated surgery. Treatment of stones also includes special care to exclude hormonal and other problems and offering dietary and medical therapy to prevent recurrence of stones.

SRMC is a central referral laboratory. Our modern clinical laboratory is one of the finest in the region with quality systems and external controls ensuring a high level of reproducibility and accuracy. Over 60,000 clinical chemistries and over 2000 hormone tests are done each month in the medical center. Complex and specialized tests including genetic tests, drug levels, etc. are done routinely. Results are available in a centralized location and soon patients can log on to a secure website and access their results.

The imaging facilities in SRMC are unparalleled in the region. The multi-slice CT system is the latest of its kind reduces time spent inside the scan room dramatically. It is ultra fast and capable of extremely thin cuts for images and is also able to provide a 3 dimensional reconstruction of the organ that will help the doctor and surgeon make accurate diagnosis and plan surgical procedures as well. This technique can also do a virtual bronchoscopy or colonoscopy without need for tubes in various orificies.

Other imaging modalities in SRMC include:

- A 1.5 tesla Magnetic resonance imaging that also provides for noninvasive angiography.
- Digital subtraction angiography.
- Doppler and ultrasound.
- Cardiac imaging including echocardiogram.
- Nuclear imaging for the heart, thyroid and bones.
- Mammography.

Partnership in Patient care

SRMC has created strategic alliances around the world that help improve its patient care delivery and education objectives. The foremost of them is the inter institutional alliance with Harvard Medical International. Signed in 1997. This first of its kind alliance brings to India through SRMC. The expertise and experience of the leader in health care and education around the world—Harvard Medical School.

Other strategic alliances include Johns Hopkins University for research in environmental health and Oshkosh University Wisconsin for nursing.

To know more about the alliance with Harvard and other partners and how it can help your care, visit www.srmc.edu

SRMC is a regional medical center attracting patients from through out India, Sri Lanka, Bangladesh, Nepal, Bhutan, South East Asia, East Africa and the Middle East. International patients are provided special care and services that include help with visa, airport transfer, special suites, customized meal plans, interpreter services and portability of international insurance. A dedicated international desk ensures that all international patients get the very best of SRMC and India.

Through a unique program that was inaugurated by the Prime Minister, SRMC provides telemedicine services to the Andaman and Nicobar Islands through a satellite link. Teleconsultation services are also offered in a cost effective internet-based system to institutions and individuals who would like this service. All of SRMC's consultants are available online and provide advice over the net for patients who desire them.

Facilities of Relative and Friends

Friends and family who accompany patients will find a beautiful and clean township with all the modern facilities that one could ask for. The campus has three multi-cuisine restaurants. ATM, gift shops, florist, ample parking, a post office, business and internet center. Expansive lawns, landscaping, running water and waterfalls add serenity to the experience.

For relatives who wish to stay close to their loved one. SRMC has a on-campus guest-house with elegant well-appointed rooms.

SRI RAMACHANDRA UNIVERSITY

(Established under Section 3 of the UGC Act, 1956)
1, Ramachandra Nagar, Porur, Chennai-600 116
Telephone: 24768031-33 Fax: 91-44-24765995/24767008
Web: www.srmc.edu

Introduction

Sri Ramachandra Medical College and Research Institute was established by Sri Ramachandra Educational and Health Trust in the year 1985 as a private not-for-profit self-financing institution and dedicated to serve the society as a centre of excellence with emphasis on medical education, research and health care. In view of its academic excellence, the Government of India declared Sri Ramachandra Medical College and Research Institute as a Deemed University in September, 1994 under the section 3 of the University Grants Commission Act, 1956. As notified by the UGC, the nomenclature of the institution has now been changed to Sri Ramachandra University. The Trust achieved the task of establishing this

Institution as a "Centre of Excellence" under the leadership of Late Shri N.P.V. Ramasamy Udayar who was the Founder and Managing Trustee of the Trust and also the first Chancellor of the Deemed University. Shri V.R. Venkatachalam is currently the Chancellor and also the Managing Trustee of the Trust.

Over two decades, it has transformed into a full-fledged university with nine constituent colleges and around 100 courses in the health care sciences. More than 3750 students call this campus their home. Over 3500 patients seek health care in the state of the art academic medical centre.

Location and Accessibility

Sri Ramachandra University is located in Porur, on the busy Chennai-Bangalore highway, a twenty minute drive from the Chennai international airport. Chennai is a busy metropolis situated at head of sixty miles of pristine beach in the Bay of Bengal. Chennai is a fast growing industrial, medical and knowledge hub in South India that retains its charm, tradition and culture. It is well connected by road, rail and air to almost any destination in the world.

Infrastructure

The infrastructure at the University has been created to provide its students the best educational environment in the country. Over two million square feet of constructed space houses technologically advanced, fully air-conditioned state of the art class rooms, modern laboratories and one of the largest medical libraries in the region—the Harvard Learning Centre.

Campus and Facilities

Spread over 175 acres, the University is housed in a refreshingly green campus. Well manicured lawns, sprawling open spaces and trees dot the campus. The campus itself is a township with colleges, the medical centre, staff and student housing, conference facilities, play grounds, multi-specialty restaurants, ATMs, gift shops, travels, railway reservation counter and a post office.

Learning experience at SRMC

SRMC takes pride in creating health care professionals who are globally competitive and locally responsive. At the forefront of this effort is the development of innovative curricula that prepare health care professionals for the demands and challenges of the 21st century. Within the framework laid by the regulatory authorities, the university has created unique learning experiences that focus on all round student development. The curriculum aims in providing a competency based patient-centered education in medical and health sciences. Extensive use of clinical material and technology enhance the value of education. The medical college in addition has developed a first of its kind education program called PRODEV that takes education beyond knowledge and concentrates on overall professional development. Every student is assessed not only in knowledge and skills but also professional attributes. A unique mentoring program that provides for personal supervision by a faculty member across the years adds to the learning experience in SRMC.

Student life at Sri Ramachandra University

The University is a youthful vibrant and colourful campus. With exceptionally well appointed student housing, manicured lawns, playgrounds, gymnasiums and restaurants, the campus is agog with student life and activity. Student housing is secure and well supervised. Designated study areas, air conditioned class rooms and small group discussion areas add value to learning. The presence of students and post-graduates across the health care spectrum enhances the interdisciplinary educational experience. Exchange students from top universities around the world provide an international flavour to student life. Beside class, social events, annual cultural, literary, fine art events and sports fill the calendar. The campus is designed to ensure that students find a safe aesthetically pleasing environment to pursue their chosen careers with maximum support.

The international student experience

Ever since its inception, international students have been a part of Sri Ramachandra University. Drawn from countries all over the globe, students have found the University a home away from home.

Separate comfortable housing is available for international students. Broadband connectivity ensures that the student is in touch with only a click. An international student office and counselor provide individualized attention to the needs of international students.

Faculty profile—a study in excellence

The faculty at the University are its greatest strength. Drawn from diverse training backgrounds from all over the country and the world over 600 plus faculty are not only experts in their fields of interest but through faculty development programs are always constantly redefining their skills in education. This translates into an education of high quality that is delivered at an individualized personal level. Our faculty take part in a unique mentorship program targeted at maximizing the educational advantage that SRMC students enjoy.

CONSTITUENT COLLEGES

Sri Ramachandra Medical College and Research Institute

Thousands of students from India and abroad have graduated and have received the MBBS degree since the medical college was initiated in 1985, in addition to several hundred who have received postgraduate degrees and diplomas in the various branches of Medicine.

The MBBS course as well as all the Postgraduate courses that come under the purview of the Medical Council of India have received full recognition from the Council. The Institution is included in the World Health Directory and is recognized by the General Medical Council, UK, Ireland Medical Council and Sri Lankan Medical Council thus giving our students an opportunity to widen their horizon in carving their careers.

The Undergraduate Medical (MBBS) programme is fine tuned to meet not only the criteria laid down by the Medical Council of India but includes the nuances of education as practised in Harvard Medical School. Postgraduate education opportunities are available in a wide spectrum of specialties and this is being further strengthened every year.

- Our institutional alliance with Harvard Medical International has grown from strength to strength. Sri Ramachandra University will complete a decade of collaboration in education, health and research with HMI in July this year. "Alliance with Sri Ramachandra deepens as milestone approaches in 2007, HMI and Sri Ramachandra Medical College and Research Institute will commemorate the tenth anniversary of an alliance that has helped the Chennai-based college become a regional leader in medical education" (quote from HMI World).
- "It is wonderful to see that Sri Ramachandra Medical College and Research Institute is now known as a center of excellence in India for education programs"—(extract from HMI Annual Report by Elizabeth Armstrong, Ph.D., Director of Education Programs, Harvard Medical International).
- Sri Ramachandra University is a "MRCP Part 2—Clinical Examination Centre" for the MRCP qualification of the Royal College of Physicians of Edinburgh, Royal College of Physicians of London. Sri Ramachandra University is the fourth such centre in South Asia where this examination is conducted outside the United Kingdom.
- The WHO has designated Sri Ramachandra Medical College and Research Institute as a WHO Collaborating Centre for Research and Training in Occupational Health.

In all 49 courses including MBBS, MD, MS, OM, M.Ch., and Diploma courses in medicine, surgery and allied subjects are offered.

Sri Ramachandra Dental College and Hospital

Shortly after the institution became a Deemed University, the Dental Faculty was included and in 1995 Sri Ramachandra Dental College and Hospital was declared open and students were admitted to the BDS course. Utilising a floor space of 2,29,000 sq. ft, the college has 330 well equipped dental chairs to fulfil the needs of the Undergraduates as well as Postgraduates in every branch of dentistry. There are specially designed laboratories and teaching facilities such as lecture halls, auditoria and departmental seminar rooms and departmental libraries which make this a well recognised institution in the country. Advanced diagnostic equipment such as Orthpantomographs, Cephalostats and maxillofacial and dental radiography have been included. In addition to the state of the art designated dental operation theatres, the vast diagnostic facilities, that are available at the medical centre are also readily accessible for the students and faculty of the dental college. Several hundred patients who visit the dental college and hospital every day appreciate the comprehensive care provided. The Courses offered are recognised by the Dental Council of India and Sri Lankan Dental Council.

BDS and MDS courses are offered.

Shri Ramachandra College of Pharmacy

Established in 1993, this constituent college is a prestigious institution located in a multilevel building with well equipped research laboratories and draws research scholars from different parts of the nation. The college offers a 4 year professional degree in pharmacy (B. Pharm.) which teaches pharmacology, medicinal chemistry, pharmaceutics and natural products chemistry as part of the course. Most prominent in the course are hospital/clinical pharmacy, health management and research. State-of-the-art equipment and up to date information on the latest drugs and therapies equip the students to practice anywhere in the world. The two years Masters program in Pharmacy Practice enables students to get hands on training in hospital, clinical and community pharmacy in close association with the clinicians. The Undergraduate and Postgraduate degree programs are approved by All India Council for Technical Education and Pharmacy Council of India, New Delhi.

B. Pharm and M. Pharm degree courses are offered.

Sri Ramachandra College of Nursing

Located in an exclusive four level building with all the infrastructure required to learn the full spectrum of nursing care, the College offers four years undergraduate degree course (B.Sc. Nursing), two years' (B.Sc. Nursing-Post-Basic) course and two years' Postgraduate degree (M.Sc. Nursing) course. The courses are split into four distinct sections that start off with preparation and development, classroom learning, simulation learning, clinical learning and field learning. Students are given real time training in nursing through community health nursing programs, rural health programs and in areas such as Medical Surgical Nursing, Child Health Nursing, Maternity Nursing, Community Health Nursing, Psychiatric Nursing, nutrition, hygiene, basic medical sciences, etc.

The courses have been designed according to the regulations of the Indian Nursing Council. Academic agreements have been made with University of Wisconsin, Oshkosh, USA, Wayne State University Detroit, USA and Queen Margaret University College, Edinburgh, Scotland, UK. Faculty and students exchange program is our strength.

Undergraduate and Master courses in Nursing are offered.

Sri Ramachandra College of Physiotherapy

The need for well programmed physiotherapy after major treatment for several movement disorders is only too well known and several problems are treated by physiotherapy using different modalities along with manual therapy in conjunction with other medical treatments in both inpatient and of patient settings.

Special central locations for various types of physiotherapy have been provided for easy access to all inpatients and outpatients. The students in training, actively participate in the management of the patients for their own learning under the guidance and supervision of the experienced faculty.

BPT and MPT are offered.

Sri Ramachandra College of Management

MBA Hospital and Health Systems Management

The vast and imposing facility of the medical centre and hospital will be under utilised if the younger generation does not get an opportunity to learn from the administration and the working systems. SRMCandRI appreciated the need for capable health care administrators who can relieve the administrative burden of the doctors and help enhance the service potentials of the hospital and came up with the idea of introducing a 2 year MBA course in Hospital and Health Systems Management. The course has already been approved by the All India Council for Technical Education, New Delhi and is popularly sought after by aspiring youngsters.

Sri Ramachandra College of Biomedical Sciences, Technology and Research

Department of Human Genetics

Opportunities to pursue the special area of Human Genetics is sought by many avid and ambitious students as they are aware of the great future that is in store for them. The Masters programme in Human Genetics has attracted students of high calibre from many parts of the country. In addition to the well structured teaching programme, they have the advantage of hands-on experience in utilising the state of the art diagnostic equipment in the field of genetics. The institution has already created a core group of committed geneticists who contribute to research in cytogenetic and connected fields.

Department of Biotechnology

Realizing the potential role of Biotechnology, this college was initiated in 1999 and offers a two year postgraduate programme in Medical Biotechnology and Ph.D. in which students receive practical training and are made to conduct guided student seminars and do dissertation work. This college is dedicated to research work in every aspect of medicine, from advanced technology to herbology.

Department of Bioinformatics

Bioinformatics is one of the major growth areas in medicine and technology. It has tremendous potential to leave its impact on the everyday lives of people from genetically engineered food to drug discovery. It is in the limelight of multifarious drug trials also.

The multidisciplinary nature of the Master's Program in Bioinformatics means that it is open to motivated candidates with appropriate qualification in science subjects. For the student who thrills at being on the cutting edge of science, with the skills to excel in two very different worlds, bio-informatics can be exciting and rewarding career.

Department of Medicinal Chemistry

Medicinal chemistry is a scientific discipline involving the identification, synthesis and development of new drugs suitable for therapeutic use. It also includes the study of existing drugs, their biological properties, and their quantitative structure-activity relationships (QSAR). Under the new WTO patent regime, Pharmaceutical companies India and elsewhere are expending their R & D activities and therefore need well trained medicinal chemists. The course is structured keeping the needs of the drug industry in mind. B.Sc. Chemistry (with organic chemistry) and B.Pharm graduates who undergo this course can look forward to an assured bright future.

Department of Biomedical Sciences

Sri Ramachandra University offers a four year B.Sc. Biomedical Sciences course from this academic year 2007-08 with an option of opting one of the three major specializations in the fourth year of the programme on Human Genetics, Biotechnology and Bioinformatics. This B.Sc. Biomedical Sciences program, which is one of its kinds in the country, has been meticulously designed keeping in mind the importance of imparting complete education with emphasis towards understanding the fundamentals of basic sciences and medical sciences, which provides a strong foundation for higher studies and professional careers. The curriculum is strongly multi-disciplinary and will sensitize students to the latest developments in the field of Biomedical Sciences like Genomics, Proteomics, Applied Biotechnology, Antibody Engineering, Medical Genetics, Medical Transcription, and Cancer Biology. The curriculum also emphasizes basic chemical, physical, mathematical sciences, computer applications and management principles. The program aims at producing highly trained and skilled biomedical scientists who have flexible career opportunities and can make valuable contributions in the field of biomedical research. Biomedical science is a continually changing, dynamic profession with long term career prospects including management, research, education and specialized laboratory work. This degree will open doors to higher studies (Master's and Doctoral program) and academic staff positions at leading universities and research institutes in India and across the globe. M.Sc. degree courses in Human Genetics, Biotechnology, Bioinformatics and Undergraduate course Biomedical Sciences.

Sri Ramachandra College of Allied Health Sciences

In the hi-tech world of modern health care, the need for a team approach in curing illness and sustaining life is essential and it takes people with varying skills and expertise to make up the team. Advanced complex instrumentation and equipment require technocrats not only to operate but also to care and maintain them as well. These experts have to possess a strong scientific foundation and be able to perform at a much higher level than the traditionally trained technicians of the past. The following undergraduate and postgraduate courses keeping the above needs of the medical profession are offered.

B.Sc. Allied Health Sciences: Sri Ramachandra University realised the significant gap in the make up of the vital medical team to care for patients in specialty areas. This led to the initiation of a Bachelor degree course in Allied Health Sciences. The 4 year course (8 semesters) requires the students to go through basic medical and allied sciences including anatomy, physiology, biochemistry, microbiology, pathology, pharmacology and disease concepts before they enter into specific specialty oriented courses. The currently available courses in Allied Health Science technology are as given below:

Anesthesia Technology
Cardiac Technology
Clinical Laboratory Technology
Gastroenterology Technology
Operation Theatre Technology
Radiology and Imaging Sciences Technology

Perfusion Technology
Respiratory Care. Technology
Renal Dialysis Technology
Neuroscience Technology
Urology Technology

Human Genetics

Emergency and Trauma Care Technology

Department of Optometry

The four year B.Sc. Optometry course (with one year Internship) trains optometrist who examines, diagnoses and helps the Ophthalmologist in the treatment and management of diseases and disorders of eye and associated structures. Optometrist is a professional who is trained to prescribe refraction corrections of the eye with high degree of competence. The course is structured to build knowledge, develop skills and expose the candidates to real-work situations in hospitals and health care organisations. It aims to meet international standards with multi-disciplinary skills. The course also trains students in aspects of management, finance and computer knowledge. The department of Ophthalmology which also runs the MS and Diploma courses in Ophthalmology offers this course.

Department of Speech, Language and Hearing Sciences

The Department of Speech, Language and Hearing Sciences was established under the Faculty of Allied Health Sciences in 1995. To date, this is the only college in the state that offers undergraduate (since 1995) and postgraduate (since 2004) degrees in the field of speech, language and hearing. The courses are recognized by the Rehabilitation Council of India. The University also offers Ph.D. in speech, language and hearing since 2002. Training in this field will enable individuals to provide diagnostic and rehabilitative services to those who are communicatively handicapped. Various facilities such as audiological suites, electrophysiology labs, speech diagnostic and therapeutic units serve as primary source for clinical and research training. The students have the opportunity to undergo training in various specialty areas including neonatal hearing screening, early intervention programs for the communicatively handicapped, cleft care, stuttering management, professional voice care, bedside evaluation of patients and routine audiological and speech evaluation and rehabilitation.

BASLP and MASLP courses are offered.

Department of Clinical Psychology

M.Phil Clinical Psychology

A two year specialty course has been introduced for the benefit of students who have a recognised Postgraduate degree in Psychology. Clinical Psychologists form an important part of the psychiatry team participating in diagnosis, psychotherapy and research programs. This course is recognized by the Rehabilitation Council of India.

Department of Clinical Nutrition

M.Sc. Clinical Nutrition

A clinical nutritionist is a specialist in the science of nutrition equipped to working in the health care system. He/she is trained to assess and evaluate nutritional deficiency or imbalance and recommend treatment through the use of specific dietary supplements, vitamins, etc., to maintain optimal health of patients and others. There is growing demand for clinical nutritionists India and Abroad.

A Postgraduate diploma course particularly to train qualified dietitians in the field of clinical nutrition has been developed for the first time in South India to meet the changing needs and nutritional challenges in treating patients.

Department of Emergency and Trauma Care Technology

For the first time in India, a 3 year Degree course leading to B.Sc. Emergency and Trauma Care Technology has been introduced in our university.

Emergency and Trauma Care Technologists are members of the emergency medical care team who use their knowledge and skills to provide basic and advanced life support to seriously ill or injured patients before these patients reach the hospital. They are involved in patient rescue and enable their safe transport by ambulance to appropriate medical centres.

The Course is accredited with Excel which is the regulatory body for paramedic education in the United Kingdom.

Sri Ramachandra Centre for Distance Education

Family Health specialists are in immediate need for the vast community in our country. SRMC initiated its distance education programme, PG Diploma in Family Health for general practitioners of this country. This is a well structured 2 year programme including contact sessions, web-based learning and assessment. There has been excellent response to this course from general practitioners all over the country, within a short period of time since its inception. The doctors enrolled into this course have been greatly benefited, as it has enabled them to change their practice styles and has helped them to be able to address the health care needs of the entire family in the ambience of the community.

The Department of Environmental Health Engineering was set-up, as a part of the Basic Science Research Wing of Sri Ramachandra University, Chennai, in 1998 with the aid of financial assistance provided by the United Nations Industrial Development Organisation. The department originally set-up to provide occupational safety and industrial hygiene monitoring services to the leather/tanning industry in Tamil Nadu, has since then been expanded to include a variety of R & D and training activities, that cover a broad spectrum of environmental health concerns. It is a recipient of extra-mural research and training grants from NIH, WHO, World Bank, UNDP, USEPA, Central and State Ministries of Government of India.

The primary focus of the department is on conduct of health risk assessments for environmental pollutants (in both the occupational and ambient environment). The department also provides routine occupational safety and health consultancy services to a wide spectrum of industries. The department is equipped with a state of the art environmental monitoring and industrial hygiene laboratory. The faculty of the department is involved in the conduct of academic courses including.

WHO has designated Sri Ramachandra Medical College and Research Institute as a WHO Collaborating Centre for Research and Training in Occupational Health with Dr. Kalpana Balakrishnan as Director of the Centre.

Our Environmental Health Engineering Department has been recognized by the International Labour Office of the United Nations, Geneva as a collaborating centre of the International Occupational Safety and Health Information Centre (HIS) Network.

SRI RAMACHANDRA UNIVERSITY CENTRAL RESEARCH FACILITY

Prof. S.P. Thyagarajan
Director and Chief Advisor (Research)

Sri Ramachandra University, a Harvard Medical International Associated Institution, has established a Central Research Facility to gain recognition as a centre of excellence in medical research. Prof. S.P. Thyagarajan, an internationally renowned medical scientist and former Vice-Chancellor, University of Madras has conducted 55 research projects during his 35 years of research career, made 326 publications and written 17 books. He holds a patent for a drug formulated from an Indian medicinal plant for chronic Hepatitis B and holds 4 more patents.

The rupees 50-crore Central Research Facility as the "A to Z gateway" for research, takes care of all logistics of research planning, research projects administration, research data analysis, storage and provides centralized sophisticated equipments facility and university-industry liaison facility on a 'ready to use platform' for all faculty members.

A Research Unit in a plinth area of 25,000 sq.ft. has been dedicated for this facility. It will have a medical informatics and modeling centre, clinical research unit, epidemiology unit, study design and project development unit, data analysis and documentation centre, traditional medicine research unit, university sophisticated instrumentation centre, all high-tech equipments for the genomics, proteomics, spectroscopy, chromatography, radioisotopy, microscopy, etc., walk-in-cold room (+4c), walk-in-incubator, cryopreservation unit (–80c to –146c), cold room -20c, central animal house, digital library, university industry liaison centre and a IPR/patents cell, besides an administrative office.

Presently there are 261 major and minor research projects operational in the University which are broadly classified as (a) international collaborative projects (6), (b) Sponsored research projects funded by national agencies like Department of Science and Technology, Department of Bio-Technology, Indian Council of Medical Research, Council of Scientific and Industrial Research, etc. (50), (c) Industry-institutional R&D consultancy projects jointly funded by DST, industries and international agencies (5), (d) Multinational and multicentric clinical trials (44), (e) Individual research projects by faculty and postgraduate students including Ph.D. students (156).

Some Major achievements of medical and allied sciences research in Sri Ramachandra University are: (i) WHO recognition for the Department of Environmental Health Engineering and its testing services, (ii) The cheaper gadget for measuring radiation exposure, developed by the Department of Genetics for DRDO currently being validated at IGCAR, Kalpaakkam, (iii) Human chondrocyte culture on thermo-reversible polymer gel by the Department of Arthroscopy and Sports Medicine, (iv) Pre-clinical validation and standardization of studies on indigenous medicines for diabetes and rheumatoid arthritis, (v) Large scale cohort studies on risk factor(s) identification for vascular disease prevalence and intervention by both traditional and modern medicines, (vi) Use of Bovine animal tissues for the preparation and characterization of collagen 3-D scaffolds for cardiomyocyte culture, and (vii) Computer model creation to evolve an ideal artificial valve.

The 'Research Vision' of the University is to evolve it as a "Centre for Excellence and Biomedical Nanotechnology."

VIDYA SUDHA

Sri Ramachandra Learning Centre for Children with Special Needs Ms. Shalini Jayanand.

Project Officer

Vidya Sudha was conceived and created by Sri Ramachandra University in the year 2004 with the aim of helping parents of children with special needs and providing optimum care, for the children. It is a uniquely designed day care centre where parents form an integral part of the plan and care process of the children with special needs. Vidya Sudha is an early intervention holistic programme where the team of experts with diverse back grounds and specialties come together to cater to the overall development of the child with special needs. At present it has about 80 children under its care.

Special rules for students

In conformity with the directives issued by the Department of Higher Education, Ministry of Human Resource Development, Government of India, storage and use of carbonated beverages and junk food are banned inside the colleges of the University.

Smoking or consumption of alcoholic beverages or drugs inside the College and Hostel premises is strictly prohibited.

D. MISSION

Sri Ramachandra Medical College and Research Institute (Deemed University

Will actively promote and preserve the higher values and ethics in education, health care and research and will pursue excellence in all these areas while consciously meeting the expectations of the people it serves without prejudice and in all fairness stay socially meaningful in its propagation of the various arts and sciences to enrich humanity at large.

Introduction

Sri Ramachandra Medical College and Research Institute was started as a medical college in 1985 with a hundred students. Over two decades, it has transformed into a deemed university with nine constituent colleges and over 75 courses in the health care sciences. 3500 students call this campus their home. Over 300,000 patients seek health care in the state of the art academic medical centre.

Location and Accessibility

SRMC is located in Porur, on the busy Chennai-Bangalore highway, a twenty minute drive from the Chennai international airport. Chennai is a busy metropolis situated at head of sixty miles of pristine beach in the bay of Bengal. Chennai is a fast growing industrial medical and knowledge hub in South India that retains its charm, tradition and culture. It is well connected by road, rail and air to almost any destination in the world.

Infrastructure

The infrastructure at SRMC has been created to provide its students the best educational environment in the country. Over two million square feet of constructed space houses technologically advanced, fully air conditioned state of the art class rooms, modern laboratories and one of the largest medical libraries in the region—the Harvard Learning Centre.

Campus and Facilities

Spread over 75 acres, SRMC is a refreshingly green campus. Well manicured lawns, sprawling open spaces and trees dot the campus. The campus itself is a township with colleges. the medical centre, staff and student housing, conference facilities, play grounds, multispecialty restaurants. ATMs, gift shops and even a post office.

The university medical centre is the focus of the clinical teaching activity of the deemed university. A 1675 bedded facility with the largest ICU in the region with state of the art cutting edge equipment, the medical centre is a tertiary care facility that provides the trainee with the opportunity to acquire knowledge and skills from the finest doctors in the country. SRMC has centres of excellence in cardiovascular sciences, interventional neuroradiology, reproductive medicine, critical care and emergency services to mention a few. The medical centre seamlessly integrates with the colleges to provide knowledge and practical application of the acquired knowledge effortlessly.

SRMC takes pride in creating health care professionals who are globally competitive and locally responsive. At the forefront of this effort is the development of innovative curricula that prepare health care professionals for the demands and challenges of the 21st century. Within the framework laid by the regulatory authorities, the university has created unique learning experiences that focus on all round student development. The curriculum aims in providing a competency-based patient centered education in the medical and health sciences. Extensive use of clinical material and technology enhance the value of education. The medical college in addition has developed a first of its kind education program called PRODEV that takes education beyond knowledge and concentrates on overall professional development. Every student is assessed not only in knowledge and skills but also professional attributes. A unique mentoring program that provides for personal supervision by a faculty member across the years adds to the learning experience in SRMC.

Student Life at SRMC

SRMC is a youthful vibrant and colourful campus. With exceptionally well appointed student housing, manicured lawns, playgrounds, gymnasiums and restaurants, the campus is agog with student life and activity. Student housing is secure and well supervised. Designated study areas, air conditioned class rooms and small group discussion areas add value to learning. The presence of students and postgraduates across the health care spectrum enhances the educational experience. Exchange students from top universities around the world provide an international flavour to student life. Beside class, social events, annual cultural, literary, fine art events and sports fill the calendar. The campus is designed to ensure that students find a safe aesthetically pleasing environment to pursue their chosen careers with maximum support.

The international student experience

Ever since its inception, international students have been a part of SRMC. Drawn from countries all over the globe, students have found SRMC a home away from home. Separate comfortable housing is available for the international students. Broadband connectivity ensures that the student is in touch with only a click. An international student office and counselor provide individualized attention to the needs of international students.

Faculty profile—A study in excellence

The faculty at SRMC are its greatest strength. Drawn from diverse training backgrounds from all over the country and the world over 600 plus faculty are not only experts in their field of interest but through faculty development programs are always constantly redefining their skills in education. This translates into an education of high quality that is delivered at an individualized personal level. Our faculty take part in a unique mentorship program targeted at maximizing the educational advantage that SRMC students enjoy.

Sri Ramachandra and Harvard Medical International—An Enduring Relationship

The pride of SRMC is the close collaboration it has with Harvard Medical International. The relationship with one of the top medical schools in the world has placed SRMC as one of the leaders in medical education in India. Student and faculty exchanges are an integral part of this relationship as are sharing of resources. The annual Shri N.P.V. Ramasamy Udayar Student Enrichment Scholarship places two students each year into coveted c1erkships at Harvard. As one of HMIs long-term partners, SRMC is working closely with Harvard in creating a competency-based medical curriculum.

Milestones 1985

Inauguration of Sri Ramachandra Medical College and Research Institute; MBBS (Bachelor of Medicine and. Bachelor of Surgery) course was started.

1993

New courses started: Diploma in Nursing, B.Sc. Nursing, BPT (Bachelor of Physiotherapy) and B.Pharm.

1994

Conferment of Deemed University status (September 1994).

1995

Postgraduate courses started: M.D. General Medicine, Obstetrics and Gynaecology, Paediatrics and Anaesthesiology.

M.S. General Surgery and Orthopaedics Postgraduate Diploma courses started:

Diploma in Obstetrics and Gynaecology, Child Health, Anaesthesiology and. Orthopaedics. Undergraduate Courses started: B.D.S. (Bachelor of Dental Surgery), B.Sc. (Allied Health Sciences) and Bachelor in Audiology and Speech-Language Pathology.

1996

40,000 square feet centrally air-conditioned University library known as Harvard Ramachandra Learning Centre was inaugurated; Registration of Ph.D. candidates started: Higher Speciality and Postgraduate Degree Courses started: D.M. Cardiology, M.D. Radio-Diagnosis, M.S. Ophthalmology and Otorhinolaryngology.

Postgraduate Diploma Courses: Diploma in Otorhinolaryngology, Ophthalmology and. Medical Radio-Diagnosis.

1997

Other job-oriented Courses started: Postgraduate Diploma in Clinical Nutrition and Certificate in Hospital Ward Technician Course.

Inter-institutional Alliance with Harvard Medical International, Boston, USA was established.

Genetics Research Cell and Basic Research Cell was inaugurated.

Medical Education Unit was established.

1998

M.Sc. (Human Genetics) Degree course was started.

1999

Higher Specialty courses started: D.M. Neurology, M.Ch. Neuro Surgery, Genito-Urinary Surgery and Cardio-Thoracic Surgery.

M.Sc. Nursing and M.P.T. (Master of Physiotherapy) and Diploma in Family Health.

2000

Postgraduate Courses started: M.D. Anatomy, Physiology, Biochemistry, Pathology, Microbiology, Pharmacology Community Medicine and Dermatology, Venereology and Leprosy and Diploma in Dermatology, Venereology and Leprosy Postgraduate Dental Courses: M.D.S. Conservative Dentistry and Endodontics. Oral and Maxillofacial Surgery, Orthodontics. Oral Pathology, Periodontics. Oral Medicine and Radiology and Prosthodontcis.

Postgraduate Diploma in Accident and Emergency Medicine. M.Phil (Clinical Psychology) and B.Sc. (Emergency and Trauma Care Technology).

2001

M.D.S (Pedodontics). M.BA (Hospital and Health Systems Management). M.Sc. Biotechnology course.

2002

B.Sc. Nursing for Trained Nurses; Higher Specialty and Postgraduate degree courses: D.M. (Nephrology) and.. M.D. Accident and Emergency Medicine.

2003

M.Pharm (Pharmacy Practice). M.Sc. Industrial Hygiene and Safety and Postgraduate Certificate Course in Industrial Health.

2004

Higher Specialty courses: D.M. Medical Gastroenterology. Cardiothoracic Anaesthesiology and Critical Care M.Ch. Surgical Gastroenterology. Plastic and Reconstructive Surgery and Post Doctoral Certificate Course in Interventional Vascular and Neuro Radiology.

M.Sc. Bioinformatics, M.Sc. Neuroscience, M.Sc. Medical Laboratory Technology and Master in Audiology and Speech-Language Pathology.

2005

Higher Specialty and Postgraduate courses started: M.Ch. Paediatric Surgery. M.D. Psychiatry. Diploma in Psychiatry and Diploma in Public Health.

SRMC alumni—a profile of success

SRMCs alumni are its pride and a measure of its success. Our students find their way into the top training programs in the world for further education. Our paramedical science students are grabbed off the shelf into top hospitals in the country and around the world. Profiled below are some success stories:

I feel proud and will always feel proud to be a part of Sri Ramachandra Medical College and Research Institute. SRMC has something special (home touch) which no other place can boast of.

Dr. R. Senthil Kumar
M.D. Pharmacology
(Currently working in National University, Ireland)

It was during my undergraduate course in Sri Ramachandra Medical College and Research Institute that my conviction for a research career was reinforced and after completing M.Tech Biotechnology, I am pursuing my aspiration of establishing my career in research.

R. Maheswari
B. Pharm
(Completed: M.Tech Biotech from Anna University)

I thank you for designing the curriculum for Human Genetics. Though it was intensive. it was only because of that I am able to cope up in my Master's in Clinical Embryology at Monash University, Australia.

Jayaprakash R.
M.Sc. Human Genetics

I am happy to inform you that I have been accepted for admission to the Diagnostic Medical Sonography course at New York University. The program director was very impressed with the Allied Health Sciences Course curriculum and allowed me to transfer a lot of credits from my Allied Health Sciences degree, so that I was admitted directly into the professional course.

Sanjana
B.Sc. Allied Health Sciences
Research Design
Methodology
Research Design

References

Aaron, Henry J., William B. Schwartz, and Melissa Cox. Can we say no? the challenge of rationing health care.

Access Project, The Consequences of Medical Debt: Evidence from Three Communities, February 2003, www.accessproject.org/downloads/med_consequences.pdf (13 December 2004).

Administrative Office of the U.S. Courts, "Bankruptcy Cases Continue to Break Federal Court Case Records: Total Bankruptcy Filings and Non-Business Filings Hit

Highs," Press Release, 18 August 2003, www.uscourts.gov/Press_Releases/603b.pdf (13 December 2004).

American Autoimmune and Related Diseases Association, 2006. Accessed on 12/2006-2/19/2006 at: http://www.aarda.org

American Medical Association Online. "Physicians react to projected Medicare physician payment cuts". 16 March 2006. 11 September 2006. http://www.ama-assn.org/ama/pub/category/16122.html

Barmeyer, Robert A. Personal Interview. 12 September 2006. Cannon, Michael F. and Michael D. Tanner.

Brooklings Institution Press: Washington, 2005.

Chrisler, Joan C. and O'hea, Erin L. 2000 Gender, Culture, and Autoimmune Disorders in Handbook of Gender, Culture and Health. Richard M. Eisler and Michael Hersen. pp. 321-342. First Edition. Mahwah: Lawrence Erlbaum Associates, Inc.

Cogan, John F., R. Glenn Hubbard, and Daniel P. Kessler. Healthy, Wealthy, and Wise: five steps to a better health care system. AEI Press: Washington, 2005.

E. Warren and A.W. Tyagi, The Two-Income Trap (New York: Basic Books, 2003). U.S. Bureau of the Census, Statistical Abstract of the United States, 1982–83 (Washington: U.S. Department of Commerce, 1983); and Administrative Office of the U.S. Courts, "Record Breaking Bankruptcy Filings Reported in Calendar Year 2001," Press Release (Washington: Administrative Office, 19 February 2002).

E.J. Emanuel et al., "Understanding Economic and Other Burdens of Terminal Illness: The Experience of Patients and Their Caregivers," Annals of Internal Medicine 132, No. 6 (2000): 451–459.

E.M. Kennedy, In Critical Condition: The Crisis in America's Health Care (New York: Simon and Schuster, 1972).

Farquhar, Judith 1996: Knowing Practice: The Clinical Encounter of Chinese Medicine (Studies in and belief graphic Imagination). First Edition. Boulder, CO: Westview Press.

Greenberg, Brad A. "Have Ailment, Will Travel". *The Los Angeles Daily News*. 7 August 2006. 8 September 2006. www.planethospital.com.

Hadady, Letha 1996 Asian Health Secrets: The Complete Guide to Asian Herbal Medicine. First Edition. New York: Three Rivers Press.

Han, Henry, Miller, Glenn E, Deville, Nancy 2003: Ancient Herbs, Modern Medicine. First Edition. New York: Bantam Books.

Harvard University Press: Cambridge, 2005.

Health Care Tourist.com. "The Process". 7 November 2006. www.healthcaretourist.com/main.php?page=process

J. Guest, "High Rate Robbery," Consumer Reports 67, No. 10 (2002): 7.

J.S. Ziegel, "A Canadian Perspective," *Texas Law Review* 79, No. 5 (2001): 241–256. Rome/Vatican City (Clermont-Ferrand, France: Michelin Travel Publications, 2001).

Kasturi Dewi, K. "Hospitals set fees for health tourism". *The Star*. 28 Oct. 2003. The Association of Private Hospitals of Malaysia. http://www.hospitals-malaysia.org/

Kher, Unmesh. "Outsourcing Your Heart". Time.com. 21 May 2006. 6 September 2006. http://www.time.com/time/magazine/article/0,9171,1196429,00.html

Lancaster, John. "Surgeries, Side Trips for Medical Tourists". *The Washington Post Online*. 21 October 2004. 7 September 2006. www.washingtonpost.com

M. Merlis, Family Out-of-Pocket Spending for Health Services (New York: Commonwealth Fund, June 2002).

Marcelo, Ray. "India Fosters Growing Medical Tourism Sector". *The Financial Times*. 2 July 2003. 8 September 2006. http://yaleglobal.yale.edu/display.article?id=2016.

Marcelo, Ray. "India Fosters Growing Medical Tourism Sector". *The Financial Times*. 2 July 2003. 8 September 2006. http://yaleglobal.yale.edu/display.article?id=2016

Mc Curdy, David W. 1995: Using Anthropology in Conformity and Conflict: Readings in Cultural Anthropology. James Spradley and David W. McCurdy, eds. pp. 415-427. Eleventh edition. Boston: Allyn and Bacon. Penn, Nolan E., Kramer, Joyce, Skinner, John F., Velasquez, Roberto J., Yee, Barbara, W.K., Arellano, Letticia M., Williams, Joyce P. 2000 Health Practices and Health Care Systems Among Cultural Groups in Handbook of Gender, Culture and Health. Richard M. Eisler and Michael Hersen. pp. 105-138. First Edition. Mahwah: Lawrence Erlbaum Associates, Inc.

Ming, Dr. 2006: The Huai Hua Red Cross Hospital Accessed on 12/2006-2/19/2006 at: <http://www.tcmtreatment.com/hospital.htm>

NBC News. NBC. 20 February 2006. 11 September 2006. www.planethospital.com Thai Websites. "Health Care in Thailand" 7 November 2006 www.thaiwebsites.com/ health care.asp

NPR/Kaiser Family Foundation/Kennedy School of Government, "National Survey on Health Care (chartpack)," June 2002, www.kff.org/kaiserpolls/upload/ 14064_1.pdf (27 January 2005); J.H. May and P.J. Cunningham, Tough Trade-Offs: Medical Bills, Family Finances, and Access to Care (Washington: Center for Studying Health System Change, June 2004); and S.R. Collins *et al.*, The Affordability Crisis in U.S. Health Care: Findings from the Commonwealth Fund, Biennial Health Insurance Survey (New York: Commonwealth Fund, March 2004).

P.F. Short and J.S. Banthin, "New Estimates of the Underinsured Younger than Sixty-five Years," *Journal of the American Medical Association* 274, No. 16 (1995): 1302–1306.

Provides research information, statistics, NIH and legislative updates. Angrosino, Michael 1986 Health and Illness in Sociocultural Perspective in A Health Practitioner's Guide to the Social and Behavioural Sciences. pp. 53-64. Auburn Press.

Richmond, Julius B., and Rashi Fein. The Health Care Mess: how we got into it and what it will take to get out.

S. Fay, E. Hurst, and MJ. White, "The Household Bankruptcy Decision," *American Economic Review* 92, No. 3 (2002): 706-711.

M.B. Jacoby, T.A. Sullivan, and E. Warren, "Rethinking the Debates over Health Care Financing: Evidence from the Bankruptcy Courts," *New York University Law Review* 76 (2001): 375–418.

Statistical Abstract of the United States: 1986 (Washington: GPO, 1985). The estimate that 8 percent of these were medical is from T.A. Sullivan, E. Warren, and J.L. Westbrook, The Fragile Middle Class: Americans in Debt (New Haven, Conn.: Yale University Press, 2000).

Thai Websites. "Health Care in Thailand". 7 November 2006 www.thaiwebsites.com/ health care.asp

The New Bankruptcy Epidemic (Hackettstown, N.J.: SMR, 2001), 127. A high incidence of collection agency calls was reported in NPR/Kaiser *et al.*, "National Survey on Health Care"; May *et al.*, Tough Trade-Offs; and Collins *et al.*, The Affordability Crisis.

The White House Domestic Policy Council. Health Security: the President's Report to the American People, October 1993.

Todd, Stephen. "Medical Tourism Saves You Money, But Which One Is Best?". Ezine Articles.com. 7 September 2006. http://ezinearticles.com/

U.S. Census Bureau. "Poverty: Health Insurance Coverage in the United States". 13 October 2004. 11 September 2006. http://factfinder.census.gov/jsp/saff/ SAFFInfo.jsp?_pageId=tp8_poverty

Uncontrolled gambling is classified as a psychiatric disorder in the Diagnostic and Statistical Manual of Mental Disorders, Fourth Edition (DSM-IV) and contributed to about 1 percent of the bankruptcies. E. Flynn *et al.*, "Bankruptcy by the Numbers," *ABI Journal* 20, No. 10 (2002): 28-29; 21, No. 3 (2002): 22, 49; and 20, No. 8 (2001): 20.

Uretsky, Samuel D. "The 'Thailand Tuck'". MedHunters.com. 9 May 2005, 10 September 2006. http://www.medhunters.com/articles/medicalTourism.html

US Census Bureau. "Poverty: Health Insurance Coverage in the United States". 13 October 2004. 11 September 2006. http://factfinder.census.gov/jsp/saff/SAFFInfo.jsp?_pageId=tp8_poverty

Wikipedia: the free encyclopedia. "Health Care System". 11 Sept 2006. www.wikipedia.org

1. Lancaster. "Surgeries, Side trips for Medical Tourists".
2. "Medical Tourism". Wikipedia.org.
3. Uretsky. "The Thailand Tuck".
4. Kasturi Dewi. "Hospitals set fees for health tourism".
5. Lancaster. "Surgeries, side trips for medical tourists".
6. Uretsky. "The 'Thailand Tuck'".
7. Robert Barmeyer. Personal Interview.
8. Kher. "Outsourcing Your Heart".

   2001 Traditional Medicine: Growing Needs and Potential.

   2006 Traditional Chinese Medicine Could Make "Health for One" True (Jia) (WHO Traditional Terms 2006, *et. al*).

   2006 Accessed on: 12/2005-2/19/2006 at: <http://www.who.int>

   2006 Traditional Medicine: Definitions.
9. Todd . "Medical tourism saves...".
10. Kher. "Outsourcing Your Heart"
11. U.S. Census Bureau.
12. Marcelo. "India fosters Medical tourism".
13. *Ibid.*
14. Lancaster. "Surgeries, side trips...".
15. Cannon, pp. 27, 139.
16. Robert Barmeyer. Personal Interview.
17. Thai Websites. "Health Care in Thailand". 7 November 2006.

World Health Organisation 1978: The Promotion and Development of Traditional Medicine:

Index

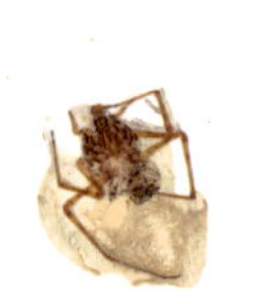